Rheumatic Diseases: Pathophysiology, Targeted Therapy, Focus on Vascular and Pulmonary Manifestations

Rheumatic Diseases: Pathophysiology, Targeted Therapy, Focus on Vascular and Pulmonary Manifestations

Editors

Barbara Ruaro
Francesco Salton
Paola Confalonieri

MDPI • Basel • Beijing • Wuhan • Barcelona • Belgrade • Manchester • Tokyo • Cluj • Tianjin

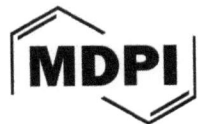

Editors
Barbara Ruaro
SC Pneumoogia, Cattinara Hospital,
University of Trieste
Trieste, Italy

Francesco Salton
SC Pneumoogia, Cattinara Hospital,
University of Trieste
Trieste, Italy

Paola Confalonieri
SC Pneumoogia, Cattinara Hospital,
University of Trieste
Trieste, Italy

Editorial Office
MDPI
St. Alban-Anlage 66
4052 Basel, Switzerland

This is a reprint of articles from the Special Issue published online in the open access journal *Pharmaceuticals* (ISSN 1424-8247) (available at: https://www.mdpi.com/journal/pharmaceuticals/special_issues/Rheumatic_Diseases).

For citation purposes, cite each article independently as indicated on the article page online and as indicated below:

LastName, A.A.; LastName, B.B.; LastName, C.C. Article Title. *Journal Name* **Year**, *Volume Number*, Page Range.

ISBN 978-3-0365-3641-5 (Hbk)
ISBN 978-3-0365-3642-2 (PDF)

© 2022 by the authors. Articles in this book are Open Access and distributed under the Creative Commons Attribution (CC BY) license, which allows users to download, copy and build upon published articles, as long as the author and publisher are properly credited, which ensures maximum dissemination and a wider impact of our publications.

The book as a whole is distributed by MDPI under the terms and conditions of the Creative Commons license CC BY-NC-ND.

Contents

About the Editors ix

Preface to "Rheumatic Diseases: Pathophysiology, Targeted Therapy, Focus on Vascular and
Pulmonary Manifestations" xi

Mattia Bellan, Ailia Giubertoni, Cristina Piccinino, Mariachiara Buffa, Debora Cromi,
Daniele Sola, Roberta Pedrazzoli, Ileana Gagliardi, Elisa Calzaducca, Erika Zecca,
Filippo Patrucco, Giuseppe Patti, Pier Paolo Sainaghi and Mario Pirisi
Cardiopulmonary Exercise Testing Is an Accurate Tool for the Diagnosis of Pulmonary Arterial
Hypertension in Scleroderma Related Diseases
Reprinted from: *Pharmaceutical* **2021**, *14*, 342, doi:10.3390/ph14040342 1

Mattia Bellan, Cristina Piccinino, Stelvio Tonello, Rosalba Minisini, Ailia Giubertoni,
Daniele Sola, Roberta Pedrazzoli, Ileana Gagliardi, Erika Zecca, Elisa Calzaducca,
Federica Mazzoleni, Roberto Piffero, Giuseppe Patti, Mario Pirisi and Pier Paolo Sainaghi
Role of Osteopontin as a Potential Biomarker of Pulmonary Arterial Hypertension in Patients
with Systemic Sclerosis and Other Connective Tissue Diseases (CTDs)
Reprinted from: *Pharmaceutical* **2021**, *14*, 394, doi:10.3390/ph14050394 11

Elena P. Calandre, Javier Hidalgo-Tallon, Rocio Molina-Barea, Fernando Rico-Villademoros,
Cristina Molina-Hidalgo, Juan M. Garcia-Leiva, Maria Dolores Carrillo-Izquierdo and
Mahmoud Slim
The Probiotic VSL#3® Does Not Seem to Be Efficacious for the Treatment of Gastrointestinal
Symptomatology of Patients with Fibromyalgia: A Randomized, Double-Blind,
Placebo-Controlled Clinical Trial
Reprinted from: *Pharmaceutical* **2021**, *14*, 1063, doi:10.3390/ph14101063 21

Satoshi Mizutani, Junko Nishio, Kanoh Kondo, Kaori Motomura, Zento Yamada,
Shotaro Masuoka, Soichi Yamada, Sei Muraoka, Naoto Ishii, Yoshikazu Kuboi,
Sho Sendo, Tetuo Mikami, Toshio Imai and Toshihiro Nanki
Treatment with an Anti-CX3CL1 Antibody Suppresses M1 Macrophage Infiltration in
Interstitial Lung Disease in SKG Mice
Reprinted from: *Pharmaceutical* **2021**, *14*, 474, doi:10.3390/ph14050474 37

Francesco Tona, Elisabetta Zanatta, Roberta Montisci, Denisa Muraru, Elena Beccegato,
Elena De Zorzi, Francesco Benvenuti, Giovanni Civieri, Franco Cozzi, Sabino Iliceto and
Andrea Doria
Higher Ventricular-Arterial Coupling Derived from Three-Dimensional Echocardiography Is
Associated with a Worse Clinical Outcome in Systemic Sclerosis
Reprinted from: *Pharmaceutical* **2021**, *14*, 646, doi:10.3390/ph14070646 51

Jacob Venborg, Anne-Marie Wegeberg, Salome Kristensen, Birgitte Brock, Christina Brock
and Mogens Pfeiffer-Jensen
The Effect of Transcutaneous Vagus Nerve Stimulation in Patients with Polymyalgia
Rheumatica
Reprinted from: *Pharmaceutical* **2021**, *14*, 1166, doi:10.3390/ph14111166 71

Salvatore Di Bartolomeo, Alessia Alunno and Francesco Carubbi
Respiratory Manifestations in Systemic Lupus Erythematosus
Reprinted from: *Pharmaceutical* **2021**, *14*, 276, doi:10.3390/ph1403027 81

Eun Ha Kang and Yeong Wook Song
Pharmacological Interventions for Pulmonary Involvement in Rheumatic Diseases
Reprinted from: *Pharmaceutical* **2021**, *14*, 251, doi:10.3390/ph14030251 . . . . **99**

**Barbara Ruaro, Marco Confalonieri, Francesco Salton, Barbara Wade, Elisa Baratella,
Pietro Geri, Paola Confalonieri, Metka Kodric, Marco Biolo and Cosimo Bruni**
The Relationship between Pulmonary Damage and Peripheral Vascular Manifestations in
Systemic Sclerosis Patients
Reprinted from: *Pharmaceutical* **2021**, *14*, 403, doi:10.3390/ph14050403 . . . . **121**

**Barbara Ruaro, Marco Confalonieri, Marco Matucci-Cerinic, Francesco Salton,
Paola Confalonieri, Mario Santagiuliana, Gloria Maria Citton, Elisa Baratella and Cosimo
Bruni** The Treatment of Lung Involvement in Systemic Sclerosis
Reprinted from: *Pharmaceutical* **2021**, *14*, 154, doi:10.3390/ph14020154 . . . . **137**

**José M. Serra López-Matencio, Manuel Gómez, Esther F. Vicente-Rabaneda,
Miguel A. González-Gay, Julio Ancochea and Santos Castañeda**
Pharmacological Interactions of Nintedanib and Pirfenidone in Patients with Idiopathic
Pulmonary Fibrosis in Times of COVID-19 Pandemic
Reprinted from: *Pharmaceutical* **2021**, *14*, 819, doi:10.3390/ph14080819 . . . . **149**

About the Editors

Barbara Ruaro, MD, European PhD, is a Senior Researcher at the Pulmonology Department, University Hospital of Cattinara, University of Trieste, Trieste, Italy. Barbara is a licensed Medical Doctor at the University of Turin (Italy). SShe obtained her specialization in Genoa (Italy) and after a period of fellowship in Ghent (Belgium) and in Chicago (USA) she received her European PhD. She was then a Postdoctoral Research Fellow at the University of Genoa. She was awarded an Investigator Starting Grant at the National Congress of Medicine. Barbara is a frequent speaker at national and international events. Currently, she is a professor of the Specialization Course on Respiratory Diseases at the University of Trieste. She coordinates many research projects. Barbara has authored several papers, posters, and book chapters. Her research activities have been reported in more than 80 publications (h-index 24) and she has been a speaker at more than 30 invited lectures in international and national symposia. Her areas of research interest encompass autoimmune diseases with lung involvement, telemedicine, imaging in pulmonary and rheumatic diseases, and COVID-19.

Francesco Salton, MD, is a physician at the Pulmonology department at the University Hospital of Trieste (Trieste, Italy) and a guest scientist at the International Center for Genetic Engineering and Biotechnology (ICGEB, Trieste, Italy) since 2016. Francesco's research interests involve lung epithelial biology and regeneration with special regard to idiopathic pulmonary fibrosis, which he studied in cooperation with the Temple Lung Center (Philadelphia, PA, USA). He has also designed and coordinated two international multicenter clinical trials on the use of glucocorticoids in severe COVID-19 pneumonia and acute respiratory distress syndrome (ARDS). FS is the author or co-author of 34 international indexed publications. He has served as a guest editor for international scientific journals and as a speaker in several national and international conferences. FS is a member of the American Thoracic Society (ATS), European Respiratory Society (ERS), World Association for Bronchology and Interventional Pulmonology (WABIP), Associazione Italiana Pneumologi Ospedalieri (AIPO), and Società Italiana di Pneumologia (SIP).

Paola Confalonieri, MD, is a Physician at the Pulmonology Department of the University Hospital of Trieste (Trieste, Italy). She earned her degree with honors in Medicine and Surgery at the University of Trieste in 2017. Since 2019, she has been a resident in Respiratory Medicine at the University of Trieste. She is the author and coauthor of 18 scientific articles published in international journals in the field of lung diseases. She is the coauthor of the chapter "Alveolar Epithelial Type II Cells" in the book "Encyclopedia of Respiratory Medicine, 2nd ed." She has attended national and international conferences and she has given oral presentations at national events. She is a member of the European Respiratory Society (ERS) and Associazione Italiana Pneumologi Ospedalieri (AIPO).

Preface to "Rheumatic Diseases: Pathophysiology, Targeted Therapy, Focus on Vascular and Pulmonary Manifestations"

This book aims to summarize the latest advances in the rheumatic diseases, particularly regarding their pathophysiology and targeted therapy, with a focus on the recent efforts of vascular and pulmonary manifestations in order to anticipate new and future directions of these research topics.

Rheumatic diseases represent a heterogeneous group of severe autoimmune disorders. The present Special Issue aims to provide an overview of the diversity and complexity of vascular and pulmonary manifestations of rheumatic diseases and to highlight gaps in our knowledge of how to effectively manage them. Despite their significant morbidity, we have a limited understanding of their pathogenesis. The eleven published articles reported here underline the complexity of rheumatic diseases and the difficulty of managing them. The manuscripts provide an overview of the pathophysiology and current management approach of these disorders, highlighting tools that assist with diagnosis, risk stratification, and therapy.

A significant number of articles have reported innovative and effective treatments for the most frequent and debilitating complications of rheumatic diseases. The book emphasizes the importance of multidisciplinary teams using the skills of laboratory researchers, clinicians, radiologists, and pathologists.

Furthermore, recent findings are presented and discussed, highlighting strategies to combat worsening symptoms of rheumatic diseases. The research described in this book provide an extremely useful example of the results achieved in the field of anti-rheumatic drug development. Detailed information on new breakthroughs can be found in this book. We strongly encourage a wide group of readers to explore the book that we are presenting for inspiration to develop new approaches to the diagnosis and treatment of rheumatic diseases.

We are grateful to all the authors for their contributions. We would also like to thank all reviewers for their help with evaluating manuscripts. We thank MDPI for their decision to publish this book and Ms. Fendy Fan for her kind assistance and technical support.

Barbara Ruaro, Francesco Salton, and Paola Confalonieri
Editors

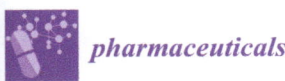

Article

Cardiopulmonary Exercise Testing Is an Accurate Tool for the Diagnosis of Pulmonary Arterial Hypertension in Scleroderma Related Diseases

Mattia Bellan [1,2,3,*], Ailia Giubertoni [1,2], Cristina Piccinino [2], Mariachiara Buffa [1], Debora Cromi [1], Daniele Sola [2], Roberta Pedrazzoli [2], Ileana Gagliardi [1], Elisa Calzaducca [1], Erika Zecca [1], Filippo Patrucco [1,2], Giuseppe Patti [1,2], Pier Paolo Sainaghi [1,2,3] and Mario Pirisi [1,2,3]

1. Department of Translational Medicine, Università del Piemonte Orientale UPO, 28100 Novara, Italy; AiliaGiubertoni@hotmail.com (A.G.); mariachiarabuffa@gmail.com (M.B.); 20008635@studenti.uniupo.it (D.C.); ileanagagliardi91@gmail.com (I.G.); elisa.calzaducca91@gmail.com (E.C.); erikazecca24@yahoo.it (E.Z.); filippo_patrucco@hotmail.it (F.P.); giuseppe.patti@med.uniupo.it (G P.); pierpaolo.sainaghi@med.uniupo.it (P.P.S.); mario.pirisi@med.uniupo.it (M.P.)
2. "AOU Maggiore della Carità" Hospital, 28100 Novara, Italy; cristina.piccinino@maggioreosp.novara.it (C.P.); daniele.sola@med.uniupo.it (D.S.); robepedra@gmail.com (R.P.)
3. CAAD, (Center for Translational Research on Autoimmune and Allergic Diseases Maggiore della Carità Hospital and Università del Piemonte Orientale UPO, 28100 Novara, Italy
* Correspondence: mattia.bellan@med.uniupo.it

Abstract: The early diagnosis of pulmonary arterial hypertension (PAH) is a major determinant of prognosis in patients affected by connective tissue diseases (CTDs) complicated by PAH. In the present paper we investigated the diagnostic accuracy of cardiopulmonary exercise testing (CPET) in this specific setting. We recorded clinical and laboratory data of 131 patients who underwent a CPET at a pulmonary hypertension clinic. Out of them, 112 (85.5%) had a diagnosis of CTDs; 8 (6.1%) received a diagnosis of CTDs-PAH and 11 (8.4%) were affected PH of different etiology. Among CPET parameters the following parameters showed the best diagnostic performance for PAH: peak volume of oxygen uptake (VO$_2$; AUC: 0.845, CI95% 0.767–0.904), ratio between ventilation and volume of exhaled carbon dioxide (VE/VCO$_2$ slope; AUC: 0.888, CI95%: 0.817–0.938) and end-tidal partial pressures (PetCO$_2$; AUC: 0.792, CI95%: 0.709–0.861). These parameters were comparable among CTDs-PAH and PH of different etiology. The diagnostic performance was even improved by creating a composite score which included all the three parameters identified. In conclusion, CPET is a very promising tool for the stratification of risk of PAH among CTDs patients; the use of composite measures may improve diagnostic performance.

Keywords: pulmonary arterial hypertension; systemic sclerosis; scleroderma; cardiopulmonary exercise testing

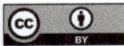

1. Introduction

Pulmonary arterial hypertension (PAH) is a progressive disease affecting the precapillary pulmonary vascular bed, leading to an increase in pulmonary vascular resistance and right ventricular failure, burdened by a high mortality rate [1]. PAH is a severe complication of different connective tissue disease (CTDs), particularly: systemic sclerosis (SSc), mixed connective tissue diseases (MCTD) and SSc overlapping with other CTDs [2]. The early diagnosis of SSc-PAH is difficult, since PAH is initially minimally symptomatic or asymptomatic, but absolutely pivotal: indeed, the early initiation of an effective treatment is the most relevant prognostic factor in patients affected by PAH [3]. This is why patients diagnosed with CTDs are commonly followed-up and screened for the development of PAH; the two-step algorithm DETECT is the most commonly used screening tool [4]. The DETECT algorithm includes a first step in which patients are indicated to echocardiography according to a composite score derived from the following variables: forced vital capacity (FVC) and diffusing capacity of the lung for carbon monoxide (DLCO); presence of teleangectasias and anti-centromere antibody; serum urate; N-terminal probrain natriuretic peptide and presence of right axis deviation on electrocardiogram. On the basis of the result of echocardiography, at risk patients will be further tested with right heart catheterization (RHC). The detect score well performs in this setting, showing a very high sensitivity (96%), as required by any screening tool; however, the specificity is low (48%) having as a direct consequence the need for a high number of unnecessary invasive measurement of pulmonary pressure, by RHC [5]. This is why there is an unmet need of novel biomarkers able to refine the PAH risk stratification among CTDs patients [6,7]. In the last years, cardiopulmonary exercise testing (CPET) has been proposed as a novel tool to better select those patients at higher risk of PAH, thus requiring RHC [8]. CPET provides an important insight into exercise physiology and, according to recent data, may contribute to the identification of PAH among SSc patients [9]. In the present study we aimed to confirm this observation and to evaluate whether CPET findings among PAH-CTDs patients differ from patients affected by PH of a different etiology, in a pilot study.

2. Results

We recruited 131 patients, 115 (87.8%) females; the median age was 61.5 (52.0–69.5) years. Out of them, 112 (85.5%) had a diagnosis of CTDs alone: 84 were affected by SSc, 15 by overlap syndrome, 5 by MCTD and 8 by Undifferentiated connective tissue disease (UCTD). The median disease duration of CTDs was 5 (2–11) years; antirheumatic treatment mainly included hydroxychloroquine (N = 57, 50.9%) and methotrexate (N = 15, 13.4%). 37 patients (33.0%) were receiving steroids when CPT was performed.

8 (6.1%) received a diagnosis of CTDs-PAH: 6 were affected by SSc, 1 by overlap syndrome and 1 by MCTD; 6 patients were on endothelin receptor antagonists, 5 patients were receiving phosphodiesterare 5 inhibitors. Moreover 1 patient was receiving riociguat and 1 patient selexipag. The median time to pulmonary hypertension diagnosis was 5 (3–6) years.

Finally, 11 (8.4%) patients received a diagnosis of PH of different etiology (5 PAH, 4 chronic thromboembolism, 1 unknown).

In Table 1 we report the main clinical and laboratory features of the three study groups:

Table 1. Main general features of the study population and comparison between groups. For abbreviation: CTDs, connective tissue diseases; PAH, pulmonary arterial hypertension; PH, pulmonary hypertension; M, males; F, females; FVC, forced vital capacity; FEV1, forced expiratory volume in the 1st second; DLCO, diffusing capacity of the lung for carbon monoxide; LVEF, left ventricular ejection fraction; sPAP, systolic pulmonary arterial pressure. * A vs. B; § A vs. B and C.

	Group A CTDs	Group B CTDs-PAH	Group C PH	p
Gender, M/F	11/101	1/7	4/7	0.04
Age, years	61 (50–68)	70.5 (68–73.5)	65 (56–78)	0.01 *
FVC, % of predicted value	104 (92–116)	99 (89–126)	87 (67–106)	0.21
FEV1, % of predicted value	104 (91–115)	117 (90–124)	87 (74–111)	0.16
DLCO, % of predicted value	89 (77–96)	48 (46–62)	76 (64–79)	<0.0001 §
LVEF, %	63 (59–66)	64 (63–66)	57 (54–65)	0.18
sPAP, mmHg	26 (23–30)	46 (38–65)	47 (39–53)	<0.0001 §

As shown in the Table 1, patients affected by PH show higher sPAP and lower DLCO, as expected. Among CTD patients, those with PAH are significantly older. Looking at the CPET parameters, we compared the results of the test among groups. The results are shown in Table 2:

Table 2. Comparison of the main CPET parameters among groups between groups. For abbreviation: VO_2, volume of oxygen uptake; VE, ventilation; VCO_2, volume of exhaled carbon dioxide; $PetCO_2$, end-tidal partial pressures for CO_2. * A vs. B; § A vs. B and C; ° C vs. A and B.

	Group A CTDs	Group B CTDs-PAH	Group C PH	p
Peak VO2 (ml/kg/min)	18.4 (15.1–21.8)	12.5 (12.0–14.0)	11.6 (9.2–17.0)	<0.0001 §
VO2 at first ventilator threshold (% of peak VO2)	56 (49–64)	55 (48–58)	64 (24–73)	0.25
VE/VCO2 slope	29.1 (26.4–32.6)	40.4 (36.3–41.2)	37.1 (31.6–51.5)	<0.0001 §
PetCO2 basal (mmHg)	29.2 (26.1–31.0)	25.0 (23.2–26.9)	25.9 (22.9–27.6)	0.005 §
Pulse O2 peak (%)	82 (73–92)	66 (63–75)	89 (52–92)	0.04 *
EQCO2 basal	37 (34–42)	42 (38–45)	41 (38–48)	0.04
Duration of exercise, minutes	10 (8.5–12)	7 (4.5–9.5)	8 (6.5–10)	0.004 §
Maximal workload, watts	68.5 (52.0–89.0)	37.0 (32.5–50.0)	56.0 (35.5–88.0)	0.02 *
Respiratory exchange ratio	1.0 (1.0–1.0)	1.0 (0.5–1.0)	1.1 (1.0–1.2)	0.004 °

Patients with PH have a significantly lower peak VO_2 and basal $PetCO_2$, and a significantly higher VE/VCO2 slope. These parameters were comparable among CTDs-PAH patients and PH patients with different etiologies. We finally evaluated the diagnostic accuracy of the different CPET parameters considered. In Figure 1 we reported the ROC curve for peak VO_2 for the diagnosis of PAH in patients affected by CTDs. As shown, this parameter has very good diagnostic performance (AUC: 0.845; CI 0.767–0.904); a value ≤ 14.1 is 87.5% sensitive (LR− 0.15, CI95% 0.02–0.90) and 83.05% specific (LR+ 5.16, CI95%: 3.2–8.4) for PAH. The NPV is 98.4% (CI 95% 90.5–99.7%), while the PPV is 36.4% (CI 95% 26.1–48.2%).

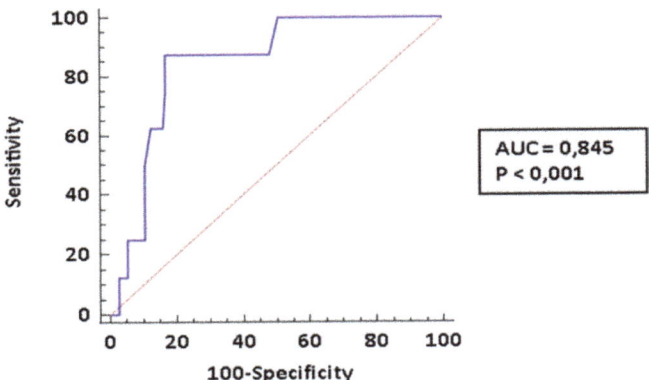

Figure 1. ROC curve for peak VO_2. We diagnosed 8 CTD-PAH.

In Figure 2 we reported the ROC curve for VE/VCO2 slope, which again demonstrates a very good diagnostic accuracy (AUC: 0.888; CI95%: 0.817–0.938); a threshold > 33.96 is 87.5% sensitive (LR− 0.15, CI95% 0.02–1.0) and 82.14% specific (LR+ 4.9, CI95%: 3.0–7.9) specific for PAH. The NPV is 98.3% (CI95% 90.4–99.7) and the PPV is 35.3 (CI95%: 25.3–46.7).

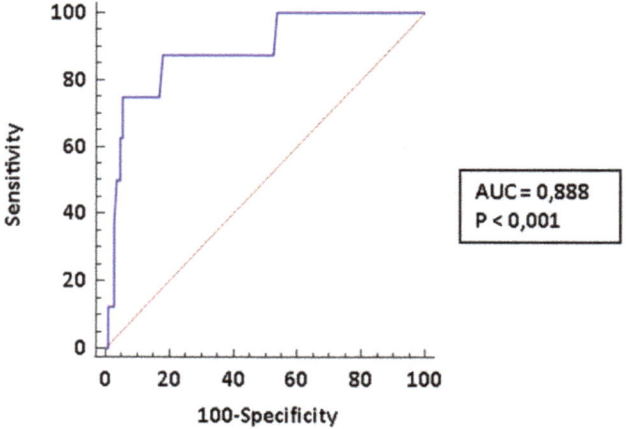

Figure 2. ROC curve for peak VE/VCO$_2$ slope. We diagnosed 8 CTD-PAH. For abbreviation: AUC, Area under the curve.

Moreover, in Figure 3 we reported the ROC curve for basal PetCO2; a threshold ≤ 27.2 is 87.5% sensitive (LR− 0.18; CI95% 0.03–1.1) and 71.43% specific (LR+ 3.1; CI95%: 2.1–4.5) specific for PAH, while the AUC is: 0.792 (CI95%: 0.709–0.861). The PPV is 25.4% (CI 95% 18.7–33.5) and the NPV is 98.1% (89.1–99.7).

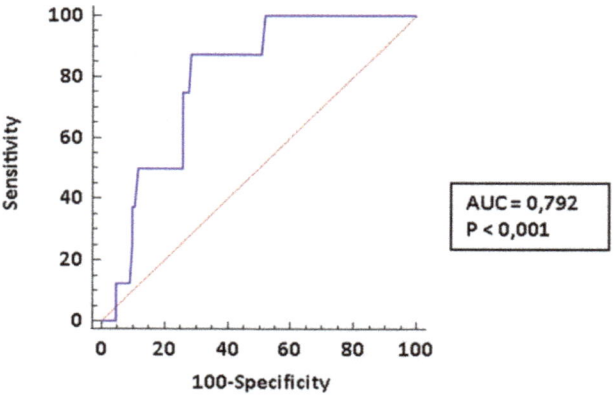

Figure 3. ROC curve for basal PetCO$_2$. We diagnosed 8 CTD-PAH.

We finally tried to evaluate the diagnostic accuracy of a composite predictive model including all these three parameters. We scored 1 point for each parameter considered: a peak VO$_2$ $\leq$ 14.1; a VE/VCO$_2$ slope > 33.96; a basal PetCO$_2$ $\leq$ 27.2. In Table 3 we report the different scores according to the presence/absence of PAH among CTDs patients. The distribution was significantly different (χ^2 for trend; 34.3 $p < 0.0001$).

Table 3. Application of the CPET scoring system among CTDs patients.

	Score = 0	Score = 1	Score = 2	Score = 3
CTDs	60 (53.6%)	34 (30.4%)	17 (15.2%)	1 (0.9%)
CTDs-PAH	1 (12.5%)	0	0	7 (87.5%)

As shown in the ROC curve (Figure 4), a score of 3 is 87.5% (CI95% 47.3–99.7) sensitive and 99.1% (CI95%:95.1–100.0) specific for PAH. The LR− is 0.13 (CI95%: 0.02–0.8) and the LR+ 98 (CI 95%: 13.7–701.8). The PPV is 91.6% (CI 95%: 60.3–98.7) and the NPV is 98.6% (CI 95%: 91.9–99.8).

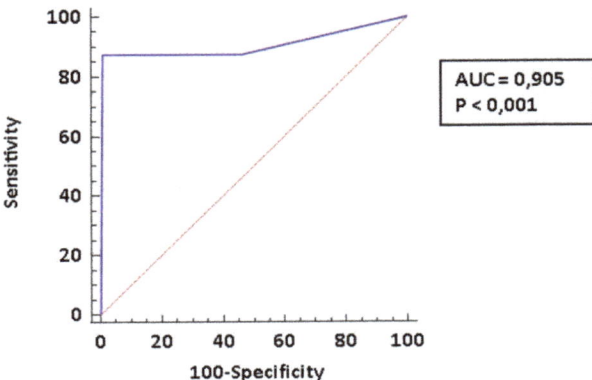

Figure 4. ROC curve for the composite model. We diagnosed 8 CTD-PAH.

3. Discussion

In the present paper we aimed at preliminary evaluating the diagnostic accuracy of CPET in the diagnosis of PAH among CTDs patients. According to our data, CPET is a potentially sensitive and specific tool for the diagnosis of pulmonary hypertension, independently from the underlying etiology. The use of composite, CPET-based scores might improve the diagnostic accuracy and should be evaluated on a larger scale, since our pilot study provides only preliminary data. These findings will be herein discussed on the basis of the current literature.

SSc is a potentially severe condition; according to a meta-analysis published in 2012, which pooled data from different cohort studies covering over 50 years of observation, patients affected by SSc have a standardized mortality ratio 3.5 times higher than the general population [10]. PAH is a major determinant of this excess of deaths; in fact, according to the EUSTAR cohort study, more than half SSc patients dies because of a condition related to their underlying CTD; more specifically, around 15% of deaths are related to the development of PAH [11]. Patients affected by PAH have a severe prognosis; the annual mortality is around 10% in idiopathic PAH [3] and even worse in CTDs-related PAH, particularly when SSc is the underlying rheumatic condition [12]. Indeed, according to Mukerjee et al., the survival rate at 1-, 2- and 3-years was respectively 81%, 63%, and 56% [13] and a comparable prognosis has been reported more recently in different registry based studies [14,15].

The degree of hemodynamic impairment is universally considered a main prognostic predictor in PAH [3,14–16]; being available different therapeutic strategies effective in the management of PAH, it is reasonable to consider early diagnosis fundamental to impact on patients' prognosis. This is why SSc patients should undergo a regular screening strategy to early identify cardiopulmonary involvement and to start the treatment as soon as possible. According to the lastly updated Eular guidelines for the management of SSc-PAH, the treatment of this condition should include the same classes of drugs used in the other forms of PAH; this recommendation belongs to the results of different high quality clinical trials including heterogeneous population of PAH patients among whom CTDs-PAH was included [17].

The most commonly used screening protocol is the DETECT algorithm, firstly described by Coghlan et al. in 2014; it is a very well performing diagnostic tool, particularly in the context of a screening strategy, because of its optimal sensitivity. However, it should be acknowledged that its specificity is quite low. This is not negligible; in fact, the relatively low positive predictive value accounts for an excess of patients needing to be tested with the gold standard for PAH diagnosis, the RHC. This test is invasive and burdened by potential complications which, although rare, may be severe and even fatal [18]; thus, a better tailoring of screening strategy and individual's risk stratification may allow to reduce the costs and limit the risk for patients, by reducing the number of patients unnecessary tested.

In the last few years an increasing number of papers investigated the diagnostic role of CPET in the identification of those CTDs patients with PAH [19]. Although this test is not currently included in the guidelines for the management of SSc, the current literature is highly consistent in confirming its potential in the identification of PAH in this specific group of individuals.

In our study, we selected the best performing parameters and finally we built a composite score to improve their diagnostic accuracy. We reported that peak VO_2 is significantly reduced in CTDs-PAH, with respect to CTDs alone; this reduction is comparable to what observed in patients affected by PH with different etiologies. Similar results were previously reported by Dumitrescu et al. and may be explained by the fact that peak VO_2 is closely related to cardiac output during exercise; therefore, a high peak VO_2 reflects a good hemodynamic adaptation to exercise and is able to rule out PAH with high accuracy. The authors also evaluated the best performing threshold for this parameter, identifying a cut-off of 13.8, very close to our one [8]. Another common finding is the good clinical performance of VE/VCO_2 slope. In a recent paper of an Italian group, VE/VCO_2 slope was the best parameter able to identify PAH at RHC, on top of a positive DETECT screening. Interestingly, once more, the cut-off used was quite close to the one that we identified (35.5 vs. 33.9) and showed an optimal sensitivity and a good specificity yielding a PPV of 0.636 (0.556–0.750) [9]. We also tested the role of $PetCO_2$; as already reported by Dumitrescu et al. [8], this marker of ventilator efficiency is predictive of PAH, although its diagnostic power is lower than peakVO_2. Interestingly, these alterations are not specific for CTDs-PAH; we, indeed, included a subgroup of subjects suffering for PH of different etiologies, demonstrating that the CPET is more generally able to detect cardiopulmonary involvement. A major novel finding of our work is the observation that combining different CPET parameters may improve the diagnostic accuracy of the test; in particular, we propose a 3-points score based on the three previously discussed parameters which very well fits to our population. Despite having a sensitivity which is similar to the one of any single parameter tested, the use of a composite score significantly enhances the specificity and the PPV. This may, finally, significantly increase the diagnostic accuracy of the present tool. On this basis, we can postulate that CPET may contribute to a better stratification of those patients really requiring a RHC; it can be argued that, in the context of a screening procedure, the use of less sensitive tools than DETECT algorithm can cause the loss of some PAH cases with relevant clinical implications; however, RHC is an invasive procedure. Thus, we might hypothesize that RHC may be postponed in those patients with an indication according to DETECT but with a normal CPET. These subjects may be addressed to a stricter follow-up to early identify clinical deterioration. Moreover, we can also postulate that, giving the very high PPV of CPET, it could even represent an alternative to RHC in those patients at higher procedural risk. However, we acknowledge that the low number of cases and the cross-sectional design of the study limit the possibility to truly test our score as a diagnostic tool. Prospective studies are indeed required to evaluate its potential clinical application.

A further element of discussion belongs to the observation that SSc patients may have less marked alteration of CPET even in absence of PAH; according to previous findings, in fact, patients with SSc may show increased VE/VCO_2 slope and decreased peak VO_2 with respect to the general population [20]. It will be interesting to evaluate, in the next future, whether those patients with an altered CPET may represent a subset of individuals at higher risk for PAH development. Obviously, our study because of its cross-sectional design is not able to give an answer to this relevant research question.

Our paper has some limitations: first of all, the number of patients affected by PAH included in the final analysis is low; our study should be, in fact, considered for what it actually is: a pilot study with preliminary results that, although promising, require a confirmation on a larger scale. Furthermore, some of the patients received a diagnosis of pulmonary hypertension on the basis of the echocardiographic findings, being RHC contraindicated. Despite this is in line with the current international guidelines, we should acknowledge that RHC is the gold standard for the diagnosis of pulmonary hypertension. Moreover, the diagnostic efficacy of this CPET-based score should be tested in a more comprehensive strategy, as integration of the standard DETECT algorithm. A further relevant limitation is that we considered prevalent PAH, rather than incident PAH; patients were not naïve to treatment, which might have affected our findings.

4. Materials and Methods

We performed a cross-sectional, observational study on patients evaluated at the Pulmonary Hypertension Clinic of the Cardiology Division, University Hospital of Novara from 3 October 2016 to 12 December 2019. The clinic was the main referral for Rheumatology Units of the geographic area, representing a major facility for PAH screening of CTDs patients. The study protocol was approved by the local ethical committee and conducted in strict accordance with the principles of the Declaration of Helsinki. Written informed consent was obtained from all individual participants included in the study.

We included all the patients older than 18 years who underwent, under clinical indication a CPET. We excluded from the study those who refused to sign the informed consent. We included in the study both CTDs patients and patients with a diagnosis of PH with a different etiology. The following criteria were applied to classify the different rheumatic conditions:

- SSc: 2013 ACR/Eular classification criteria [21];
- MCTD: Kasukawa's criteria [22];
- Overlap syndrome: patients fulfilling the classification criteria for SSc along with those of other rheumatic conditions [23];
- UCTD was made when patients with a connective tissue disease did not meet the classification criteria of any specific syndrome [24].

All the included patients also underwent a comprehensive clinical evaluation and a biochemistry panel; moreover, respiratory function and echocardiography were performed as described in previous papers belonging to the same project [6,7].

We recorded the following standardized measurements: forced vital capacity (FVC), forced expiratory volume in one second (FEV1), and FEV1/FVC%), diffusing capacity of the lung for carbon monoxide adjusted for alveolar volume (DLCO VA), measured with the single-breath Jones-Meade protocol, corrected for alveolar ventilation, systolic pulmonary pressure (sPAP), right atrium area (RAA), right ventricle diameter (RVD), and ejection fraction (EF).

According to the application of international guidelines, those patients with a suspected PAH underwent right heart catherization. PAH was defined by mean pulmonary artery pressure (mPAP) ≥ 25 mmHg, pulmonary capillary wedge pressure ≤ 15 mmHg, and pulmonary vascular resistance >3 wood units. Whenever contraindications to RHC occurred, pulmonary hypertension was diagnosed based on echocardiography-estimated sPAP ≥ 35 mmHg and additional high probability criteria (1 patient in the group B and 5 patients in the group C), in agreement with the 2015 ESC/ESR guidelines [1].

CPET was performed on a stationary bicycle ergometer, within two weeks from echocardiographic assessment and PFTs. The exercise protocol consists of 3 min of rest followed by the incremental work rate to the patients' maximum tolerance, then 5 min of recovery. The incremental work rate was selected according to the patient's exercise capacity to aim for 8–12 min in length. Gas exchange was measured breath-by-breath during the test using a Schiller Cardiovit CS-200 Ergo-Spiro System (Baar, Switzerland); we used the Ganshorn Medizine Eletronic software for pulmonary function testing (v. LF8.5M

SR3, Niederlauer, Germany). Equipment was calibrated before each exam. ECG and pulse oximetry were continuously monitored, and blood pressure was measured every three minutes. Minute ventilation (VE), heart rate (HR), oxygen uptake (VO_2), carbon dioxide production (VCO_2), CO_2 ventilatory equivalent (VE/VCO_2 or $EQCO_2$), O_2 ventilatory equivalent (VE/VO_2 or EQO_2), end tidal O_2 ($PetO_2$), end tidal CO_2 ($PetCO_2$), tidal volume and $PulseO_2$ were averaged every 10 s. Predicted value for peak VO_2 were calculated according to the standard formula. The first ventilatory threshold was determined from gas exchange by the V-slope method, derived from the plot with VO_2 and VCO_2 recognizing the point where VCO_2 started increasing faster than VO_2, in all patients. The relationship between VE and VCO2 (VE/VCO_2 slope) was calculated as the slope of the linear relationship between VE and VCO_2 from one minute after the beginning of loaded exercise to the end of the isocapnic buffering period. We considered maximal effort ad achieved if the respiratory exchange ratio (RER) calculated as the ratio between VO_2 and VCO_2 was above 1,10. All CPET were executed and analyzed by one physician's blinded to patients' clinical features.

Statistical Analysis

All the data were recorded in a database and analyzed by the statistical software package MedCalc v.19.6.4 (MedCalc Software, Broekstraat 52, 9030, Mariakerke, Belgium). Continuous variables are presented as medians and interquartile range [IQR]. We compared continuous variables among groups by Kruskal-Wallis test, while categorical distribution was tested by Pearson's χ^2.

To test the diagnostic performance of different CPET parameters among CTDs patients, receiver operating characteristics curves were built, with calculation of the areas under the curve (AUC). Moreover, we calculated the sensitivity, specificity, positive and negative likelihood ratio (LR+ and LR−), negative predictive value (NPV) and positive predictive value (PPV) for the different thresholds. NPV and PPV were calculated on the basis of an estimated rate of CTDs-PAH of 10%. The best diagnostic thresholds were identified according to the Youden index J and used to build a composite score which was tested for its diagnostic performance.

The level of significance chosen for all statistical analysis was 0.05 (two-tailed).

5. Conclusions

In conclusion, our paper supports the idea that CPET should be considered for the extensive use in the follow-up of CTDs patients at risk for PAH; a multiparametric diagnostic strategy might be more effective to improve the diagnostic performance of this examination.

Author Contributions: Conceptualization, M.B. (Mattia Bellan), A.G., C.P., P.P.S. and M.P.; data curation, M.B. (Mariachiara Buffa), A.G., C.P., M.B. (Mattia Bellan), D.C., D.S., R.P., I.G., E.C., E.Z. and F.P.; formal analysis, M.B. (Mattia Bellan), G.P. and M.P.; investigation, M.B. (Mattia Bellan), A.G., C.P., D.S., R.P., I.G., E.C., E.Z., F.P. and G.P.; methodology, M.B. (Mattia Bellan), A.G., C.P. and P.P.S.; project administration, P.P.S.; writing—original draft, M.B. (Mattia Bellan); writing—review and editing, M.B. (Mattia Bellan), G.P., P.P.S. and M.P. All authors have read and agreed to the published version of the manuscript.

Funding: This research received no external funding.

Institutional Review Board Statement: The study was conducted according to the guidelines of the Declaration of Helsinki, and approved by the Ethics Committee of Novara (protocol code 105/16, approved on 09/09/2016).

Informed Consent Statement: Informed consent was obtained from all subjects involved in the study.

Data Availability Statement: Data are available upon reasonable request to the corresponding author.

Conflicts of Interest: The authors declare no conflict of interest.

References

1. Galiè, N.; Humbert, M.; Vachiery, J.L.; Gibbs, S.; Lang, I.; Torbicki, A.; Simonneau, G.; Peacock, A.; Vonk Noordegraaf, A.; Beghetti, M. Guidelines for the diagnosis and treatment of pulmonary hypertension: The joint task force for the diagnosis and treatment of pulmonary hypertension of the European Society of Cardiology (ESC) and the European Respiratory Society (ERS): Endorsed by: Association for European Paediatric and Congenital Cardiology (AEPC), International Society for Heart and Lung Transplantation (ISHLT). *Eur. Heart J.* **2016**, *37*, 67–119. [CrossRef] [PubMed]
2. Jawad, H.; McWilliams, S.R.; Bhalla, S. cardiopulmonary manifestations of collagen vascular diseases. *Curr. Rheumatol. Rep.* **2017**, *19*, 71. [CrossRef] [PubMed]
3. Humbert, M.; Sitbon, O.; Yaïci, A.; Montani, D.; O'Callaghan, D.S.; Jaïs, X.; Parent, F.; Savale, L.; Natali, D.; Günther, S. French pulmonary arterial hypertension network. Survival in incident and prevalent cohorts of patients with pulmonary arterial hypertension. *Eur. Respir. J.* **2010**, *36*, 549–555. [CrossRef] [PubMed]
4. Coghlan, J.G.; Denton, C.P.; Grünig, E.; Bonderman, D.; Distler, O.; Khanna, D.; Müller-Ladner, U.; Pope, J.E.; Vonk, M.C.; Doelberg, M.; et al. Evidence-based detection of pulmonary arterial hypertension in systemic sclerosis: The DETECT study. *Ann. Rheum. Dis.* **2014**, *73*, 1340–1349. [CrossRef]
5. Hao, Y.; Thakkar, V.; Stevens, W.; Morrisroe, K.; Prior, D.; Rabusa, C.; Youssef, P.; Gabbay, E.; Roddy, J.; Walker, J. A comparison of the predictive accuracy of three screening models for pulmonary arterial hypertension in systemic sclerosis. *Arthritis Res. Ther.* **2015**, *17*, 7. [CrossRef] [PubMed]
6. Bellan, M.; Dimagli, A.; Piccinino, C.; Giubertoni, A.; Ianniello, A.; Grimoldi, F.; Sguazzotti, M.; Nerviani, A.; Barini, M.; Carriero, A. Role of Gas6 and TAM receptors in the identification of cardiopulmonary involvement in systemic sclerosis and scleroderma spectrum disorders. *Dis. Markers* **2020**, *2020*, 2696173. [CrossRef]
7. Bellan, M.; Giubertoni, A.; Piccinino, C.; Dimagli, A.; Grimoldi, F.; Sguazzotti, M.; Burlone, M.E.; Smirne, C.; Sola, D.; Marino, P. Red cell distribution width and platelet count as biomarkers of pulmonary arterial hypertension in patients with connective tissue disorders. *Dis. Markers* **2019**, *2019*, 4981982. [CrossRef]
8. Dumitrescu, D.; Nagel, C.; Kovacs, G.; Bollmann, T.; Halank, M.; Winkler, J.; Hellmich, M.; Grünig, E.; Olschewski, H.; Ewert, R. Cardiopulmonary exercise testing for detecting pulmonary arterial hypertension in systemic sclerosis. *Heart* **2017**, *103*, 774–782. [CrossRef]
9. Santaniello, A.; Casella, R.; Vicenzi, M.; Rota, I.; Montanelli, G.; De Santis, M.; Bellocchi, C.; Lombardi, F.; Beretta, L. Cardiopulmonary exercise testing in a combined screening approach to individuate pulmonary arterial hypertension in systemic sclerosis. *Rheumatology* **2020**, *59*, 1581–1586. [CrossRef]
10. Elhai, M.; Meune, C.; Avouac, J.; Kahan, A.; Allanore, Y. Trends in mortality in patients with systemic sclerosis over 40 years: A systematic review and meta-analysis of cohort studies. *Rheumatology* **2012**, *51*, 1017–1026. [CrossRef]
11. Tyndall, A.J.; Bannert, B.; Vonk, M.; Airò, P.; Cozzi, F.; Carreira, P.; Bancel, D.F.; Allanore, Y.; Müller-Ladner, U.; Distler, O.; et al. Causes and risk factors for death in systemic sclerosis: A study from the EULAR scleroderma trials and research (EUSTAR) database. *Ann. Rheumatol. Dis.* **2010**, *69*, 1809–1815. [CrossRef]
12. Condliffe, R.; Kiely, D.G.; Peacock, A.J.; Corris, P.A.; Gibbs, J.S.; Vrapi, F.; Das, C.; Elliot, C.A.; Johnson, M.; DeSoyza, J.; et al. Connective tissue disease-associated pulmonary arterial hypertension in the modern treatment era. *Am. J. Respir. Crit. Care Med.* **2009**, *179*, 151–157. [CrossRef] [PubMed]
13. Mukerjee, D.; St George, D.; Coleiro, B.; Knight, C.; Denton, C.P.; Davar, J.; Black, C.M.; Coghlan, J.G. Prevalence and outcome in systemic sclerosis associated pulmonary arterial hypertension: Application of a registry approach. *Ann. Rheumatol. Dis.* **2003**, *62*, 1088–1093. [CrossRef] [PubMed]
14. Weatherald, J.; Boucly, A.; Launay, D.; Cottin, V.; Prévot, G.; Bourlier, D.; Dauphin, C.; Chaouat, A.; Savale, L.; Jaïs, X.; et al. Haemodynamics and serial risk assessment in systemic sclerosis associated pulmonary arterial hypertension. *Eur. Respir. J.* **2018**, *52*, 1800678. [CrossRef]
15. Chung, L.; Farber, H.W.; Benza, R.; Miller, D.P.; Parsons, L.; Hassoun, P.M.; McGoon, M.; Nicolls, M.R.; Zamanian, R.T. Unique predictors of mortality in patients with pulmonary arterial hypertension associated with systemic sclerosis in the REVEAL registry. *Chest* **2014**, *146*, 1494–1504. [CrossRef] [PubMed]
16. Xanthouli, P.; Jordan, S.; Milde, N.; Marra, A.; Blank, N.; Egenlauf, B.; Gorenflo, M.; Harutyunova, S.; Lorenz, H.M.; Nagel, C.; et al. Haemodynamic phenotypes and survival in patients with systemic sclerosis: The impact of the new definition of pulmonary arterial hypertension. *Ann. Rheumatol. Dis.* **2020**, *79*, 370–378. [CrossRef]
17. Kowal-Bielecka, O.; Fransen, J.; Avouac, J.; Becker, M.; Kulak, A.; Allanore, Y.; Distler, O.; Clements, P.; Cutolo, M.; Czirjak, L.; et al. EUSTAR coauthors. Update of EULAR recommendations for the treatment of systemic sclerosis. *Ann. Rheumatol. Dis.* **2017**, *76*, 1327–1339. [CrossRef] [PubMed]
18. Chen, Y.; Shlofmitz, E.; Khalid, N.; Bernardo, N.L.; Ben-Dor, I.; Weintraub, W.S.; Waksman, R. Right heart catheterization-related complications: A review of the literature and best practices. *Cardiol. Rev.* **2020**, *28*, 36–41. [CrossRef] [PubMed]
19. Weatherald, J.; Montani, D.; Jevnikar, M.; Jaïs, X.; Savale, L.; Humbert, M. Screening for pulmonary arterial hypertension in systemic sclerosis. *Eur. Respir. Rev.* **2019**, *28*, 190023. [CrossRef]
20. Rosato, E.; Romaniello, A.; Magrì, D.; Bonini, M.; Sardo, L.; Gigante, A.; Quarta, S.; Digiulio, M.A.; Viola, G.; Di Paolo, M.; et al. Exercise tolerance in systemic sclerosis patients without pulmonary impairment: Correlation with clinical variables. *Clin. Exp. Rheumatol.* **2014**, *32*, S103–S108.

21. Hoogen, F.V.D.; Khanna, D.; Fransen, J.; Johnson, S.R.; Baron, M.; Tyndall, A.; Matucci-Cerinic, M.; Naden, R.P.; Medsger, T.A., Jr.; Carreira, P.E.; et al. 2013 classification criteria for systemic sclerosis: An American college of rheumatolo-gy/European league against rheumatism collaborative initiative. *Ann. Rheumatol. Dis.* **2013**, *72*, 1747–1755. [CrossRef] [PubMed]
22. Kasukawa, R. Preliminary diagnostic criteria for classification of mixed connective tissue disease. In *Mixed Connective Tissue Disease and Antinuclear Antibodies*; Sharp, G., Ed.; Elsevier: Amsterdam, The Netherlands, 1987; p. 41.
23. Balbir-Gurman, A.; Braun-Moscovici, Y. Scleroderma overlap syndrome. *Isr. Med. Assoc. J.* **2011**, *13*, 14–20. [PubMed]
24. Mosca, M.; Baldini, C.; Bombardieri, S. Undifferentiated connective tissue diseases in 2004. *Clin. Exp. Rheumatol.* **2004**, *22*, S14–S18. [PubMed]

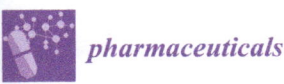

Article

Role of Osteopontin as a Potential Biomarker of Pulmonary Arterial Hypertension in Patients with Systemic Sclerosis and Other Connective Tissue Diseases (CTDs)

Mattia Bellan [1,2,3,*], Cristina Piccinino [2], Stelvio Tonello [1], Rosalba Minisini [1], Ailia Giubertoni [1], Daniele Sola [2], Roberta Pedrazzoli [2], Ileana Gagliardi [1], Erika Zecca [1], Elisa Calzaducca [1], Federica Mazzoleni [1], Roberto Piffero [1], Giuseppe Patti [1,2], Mario Pirisi [1,2,3] and Pier Paolo Sainaghi [1,2,3]

1. Department of Translational Medicine, Università del Piemonte Orientale UPO, 28100 Novara, Italy; stelvio.tonello@uniupo.it (S.T.); rosalba.minisini@uniupo.it (R.M.); ailia.giubertoni@maggioreosp.novara.it (A.G.); ileanagagliardi91@gmail.com (I.G.); erikazecca24@yahoo.it (E.Z.); elisa.calzaducca91@gmail.com (E.C.); 20009581@studenti.uniupo.it (F.M.); 20009551@studenti.uniupo.it (R.P.); giuseppe.patti@med.uniupo.it (G.P.); mario.pirisi@med.uniupo.it (M.P.); pierpaolo.sainaghi@med.uniupo.it (P.P.S.)
2. Division of Cardoilogy, "AOU Maggiore della Carità" Hospital, 28100 Novara, Italy; cristina.piccinino@maggioreosp.novara.it (C.P.); daniele.sola@med.uniupo.it (D.S.); roberta.pedrazzoli@maggioreosp.novara.it (R.P.)
3. CAAD (Center for Translational Research on Autoimmune and Allergic Disease), Maggiore della Carità Hospital, 28100 Novara, Italy
* Correspondence: mattia.bellan@med.uniupo.it

Abstract: Pulmonary arterial hypertension (PAH) is a severe complication of connective tissue diseases (CTD). Its early diagnosis is essential to start effective treatment. In the present paper, we aimed to evaluate the role of plasma osteopontin (OPN) as a candidate biomarker of PAH in a cohort of CTD patients. OPN is a pleiotropic protein involved in inflammation and fibrogenesis and, therefore, potentially promising in this specific clinical context. We performed a cross-sectional observational study on a cohort of 113 CTD patients (females N = 101, 89.4%) affected by systemic sclerosis N = 88 (77.9%), mixed connective tissue disease N = 10 (8.8%), overlap syndrome N = 10 (8.8%) or undifferentiated connective tissue disease N = 5 (4.4%). CTD-PAH patients showed significantly higher OPN plasma values than patients with CTD alone (241.0 (188.8–387.2) vs. 200.7 (133.5–281.6) ng/mL; $p = 0.03$). Although OPN levels were directly correlated with age and inversely with glomerular filtration rate, they remained associated with PAH at multivariate analysis. In conclusion, OPN was significantly associated with PAH among patients with CTD, suggesting it may have a role as a non-invasive disease biomarker of PAH.

Keywords: osteopontin; pulmonary arterial hypertension; systemic sclerosis; connective tissue diseases

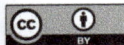

1. Introduction

Pulmonary arterial hypertension (PAH) is a relatively uncommon condition, defined by the presence of a mean pulmonary arterial pressure (mPAP) equal to or greater than 25 mmHg assessed during invasive right heart catheterization (RHC) at rest; PAH is defined precapillary when pulmonary capillary wedge pressure (PCWP) equal to or less than 15 mmHg, [1]. PAH is a severe and potentially life-threatening complication of systemic sclerosis (SS) and scleroderma spectrum disorders (SSD), a definition encompassing clinical entities sharing common features with SSc: mixed connective tissue diseases (MCTD) and SS overlap with other connective tissue diseases (CTDs) [2]. The CTD-associated PAH (CTD-PAH) carries a worse prognosis than the idiopathic PAH [3].

The early diagnosis of PAH in a patient affected by a CTD is crucial but requires a high degree of suspicion since PAH is initially minimally symptomatic or asymptomatic.

The two-step algorithm DETECT is the most widely used screening tool for SS patients [4]. However, novel diagnostic biomarkers and PAH predictors are needed [5,6], being a timely diagnosis quintessential to early treatment and improved prognosis [7].

Osteopontin (OPN) is a 32-kDa secreted, extracellular-matrix glycosylated phosphoprotein encoded by a gene located on chromosome 4 (4q13) with pleiotropic effects, among which regulation of the inflammatory response is paramount [8]. Indeed, systemic inflammatory disorders are associated with an increase in OPN plasma levels. For instance, patients with rheumatoid arthritis have high OPN concentrations [9]; similarly, OPN levels are increased in sepsis and have a prognostic value [10]. This increase follows the release of OPN by macrophages, activated T cells, endothelial and epithelial cells during the inflammatory response [8]: OPN then acts as a chemoattractant, assisting the recruitment of immune cells in the inflamed tissues [11].

Moreover, OPN is implicated in regulating fibrogenesis [12,13], with growing evidence linking this molecule specifically to the pathogenesis of dermal fibrosis in SSc [14]. Finally, OPN plays a role in the vascular remodeling process [15], and its levels are increased in patients affected by PAH. Importantly, OPN is one of the top five overregulated genes in explanted lungs of PAH patients, independently from what caused PAH, but with a direct correlation with the severity of the disease [16].

Inflammation, fibrosis and vascular remodeling are major pathogenetic mechanisms driving developing PAH during CTD clinical course. Therefore, OPN may represent a promising candidate biomarker of PAH among CTD patients; the present pilot study was built to verify this hypothesis.

2. Results

The study population included 101 females (89.4%) and 12 males (10.6%), with a median age of 65 years (54–74). These patients were classified as follows: SSc, N = 88 (77.9%); MCTD, N = 10 (8.8%); overlap syndrome, N = 10 (8.8%); UCTD, N = 5 (4.4%). Of the 88 patients with SSc, 68 (77.3%) were classified as limited cutaneous SSc and 20 (22.7%) with the diffuse variant. Table 1 presents the main clinical features and main antirheumatic ongoing treatment of the study population.

Table 1. Clinical and laboratory features of the study population. Abbreviations: CTD—connective tissue diseases; PAH—pulmonary arterial hypertension.

Clinical Features	Study Population	CTD without PAH	CTD-PAH	p
Female gender	101 (89.4)	87 (89.7)	14 (87.5)	0.68
Median age, years	65.0 (54.0–75.0)	62.0 (51.0–71.0)	74.0 (69.0–78.5)	0.0004
Hydroxychloroquine	65 (57.7)	57 (58.8)	8 (50.0)	0.59
Methotrexate	15 (13.3)	15 (15.5)	0 (0.0)	0.12
Steroids	38 (33.6)	36 (37.1)	2 (12.5)	0.08
Phosphodiesterase 5 inhibitors	6 (5.3)	2 (2.1)	6 (37.5)	<0.0001
Endothelin-1 receptors antagonists	8 (7.1)	7 (7.2)	8 (50.0)	<0.0001
Riociguat	1 (0.9)	0 (0.0)	1 (6.2)	0.14
Raynaud's phenomenon	102 (90.3)	87 (89.7)	14 (87.5)	0.61
Previous acral ulcers	49 (43.4)	43 (44.3)	7 (43.7)	1.00
Digital ulcers in the past month	5 (4.4)	4 (4.1)	1 (6.2)	0.54
Sclerodactyly	66 (58.4)	57 (58.8)	9 (56.2)	1.00
Puffy fingers	16 (14.2)	16 (16.5)	0 (0.0)	0.12
Telangiectasia	32 (28.3)	28 (28.9)	5 (31.2)	1.00
Pulmonary interstitial disease	38 (33.6)	31 (32.0)	7 (43.7)	0.40
Gastrointestinal involvement	22 (19.5)	18 (18.6)	4 (25.0)	0.51

Table 1. cont.

Clinical Features	Study Population	CTD without PAH	CTD-PAH	p
Renal involvement	3 (2.7)	2 (2.1)	1 (6.2)	0.37
Anti-nuclear antibodies (ANA)	104 (92.0)	88 (90.7)	16 (100.0)	0.35
Anti-centromere antibodies	69 (61.1)	56 (57.7)	13 (81.2)	0.10
Anti-Scl-70 antibodies	28 (24.8)	23 (23.7)	5 (31.2)	0.54
Anti-U1-RNP antibodies	21 (18.6)	16 (16.5)	5 (31.2)	0.17
Disease duration	5 (3–13)	5 (4–13)	5 (3–11)	0.66

Sixteen patients (14.2%) were diagnosed with CTD-PAH (all the patients received a diagnosis of type 1 pulmonary hypertension; however, 2/16 showed mixed pathogenesis, type 1 and 3). The diagnosis was established by RHC in 15/16 patients. The mean pulmonary arterial pressure (PAP) was 30 (26–36) mmHg, with a median pulmonary vein resistance of 4.1 (3.3–6.4) WU.

As shown in Table 1, PAH patients were significantly older than those with CTD. In Table 2, we report the differences among groups concerning laboratory and instrumental findings.

Table 2. Laboratory and instrumental data in the entire study population and in two subgroups categorized according to the presence/absence of pulmonary arterial hypertension. Abbreviations: CTD—connective tissue diseases; PAH—pulmonary arterial hypertension; WBC—white blood cells; Hb—hemoglobin—PLTs—platelets; ALT—alanine aminotransferase; AST—aspartate aminotransferase; eGFR—estimated glomerular filtration rate; CRP—C-reactive protein; ESR—erythrocyte sedimentation rate; BNP—brain natriuretic peptide; FEV1—forced expiratory volume in 1 s; FVC—forced vital capacity; TLC—total lung capacity; EF—ejection fraction; PAPS—pulmonary artery pressures; TAPSE—tricuspid annular plane excursion.

Variable	Study Population	CTD without PAH	CTD-PAH	p
WBC, $\times 10^9$/L	6.49 (5.26–7.68)	6.47 (5.26–7.63)	6.77 (5.15–7.87)	0.81
Hb, g/dL	12.8 (11.9–13.7)	12.9 (12.2–13.7)	11.3 (10.8–13.5)	0.01
PLTs, $\times 10^9$/L	228 (192–286)	234 (202–286)	188 (167–273)	0.07
ALT, U/L	17 (13–22)	18 (13–22)	13 (12–20)	0.33
AST, U/L	23 (20–26)	23 (20–26)	23 (20–27)	0.63
Creatinine, mg/dL	0.72 (0.61–0.88)	0.68 (0.6–0.81)	0.95 (0.81–1.08)	<0.0001
eGFR, mL/min	90 (63.5–101.3)	93 (72–103)	58.5 (51.5–64.5)	<0.0001
CRP, mg/dL	0.18 (0.04–0.78)	0.14 (0.04–0.34)	0.77 (0.04–0.98)	0.26
ESR, mm/h	14.5 (7–28)	13 (7–25)	25 (7–50)	0.31
C3, mg/dL	104 (90–121)	106 (91–121)	92 (84–119)	0.13
C4, mg/dL	24 (19–28)	24 (20–29)	22 (16–26)	0.11
BNP, pg/mL	46.8 (27.1–99.6)	39.6 (24.9–85.7)	177.0 (82.3–305.2)	<0.0001
FEV1, %	99 (88–114)	100.5 (88–113.5)	94 (88.5–113)	0.76
FVC, %	100 (90–112)	100 (90.5–113.5)	91 (80–104)	0.25
FEV1/FVC, %	109 (102–113.3)	109 (102–114)	107.5 (101–113)	0.74
TLC, %	98 (86.5–112)	99 (87–112)	82 (58–95)	0.07
DLCO-VA, %	86 (76–99)	87 (78–99)	54.5 (53–76)	0.008
DLCO-Hb, %	77 (61–91)	80 (62–91)	51 (43–72)	0.03
EF, %	63 (58–67)	63 (58–67)	61 (58.3–66)	0.41
PAPS, mmHg	27 (23–35)	26 (23–30)	44 (42–51)	<0.0001
TAPSE, mm	22 (19–24)	22 (20–24)	22 (18–23)	0.42

Looking at the laboratory parameters, patients with CTD-PAH showed lower Hb and eGFR; conversely, BNP was significantly higher. As expected, CTD-PAH patients have a reduced DLCO, while other pulmonary function tests were not statistically different from those observed in the other CTD patients. Moreover, CTD-PAH patients had higher PAPS.

Disease duration, years: 10.5 (4.0–14.0)

We then assessed the diagnostic role of OPN. First of all, patients with CTD-PAH have significantly higher plasma values compared to patients with CTD (241.0 (188.8–387.2) vs. 200.7 (133.5–281.6) ng/mL; $p = 0.03$; see also Figure 1).

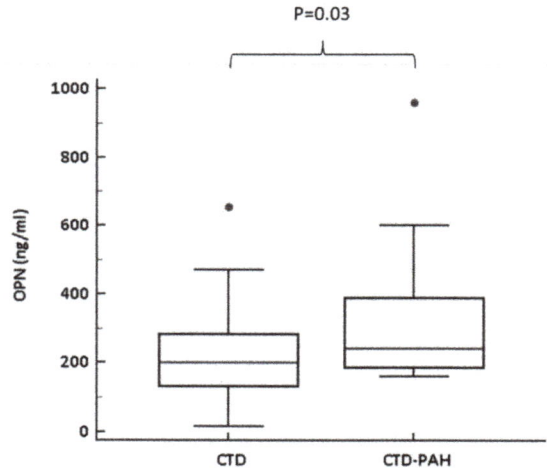

Figure 1. Plasma osteopontin (OPN) levels in CTD and CTD-associated pulmonary arterial hypertension (CTD-PAH) patients. As shown in the figure, CTD-PAH patients showed higher OPN plasma levels.

To assess the diagnostic power of measuring the OPN concentration in identifying PAH in patients with CTD, we built the corresponding ROC curve. As shown in Figure 2, OPN plasma levels had an area under the curve (AUC) = 0.662 (IC95% (0.567–0.748); $p = 0.016$).

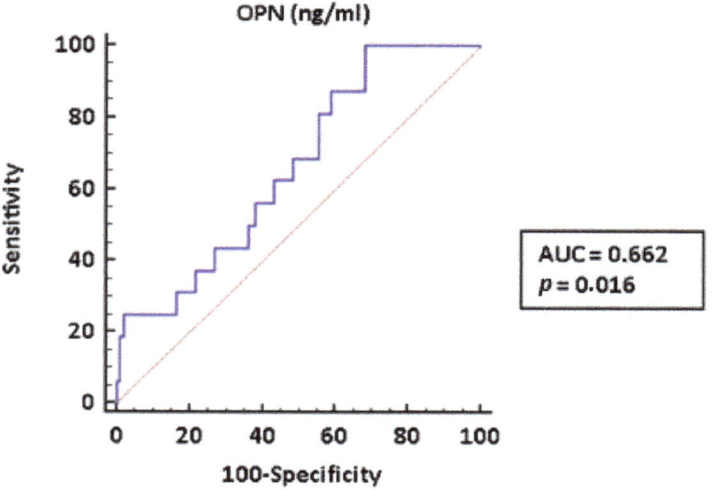

Figure 2. OPN ROC curve. Abbreviations: ROC—receiver operating characteristic; OPN—osteopontin; AUC—area under the curve.

In Table 3, we report the sensitivity/specificity table for OPN.

Table 3. Sensitivity/specificity table. Abbreviations: Sens—sensitivity; Spec—specificity; LR—likelihood ratio.

Criterion	Sens	95% CI	Spec	95% CI	+LR	95% CI	−LR	95% CI
>159.65	100.00	79.4–100.0	31.96	22.9–42.2	1.47	1.3–1.7	0.00	
>159.89	93.75	69.8–99.8	31.96	22.9–42.2	1.38	1.1–1.7	0.20	0.03–1.3
>174.01	87.50	61.7–98.4	41.24	31.3–51.7	1.49	1.2–1.9	0.30	0.08–1.1
>185.73	81.25	54.4–96.0	44.33	34.2–54.8	1.46	1.1–2.0	0.42	0.1–1.2
>188.15	75.00	47.6–92.7	44.33	34.2–54.8	1.35	1.0–1.9	0.56	0.2–1.4
>201.59	68.75	41.3–89.0	51.55	41.2–61.8	1.42	1.0–2.1	0.61	0.3–1.3
>225.16	62.50	35.4–84.8	56.70	46.3–66.7	1.44	0.9–2.2	0.66	0.3–1.3
>236.49	56.25	29.9–80.2	61.86	51.4–71.5	1.47	0.9–2.4	0.71	0.4–1.3
>243.8	50.00	24.7–75.3	63.92	53.5–73.4	1.39	0.8–2.4	0.78	0.5–1.3
>271.22	43.75	19.8–70.1	73.20	63.2–81.7	1.63	0.9–3.1	0.77	0.5–1.2
>293.54	37.50	15.2–64.6	78.35	68.8–86.1	1.73	0.8–3.6	0.80	0.5–1.2
>316	31.25	11.0–58.7	83.51	74.6–90.3	1.89	0.8–4.4	0.82	0.6–1.2
>450.44	25.00	7.3–52.4	97.94	92.7–99.7	12.12	2.4–60.8	0.77	0.6–1.0
>470.97	18.75	4.0–45.6	98.97	94.4–100.0	18.19	2.0–164.2	0.82	0.6–1.0
>564.24	12.50	1.6–38.3	98.97	94.4–100.0	12.13	1.2–126.1	0.88	0.7–1.1
>654.78	6.25	0.2–30.2	100.00	96.3–100.0			0.94	0.8–1.1

The OPN values had a direct relationship with age ($\rho = 0.249$, $p = 0.008$), while were inversely related to glomerular filtration rate ($\rho = -0.241$, $p = 0.01$). There was no association with gender or mPAP. In a multiple regression model that had PAH as the dependent variable, and OPN, age and glomerular filtration rate as independent variables, OPN was confirmed to be independently associated with PAH diagnosis (F-ratio = 11.32, $p < 0.0001$; Table 4).

Table 4. Variables associated with PAH. In the table, we show a multiple regression model of predictive factors for PAH. Abbreviations: OPN—osteopontin; eGFR—estimated glomerular filtration rate.

Variable	Coefficient	Standard Error	r	t	p
OPN	0.0005	0.0002	0.19	2.09	0.04
eGFR	−0.007	0.002	−0.32	−3.52	0.0006
Age	−0.002	0.003	−0.04	−0.49	0.62

3. Discussion

The present data, though admittedly preliminary, show that plasma OPN levels are significantly higher in CTD-PAH than in CTD patients without PAH, independently of age and renal function. Thus, they confirm that plasma OPN is a putative biomarker of PAH worth further study in this setting. The merits and limitations of this study will be discussed in light of the current literature on the topic.

In our series, we observed a prevalence of PAH (14.2%) slightly higher than expected based on other epidemiological data (8–12%) [17]. Compared to those with CTD alone, those with a PAH diagnosis were, as expected, older and had higher PAPS. Similarly, DLCO was significantly reduced. DLCO is a well-known predictor of PAH; its alterations may antedate the recognition of pulmonary hypertension of several years [18].

To the best of our knowledge, the present is the first report to suggest a potential role for OPN in this clinical context and may also be taken as a clue for a potential pathogenetic role played by this molecule in PAH. In fact, we started from what we believe is a solid rationale. First of all, OPN was related to fibrogenesis in SSc. Patients with SSc show higher OPN plasma levels; when dermal fibroblasts are challenged with pro-fibrotic stimuli, the expression of OPN is induced, suggesting a potential role in this pathogenetic process [19]. Moreover, OPN-deficient (OPN(-/-)) mice develop less dermal fibrosis compared with wild-type (WT) mice in the bleomycin-induced dermal fibrosis model, a commonly used animal model of SSc. In vitro, OPN(-/-) dermal fibroblasts have decreased migratory capacity, and TGF-β production by OPN-deficient macrophages is reduced compared with WT animals [14]. Finally, two single nucleotide polymorphisms of the OPN gene (namely, the alleles −156G in the proximal promoter and +1239C in the untranslated region) are more frequent among SSc patients suggesting that these OPN genetic variations may contribute to SSc susceptibility [20].

Second, OPN appears potentially implicated in developing pulmonary hypertension. OPN plasma concentrations increase in patients affected by idiopathic PAH concerning healthy controls, being an independent predictor of mortality [21,22]. Similarly, OPN levels are increased in the case of pulmonary hypertension related to chronic thromboembolism, supporting the idea that this biomarker is related to developing pulmonary hypertension rather than to a specific etiology [23]. Indeed, OPN is upregulated in explanted lungs of pulmonary hypertension patients, either affected by type I or type II pulmonary hypertension, being correlated to disease severity [16]. OPN seems to be involved in the pathogenesis of the vascular remodeling process accompanying developing PAH. Fibroblasts isolated from pulmonary arteries of chronically hypoxic hypertensive calves are constitutively activated, showing a high proliferative and migratory potential. These fibroblasts overexpress OPN and its receptors. This is associated with high proliferative, migratory, and invasive properties; OPN silencing is conversely paralleled by a decreased proliferation, migration and invasion [24].

OPN levels are directly related to age and inversely related to glomerular filtration rate. This is particularly important in CTD-PAH; indeed, a lower glomerular filtration rate is observed in PAH patients, as also reported in the present study. The reduction in glomerular filtration rate is partly explained by the difference in age between the two groups; however, the altered renal function could also be the consequence of altered hemodynamics due to an overloaded right ventricle, leading to progressive functional deterioration. In any case, the association between OPN and PAH remains even after correction for age and renal function, suggesting that OPN is an independent biomarker of PAH. It should be, however, acknowledged that the association between PAH and OPN has a weak statistical significance; therefore, the differences between groups may be explained by the different glomerular filtration rates, the association, of which is much stronger. Nevertheless, our study represents a proof of concept. OPN may be proposed as a diagnostic and prognostic biomarker in CTD-PAH, the clinical relevance, of which should be assessed in further, larger cohorts. Indeed, the dosage of this protein, combined with data such as red cell distribution width (RDW), diffusing capacity of the lung for carbon monoxide (DLCO), systolic pulmonary arterial pressures (sPAP), may allow better risk stratification in CTD patients. The demonstration of the prognostic role of OPN in the context of CTD-PAH goes, however, beyond the aim of the present study and should be specifically addressed by ad hoc prospective studies.

Our study has limitations. First of all, the study population is relatively small; however, it should be acknowledged that SSc is a rare and relatively small proportion of patients who develops PAH. The AUC of the ROC curve is poor, particularly if we consider OPN in a screening strategy, requiring high sensitivity; however, our study only adds a proof of concept, which requires confirmation on a larger scale and which has possibly been underpowered by the small sample size.

A further limitation is that many patients were already receiving treatment either for PAH or for CTD-ILD, and this may have partly influenced the OPN plasma values. Moreover, not all the patients included in the present cohort underwent RHC, which was limited to those with echocardiographic findings suggestive for PAH. Ideally, being RHC the gold standard for PAH diagnosis, we cannot exclude a misclassification for a minor proportion of subjects. However, this approach is supported by international guidelines for diagnosing CTDs-PAH and is used to limit unnecessary RHC, which may expose patients to potential risks.

Finally, for the present study, the diagnosis of PAH relied on the 2015 ESC/ESR guidelines, which were revised during the 2018 PH World Symposium. The new proposed cutoff for PAH diagnosis is an mPAP $\geq$ 20 mmHg with a pulmonary vascular resistance $\geq$ 3 WU at RHC. However, it should be considered that the threshold of 25 mmHg was the diagnostic cutoff when the present study was conducted.

4. Materials and Methods

We performed a cross-sectional, observational study on patients already diagnosed with CTDs, referred and consecutively evaluated at the Pulmonary Hypertension Clinic of the Cardiology Division, University Hospital of Novara, from 3 October 2016 to 12 December 2019. The study protocol (no. 108/16) was approved by the local ethical committee on 9 September 2016 and conducted in strict accordance with the principles of the Declaration of Helsinki. Written informed consent was obtained from all individual participants included in the study.

The inclusion criteria were: (1) diagnosis of SSc or other connective tissue diseases at risk for PAH (MCTD, scleroderma overlap syndromes, UCTD) defined in relation to the fulfillment of diagnostic criteria international employees currently employed; (2) Age > 18.

The exclusion criteria were: (1) refusal to give informed consent to participation; (2) impossibility to undergo the investigations included in the study Protocol.

The diagnosis of SSc has been confirmed in relation to the fulfillment of the 2013 ACR/Eular classification criteria [25], while the diagnosis of MCTD was made based on Kasukawa's criteria [26]. Patients fulfilling the classification criteria for SSc along with those of other rheumatic conditions were classified as overlap syndrome [27]. Finally, the diagnosis of UCTD was made when patients with a connective tissue disease did not meet the classification criteria of any specific syndrome [28]. We identified 113 patients who underwent:

Clinical evaluation, including a comprehensive medical history and a physical examination performed by an experienced clinician;

A biochemistry panel;

12-lead electrocardiogram with 6-limb and 6 precordial leads with paper speed set at the standard rate of 25 mm/s;

Posteroanterior and lateral chest X-rays;

Pulmonary function tests (PFTs): were performed using standardized equipment and technique with a spirometer (COSMED, Rome, Italy). The device was connected to a computer employing the software "Medisoft Expair 1.28.20". The following standardized measurements were evaluated: forced vital capacity (FVC), forced expiratory volume in one second (FEV1), and FEV1/FVC% (also known as the Tiffeneau index). We also evaluated the diffusing capacity of the lung for carbon monoxide (DLCO), measured with the single-breath Jones–Meade protocol.

Transthoracic echocardiography (TTE) was performed using the Vivid 7 or E9 cardiovascular ultrasound machine by GE Medical Systems (Horten, Norway) with a 1.7/3.4 MHz tissue harmonic transducer. All data were obtained in standardized patient positions, according to the standards of the American Society of Echocardiography. The test was performed by an expert echocardiographer with a special interest in pulmonary hypertension. The following parameters were generated: systolic pulmonary pressure (sPAP), right atrium area (RAA), right ventricle diameter (RVD), and ejection fraction (EF). Right ventricle systolic function was evaluated by estimating the tricuspid annular plane systolic excursion (TAPSE).

According to the application of international guidelines, those patients with a suspected PAH underwent right heart catheterization within one month after TTE. PAH was defined by mean pulmonary artery pressure (mPAP) $\geq$ 25 mmHg, pulmonary capillary wedge pressure $\leq$ 15 mmHg, and pulmonary vascular resistance > 3 wood units. Whenever contraindications to RHC occurred, pulmonary hypertension was diagnosed based on echocardiography-estimated sPAP $\geq$ 35 mmHg and additional high probability criteria, in agreement with the 2015 ESC/ESR guidelines [1].

For each patient, a blood sample was drawn and collected in a tube with EDTA; the samples were then centrifuged at room temperature for 10 min at 3000 rpm within one hour of collection, then stored at −80 °C at the Laboratory of the University of Eastern Piedmont, Department of Medicine Translational.

OPN concentrations were measured by a commercially available enzyme-linked immunosorbent assay (ELISA) (DUOSET® ELISA R&D System, Minneapolis, MN, USA. Code DY1433) following the manufacturer's instructions.

Statistical Analysis

Anthropometric, clinical, and biochemical data were recorded in a database and analyzed by the statistical software package MedCalc v.19.6.4 (MedCalc software, Broekstraat 52, 9030, Mariakerke, Belgium). The normality of OPN distribution was assessed by the Shapiro–Wilk test. Continuous variables are presented as medians and interquartile range (IQR). Differences in these variables between CTD and CTD-PAH patients were compared by the Mann–Whitney. Correlations between continuous variables were analyzed by Spearman's rank test. To test the diagnostic performance of OPN in identifying patients with PAH receiver operating characteristics, curves were built with the calculation of the areas under the curve (AUC). To test whether OPN was independently associated with the diagnosis of PAH we first, run a univariate analysis evaluating the association with potential confounders, such as age, gender and renal function. We then built a multiple regression model. The level of significance chosen for all statistical analyses was 0.05 (two-tailed).

5. Conclusions

In conclusion, OPN was significantly associated with PAH in patients affected by SSC, suggesting a possible role for this protein as a non-invasive disease biomarker.

Author Contributions: Conceptualization, M.B., C.P., A.G., G.P., M.P. and P.P.S.; data curation, M.B., A.G., R.P. (Roberta Pedrazzoli), E.C., F.M. and R.P. (Roberto Piffero); formal analysis, M.B. and C.P.; investigation, M.B., C.P., S.T., R.M., A.G., D.S., R.P. (Roberta Pedrazzoli), I.G., E.Z., E.C., F.M., R.P. (Roberto Piffero) and P.P.S.; methodology, M.B., C.P., D.S., R.P. (Roberta Pedrazzoli), F.M. and P.P.S.; writing—original draft, M.B.; writing—review and editing, C.P., A.G., G.P., M.P. and P.P.S. All authors have read and agreed to the published version of the manuscript.

Funding: This research received no external funding.

Institutional Review Board Statement: The study was conducted according to the guidelines of the Declaration of Helsinki and approved by the Institutional Review Board (Comitato Etico Interaziendale, Novara, Italy) (protocol code 108/16; date of approval: 9 September 2016).

Informed Consent Statement: Informed consent was obtained from all subjects involved in the study.

Data Availability Statement: All the data are available upon reasonable request to the corresponding author.

Conflicts of Interest: The authors declare no conflict of interest.

References

1. Galiè, N.; Humbert, M.; Vachiery, J.L.; Gibbs, S.; Lang, I.; Torbicki, A.; Simonneau, G.; Peacock, A.; Vonk Noordegraaf, A.; Beghetti, M.; et al. ESC Scientific Document Group. 2015 ESC/ERS Guidelines for the Diagnosis and Treatment of Pulmonary Hypertension. *Eur. Heart J.* **2016**, *37*, 67–119. [CrossRef] [PubMed]
2. Jawad, H.; McWilliams, S.R.; Bhalla, S. Cardiopulmonary Manifestations of Collagen Vascular Diseases. *Curr. Rheumatol. Rep.* **2017**, *19*, 71. [CrossRef] [PubMed]
3. Ruiz-Cano, M.J.; Escribano, P.; Alonso, R.; Delgado, J.; Carreira, P.; Velazquez, T.; Sanchez, M.A.G.; de la Calzada, C.S. Comparison of Baseline Characteristics and Survival between Patients with Idiopathic and Connective Tissue Disease–related Pulmonary Arterial Hypertension. *J. Heart Lung Transplant.* **2009**, *28*, 621–627. [CrossRef] [PubMed]
4. Coghlan, J.G.; Denton, C.P.; Grünig, E.; Bonderman, D.; Distler, O.; Khanna, D.; Müller-Ladner, U.; Pope, J.E.; Vonk, M.C.; Doelberg, M.; et al. Evidence-Based Detection of Pulmonary Arterial Hypertension in Systemic Sclerosis: The DETECT Study. *Ann. Rheum. Dis.* **2014**, *73*, 1340–1349. [CrossRef]
5. Bellan, M.; Dimagli, A.; Piccinino, C.; Giubertoni, A.; Ianniello, A.; Grimoldi, F.; Sguazzotti, M.; Nerviani, A.; Barini, M.; Carrero, A.; et al. Role of Gas6 and TAM Receptors in the Identification of Cardiopulmonary Involvement in Systemic Sclerosis and Scleroderma Spectrum Disorders. *Dis. Markers* **2020**, 2696173. [CrossRef]

6. Bellan, M.; Giubertoni, A.; Piccinino, C.; Dimagli, A.; Grimoldi, F.; Sguazzotti, M.; Burlone, M.E.; Smirne, C.; Sola, D.; Marino, P.; et al. Red Cell Distribution Width and Platelet Count as Biomarkers of Pulmonary Arterial Hypertension in Patients with Connective Tissue Disorders. *Dis. Markers* **2019**, 4981982. [CrossRef]
7. Galiè, N.; Rubin, L.J.; Hoeper, M.M.; Jansa, P.; Al-Hiti, H.; Meyer, G.; Chiossi, E.; Kusic-Pajic, A.; Simonneau, G. Treatment of Patients with Mildly Symptomatic Pulmonary Arterial Hypertension with Bosentan (EARLY study): A Dou-ble-Blind, Randomised Controlled Trial. *Lancet* **2008**, *371*, 2093–2100. [CrossRef]
8. Icer, M.A.; Gezmen-Karadag, M. The Multiple Functions and Mechanisms of Osteopontin. *Clin. Biochem.* **2018**, *59*, 17–24. [CrossRef]
9. Liu, L.N.; Mao, Y.M.; Zhao, C.N.; Wang, H.; Yuan, F.F.; Li, X.M.; Pan, H.F. Circulating Levels of Osteoprotegerin, Osteocalcin and Osteopontin in Patients with Rheumatoid Arthritis: A Systematic Review and Meta-Analysis. *Immunol. Investig.* **2019**, *48*, 107–120. [CrossRef]
10. Castello, L.M.; Baldrighi, M.; Molinari, L.; Salmi, L.; Cantaluppi, V.; Vaschetto, R.; Zunino, G.; Quaglia, M.; Bellan, M.; Gavelli, F.; et al. The Role of Osteopontin as a Diagnostic and Prognostic Biomarker in Sepsis and Septic Shock. *Cells* **2019**, *8*, 174. [CrossRef]
11. Ashkar, S.; Weber, G.F.; Panoutsakopoulou, V.; Sanchirico, M.E.; Jansson, M.; Zawaideh, S.; Rittling, S.R.; Denhardt, D.T.; Glimcher, M.J.; Cantor, H. Eta-1 (osteopontin): An Early Component of Type-1 (Cell-Mediated) Immunity. *Science* **2000**, *287*, 860–864. [CrossRef]
12. Bellan, M.; Castello, L.M.; Pirisi, M. Candidate Biomarkers of Liver Fibrosis: A Concise, Pathophysiology-oriented Review. *J. Clin. Transl. Hepatol.* **2018**, *6*, 317–325. [CrossRef]
13. Kothari, A.N.; Arffa, M.L.; Chang, V.; Blackwell, R.H.; Syn, W.K.; Zhang, J.; Mi, Z.; Kuo, P.C. Osteopontin-A Master Regulator of Epithelial-Mesenchymal Transition. *J. Clin. Med.* **2016**, *5*, 39. [CrossRef]
14. Wu, M.; Schneider, D.J.; Mayes, M.D.; Assassi, S.; Arnett, F.C.; Tan, F.K.; Blackburn, M.R.; Agarwal, S.K. Osteopontin in Systemic Sclerosis and its Role in Dermal Fibrosis. *J. Investig. Derm.* **2012**, *132*, 1605–1614. [CrossRef] [PubMed]
15. Gadeau, A.P.; Campan, M.; Millet, D.; Candresse, T.; Desgranges, C. Osteopontin Overexpression is Associated with Arterial Smooth Muscle Cell Proliferation in Vitro. *Arterioscler. Thromb.* **1993**, *13*, 120–125. [CrossRef] [PubMed]
16. Mura, M.; Cecchini, M.J.; Joseph, M.; Granton, J.T. Osteopontin Lung Gene Expression is a Marker of Disease Severity in Pulmonary Arterial Hypertension. *Respirology* **2019**, *24*, 1104–1110. [CrossRef]
17. Hachulla, E.; Gressin, V.; Guillevin, L.; Carpentier, P.; Diot, E.; Sibilia, J.; Kahan, A.; Cabane, J.; Frances, C.; Launay, D.; et al. Early Detection of Pulmonary Arterial Hypertension in Systemic Sclerosis: A French Nationwide Prospective Multicenter Study. *Arthritis Rheum.* **2005**, *52*, 3792–3800. [CrossRef]
18. Steen, V.; Medsger, T.A., Jr. Predictors of Isolated Pulmonary Hypertension in Patients with Systemic Sclerosis and Limited Cutaneous Involvement. *Arthritis Rheum.* **2003**, *48*, 516–522. [CrossRef]
19. Corallo, C.; Volpi, N.; Franci, D.; Montella, A.; Biagioli, M.; Mariotti, G.; D'Onofrio, F.; Gonnelli, S.; Nuti, R.; Giordano, N. Is Osteopontin Involved in Cutaneous Fibroblast Activation? Its Hypothetical Role in Scleroderma Pathogenesis. *Int. J. Immunopathol. Pharmacol.* **2014**, *27*, 97–102. [CrossRef]
20. Barizzone, N.; Marchini, M.; Cappiello, F.; Chiocchetti, A.; Orilieri, E.; Ferrante, D.; Corrado, L.; Mellone, S.; Scorza, R.; Dianzani, U.; et al. Association of Osteopontin Regulatory Polymorphisms with Systemic Sclerosis. *Hum. Immunol.* **2011**, *72*, 930–934. [CrossRef]
21. Lorenzen, J.M.; Nickel, N.; Krämer, R.; Golpon, H.; Westerkamp, V.; Olsson, K.M.; Haller, H.; Hoeper, M.M. Osteopontin in Patients with Idiopathic Pulmonary Hypertension. *Chest* **2011**, *139*, 1010–1017. [CrossRef] [PubMed]
22. Rosenberg, M.; Meyer, F.J.; Gruenig, E.; Schuster, T.; Lutz, M.; Lossnitzer, D.; Wipplinger, R.; Katus, H.A.; Frey, N. Osteopontin (OPN) Improves Risk Stratification in Pulmonary Hypertension (PH). *Int. J. Cardiol.* **2012**, *155*, 504–505. [CrossRef]
23. Kölmel, S.; Hobohm, L.; Käberich, A.; Krieg, V.J.; Bochenek, M.L.; Wenzel, P.; Wiedenroth, C.B.; Liebetrau, C.; Hasenfuß, G.; Mayer, E.; et al. Potential Involvement of Osteopontin in Inflammatory and Fibrotic Processes in Pulmonary Embolism and Chronic Thromboembolic Pulmonary Hypertension. *Thromb. Haemost.* **2019**, *119*, 1332–1346. [CrossRef] [PubMed]
24. Anwar, A.; Li, M.; Frid, M.G.; Kumar, B.; Gerasimovskaya, E.V.; Riddle, S.R.; McKeon, B.A.; Thukaram, R.; Meyrick, B.O.; Fini, M.A.; et al. Osteopontin is an Endogenous Modulator of the Constitutively Activated Phenotype of Pulmonary Adventitial Fibroblasts in Hypoxic Pulmonary Hypertension. *Am. J. Physiol. Lung. Cell. Mol. Physiol.* **2012**, *303*, L1–L11. [CrossRef]
25. van den Hoogen, F.; Khanna, D.; Fransen, J.; Johnson, S.R.; Baron, M.; Tyndall, A.; Matucci-Cerinic, M.; Naden, R.P.; Medsger, T.A., Jr.; Carreira, P.E.; et al. 2013 Classification Criteria for Systemic Sclerosis: An American College of Rheumatology/European League Against Rheumatism Collaborative Initiative. *Ann. Rheum. Dis.* **2013**, *72*, 1747–1755. [CrossRef]
26. Kasukawa, R.; Tojo, T.; Miyawaki, S. Preliminary Diagnostic Criteria for Classification of Mixed Connective Tissue Disease. In *Mixed Connective Tissue Disease and Antinuclear Antibodies*; Sharp, G., Ed.; Elsevier: Amsterdam, The Netherlands, 1987; p. 41.
27. Balbir-Gurman, A.; Braun-Moscovici, Y. Scleroderma Overlap Syndrome. *Isr. Med. Assoc. J.* **2011**, *13*, 14–20.
28. Mosca, M.; Baldini, C.; Bombardieri, S. Undifferentiated Connective Tissue Diseases in 2004. *Clin. Exp. Rheumatol.* **2004**, *22*, S14–S18.

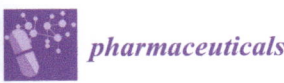

Article

The Probiotic VSL#3® Does Not Seem to Be Efficacious for the Treatment of Gastrointestinal Symptomatology of Patients with Fibromyalgia: A Randomized, Double-Blind, Placebo-Controlled Clinical Trial

Elena P. Calandre [1,*], Javier Hidalgo-Tallon [1], Rocio Molina-Barea [2], Fernando Rico-Villademoros [1], Cristina Molina-Hidalgo [3], Juan M. Garcia-Leiva [1], Maria Dolores Carrillo-Izquierdo [4] and Mahmoud Slim [5]

1 Instituto de Neurociencias, Universidad de Granada, 18100 Granada, Spain; fjht63@gmail.com (J.H.-T.); fernando.ricovillademoros@gmail.com (F.R.-V.); jmgleiva@ugr.es (J.M.G.-L.)
2 Servicio de Cirugía, Complejo Hospitalario de Jaen, 23007 Jaén, Spain; barea1984@gmail.com
3 Departamento de Psicología Médica, Universidad de Granada, 18011 Granada, Spain; cristinamolinapsico@gmail.com
4 Departamento de Enfermería, Universidad Católica de Murcia, 30107 Murcia, Spain; mariadocarrillo@gmail.com
5 Division of Neurology, The Hospital for Sick Children, Toronto, ON M5G 1X8, Canada; mahmoud.slim@gmail.com
* Correspondence: epita@ugr.es; Tel.: +34-958-246-291

Abstract: Gastrointestinal symptomatology is frequent among patients with fibromyalgia, which increases disease burden and lacks specific treatment, either pharmacological or non-pharmacological. We aimed to evaluate the efficacy and tolerability of a multi-strain probiotic, VSL#3®, for the treatment of fibromyalgia-associated gastrointestinal manifestations. This randomized, placebo-controlled trial included 12 weeks of probiotic or placebo treatment followed by 12 weeks of follow up. The primary outcome variable was the mean change from the baseline to the endpoint in the composite severity score of the three main gastrointestinal symptoms reported by patients with fibromyalgia (abdominal pain, abdominal bloating and meteorism). Secondary outcome variables were the severity of additional gastrointestinal symptoms, fibromyalgia severity, depression, sleep disturbance, health-related quality of life and patients' overall impression of improvement. No differences were found between VSL#3® (n = 54) and the placebo (n = 56) in the primary outcome (estimated treatment difference: 1.1; 95% confidence interval [CI]: −2.1, 4.2; p = 0.501), or in any of the secondary outcomes. However, responders to VSL#3 were more likely to maintain any improvement during the follow-up period compared to responders in the placebo arm. Overall, VSL#3 tolerability was good. Our data could not demonstrate any beneficial effects of VSL#3® either on the composite score of severity of abdominal pain, bloating and meteorism or in any of the secondary outcome variables. More research is needed to elucidate specific factors that may predict a favourable response to treatment in patients with fibromyalgia.

Keywords: fibromyalgia; gastrointestinal symptoms; probiotic; VSL#3®; efficacy; tolerability

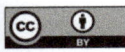

1. Introduction

Fibromyalgia is a complex syndrome in that, although its main characteristic is chronic generalized musculoskeletal pain, this is accompanied in most patients by other symptoms, the most common of which are non-restorative sleep, chronic fatigue, cognitive difficulties and anxious and/or depressive symptoms [1]. It is included within the central sensitization syndromes, such as migraine, irritable bowel syndrome (IBS) or temporomandibular disorders, with which it shows a high comorbidity [2].

Gastrointestinal symptoms are very common in patients with fibromyalgia, and could be derived from the presence of comorbid IBS or other underlying pathophysiological mechanisms [3]. A systematic review reported a pooled prevalence of 51% for functional gastrointestinal disorders and 46% for IBS among patients with fibromyalgia [4]. On the other hand, even among patients with fibromyalgia who do not meet the criteria to diagnose IBS, the presence of gastrointestinal symptomatology is frequently observed [3]. The cause of these symptoms remains unknown, although some studies suggest that they could be due to intestinal bacterial overgrowth or intestinal permeability alterations [5–7]. A recent study in patients with chronic fatigue syndrome, a pathology that shows a broad overlap with fibromyalgia, described an increased likelihood of intestinal dysbiosis for these patients [8]. Patients with fibromyalgia also showed an alteration in gut microbiota, although the role of these alterations should be further elucidated [9,10].

No specific treatment for alleviating the gastrointestinal symptoms associated with fibromyalgia has been studied, despite their frequency and most patients describing them as extremely annoying [3,11]. This may explain the frequency with which these patients resort to different types of diets, even though their benefits have not been previously demonstrated [12–14]. In this regard, the use of probiotics, alone or associated with prebiotics (synbiotics), could be an interesting therapeutic approach for managing gastrointestinal symptoms in patients with fibromyalgia. Probiotics have been studied in a variety of clinical conditions, including gastrointestinal disorders, dermatological disorders and metabolic diseases [15,16]. Among gastrointestinal disorders, the most studied condition is IBS, where probiotics seem to exert a favourable response in global symptoms, although there are not still enough data to specify which individual probiotics could be more effective [17]. Probiotics seem to be well tolerated in general [17].

Considering the frequent presence of gastrointestinal symptoms in patients with fibromyalgia who might be susceptible to treatment with probiotics, the objective of this trial was to assess the efficacy and tolerability of VSL#3®, a multi-strain probiotic, which has demonstrated a trend for an overall improvement in the treatment of IBS [18,19] in patients with fibromyalgia and gastrointestinal symptomatology.

2. Results

2.1. Patient Disposition and Characteristics

One hundred and ten patients were recruited from May 2018 to November 2019 and allocated to either placebo (n = 56) or VSL#3® (n = 54). Twenty-five subjects (44.6%) in the placebo group and 28 (51.8%) subjects in the VSL#3® group did not complete the study (Figure 1). Fifty-three subjects in each study group were included in the analysis of the primary outcome and that of a proportion of responders according to the composite score of abdominal pain, bloating and meteorism; secondary efficacy outcomes, including the proportion of responders according to the Patient Global Improvement scale (PGI), were evaluated in 35 subjects in the placebo group and 28 subjects in the VSL#3® group. All randomised subjects were included in the safety analysis.

Subjects were middle-aged, and the vast majority were women (Table 1). Comorbidity was high, with anxiety/depressive disorder, tension-type headache, craniomandibular dysfunction, chronic fatigue syndrome and irritable bowel syndrome present in over 50% of the patients (Table 1). Most patients were receiving pharmacological treatment with some activity for the symptoms of fibromyalgia. Benzodiazepines, antidepressants, NSAIDs, paracetamol and tramadol were mainly used, each in over 30% of the patients; one-third of patients were receiving gastroprotectant drugs (Table 1). At baseline, the study groups were generally well-balanced regarding demographics and clinical characteristics (Table 1), including the individual gastrointestinal symptoms of abdominal pain, abdominal bloating, meteorism, and the composite score of these three symptoms (Table 2). However, the impact of fibromyalgia as evaluated with the revised fibromyalgia impact questionnaire (FIQR) was greater among placebo-treated patients than in VSL#3®-treated patients (FIQR total score 75.5 ± 12.3 vs. 70.0 ± 17.8), although the difference was not statistically significant.

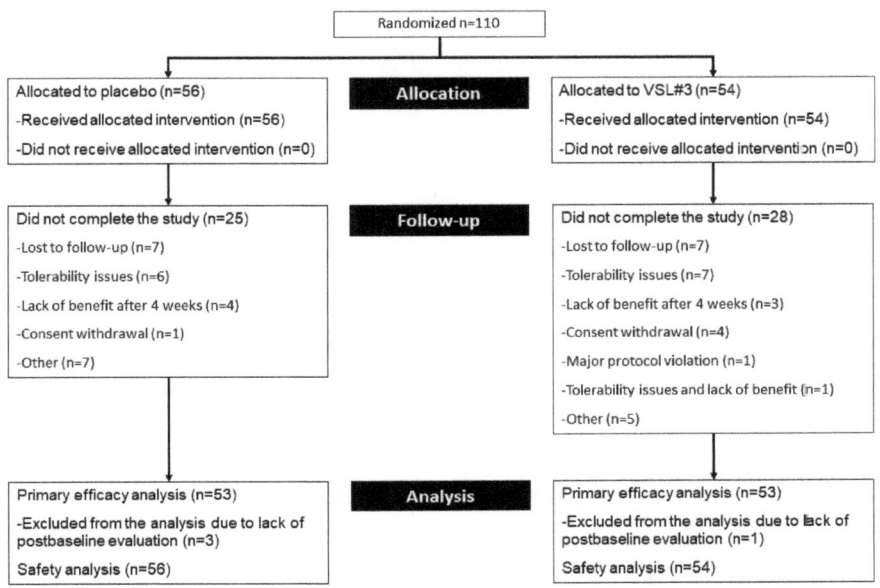

Figure 1. Disposition of trial participants.

Table 1. Demographic and clinical characteristics.

Variable	Placebo N = 56	VSL#3® N = 54
Age (years), mean (SD)	55.5 (8.6)	56.0 (7.5)
Sex (females), n (%)	55 (98.2)	52 (96.3)
Weight (kg),	71.2 (13.4)	73.3 (17.7)
Comorbidities [a], n (%)		
Anxiety/depressive disorder	48 (85.7)	45 (83.3)
Tension-type headache	40 (71.4)	36 (66.7)
Craniomandibular dysfunction	36 (64.3)	36 (66.7)
Chronic fatigue syndrome	35 (62.5)	28 (51.9)
Irritable bowel syndrome	33 (58.9)	32 (59.3)
Migraine	24 (42.9)	30 (55.6)
Hypothyroidism	25 (44.6)	15 (27.8)
Osteoarthritis	21 (37.5)	15 (27.8)
Rheumatoid arthritis	10 (17.9)	10 (18.5)
Hypercholesterolemia	4 (7.1)	9 (16.7)
Hypertension	9 (16.1)	9 (16.7)
Diabetes mellitus	7 (12.5)	4 (7.4)

Table 1. Cont.

Variable	Placebo N = 56	VSL#3® N = 54
Fibromyalgia diagnosis, mean (SD)		
Widespread Pain Index (WPI) [range 0–19]	16.5 (2.6)	15.9 (3.0)
Symptom Severity Score (SSS) [0–12]	9.7 (1.7)	9.3 (2.0)
Fibromyalgia Score (WPI + SSS) [0–31]	26.2 (3.5)	25.3 (4.3)

[a] Those with a frequency equal to or greater than 10% in any of the trial arms. SD, standard deviation.

2.2. Primary Outcome

In the intent-to-treat last observation carried forward (LOCF) analysis, at week 12, the severity of pain, bloating and meteorism as measured with the composite score was reduced by 6.5 points among VSL#3®-treated patients and 5.4 points among placebo-treated patients; this difference was not statistically different (estimated treatment difference (ETD): 1.1; 95% confidence interval [CI]: −2.1 to 4.2; p = 0.501) nor clinically relevant (Cohen's d = 0.13).

2.3. Secondary Outcomes

2.3.1. Gastrointestinal Symptoms

There were no statistically significant differences between VSL#3® and placebo in any of the individual gastrointestinal symptoms (Table 2). The largest difference was observed in diarrhoea, in favour of VSL#3® (ETD: 1.3; 95% CI: −0.4 to 2.9; p = 0.131). All effect sizes for the differences between VSL#3® and placebo in the gastrointestinal symptoms were trivial, except for a small effect size for abdominal pain and diarrhoea in favour of VSL#3 and a small effect size for constipation in favour of the placebo. Results of the complete case analysis for the primary outcome and the gastrointestinal symptoms were generally similar to those of the LOCF approach, except for the largest mean within-group changes in the scores (Table 3).

In the intent-to-treat population and using an LOCF approach, by week 12, 27 out of the 53 (50.9%) patients showed a reduction equal to or greater than 30% in the composite score of abdominal pain, bloating and meteorism in the VSL#3® group, compared to 22 of the 53 (41.5%) in the placebo group (relative risk [RR]: 1.23; 95% CI: 0.81 to 1.86). The proportion of responders according to the PGI was 22.2% and 26.4% for VSL#3- and placebo-treated patients, respectively (RR: 0.86; 95% CI: 0.44 to 1.68) (Figure 2).

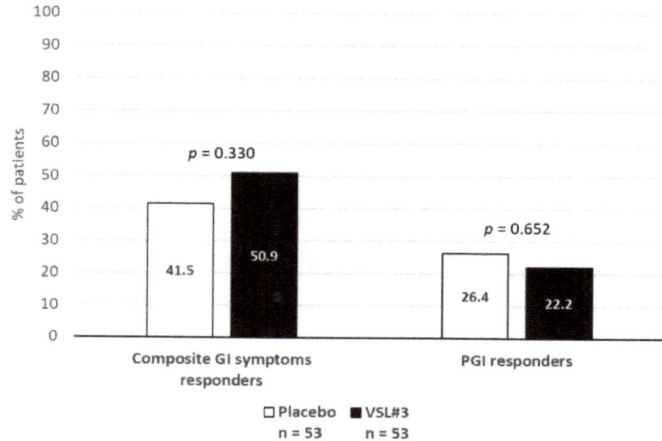

Figure 2. Proportion of responders to treatment.

Among the patients who responded to treatment at week 12 according to the reduction in the composite score of abdominal pain, bloating and meteorism, after discontinuing the study treatment, the composite score increased by over four points during the 12-week follow-up extension in the placebo group and by over one point in the VSL#3® group, with an ETD of 2.8 points (95% CI: 0.0 to 5.6; $p = 0.048$) (Figure 3).

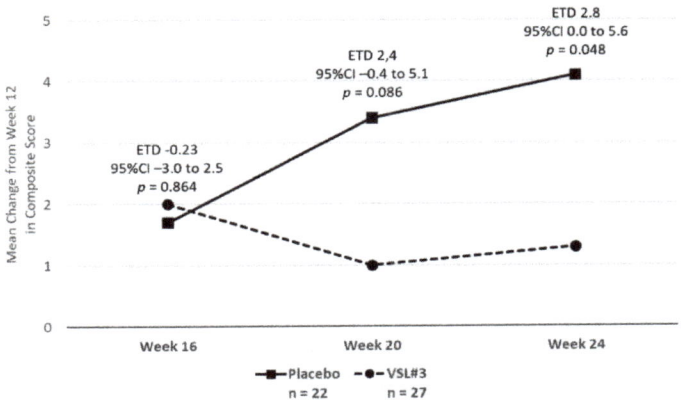

Figure 3. Composite score of abdominal pain, bloating and meteorism after discontinuing the study treatment.

There were no relevant differences in the baseline characteristics between responders and non-responders in either the total sample or in the VSL#3® and placebo groups (data not shown).

2.3.2. The Effect on Other Symptoms of Fibromyalgia and Quality of Life

Overall, the severity of fibromyalgia was reduced in both study groups, but to a greater extent among placebo-treated patients, although the differences between the two study groups were not statistically significant (ETD: −5.2; 95% CI: −12.0 to 1.6; $p = 0.128$; Cohen's d: 0.40). Except for stiffness, which improved to a significantly greater extent with the placebo than with VSL#3® (ETD: −1.5; 95% CI: −2.8 to 0.1; $p = 0.0304$; Cohen's d: 0.56), there were no significant differences in the changes from baseline in the core symptoms of fibromyalgia, sleep impairment, depressive symptoms or quality of life between VSL#3® and the placebo (Table 4).

Table 2. Comparison of the impact of VSL#3® and placebo on gastrointestinal symptoms (ITT-LOCF analysis).

Gastrointestinal Symptom	Baseline Mean ± SD		Mean Change (±SD) from Baseline to Week 12			Treatment Difference (Placebo Minus VSL#3)			
	Placebo N = 56	VSL#3® N = 54	Placebo N = 53	VSL#3® N = 53	ETD	95% CI	p-Value	Cohen's d
Primary outcome: composite score of Pain + Bloating + Meteorism	20.9 ± 5.6	20.7 ± 5.0	−5.4 ± 6.6	−6.5 ± 9.5	1.1	−2.1 to 4.2	0.501	0.13
Abdominal pain	6.2 ± 2.5	6.1 ± 2.5	−1.6 ± 3.2	−2.4 ± 3.8	0.8	−0.5 to 2.2	0.228	0.24
Abdominal bloating	7.8 ± 2.2	7.4 ± 2.1	−2.1 ± 2.9	−2.1 ± 3.6	−0.0	−1.3 to 1.3	0.976	0.01
Meteorism	6.9 ± 2.8	7.2 ± 2.5	−1.7 ± 2.8	−2.0 ± 3.5	0.3	−1.0 to 1.5	0.668	0.08
Flatulence	6.5 ± 2.9	6.0 ± 2.3	−1.3 ± 3.2	−1.1 ± 4.0	−0.2	−1.6 to 1.2	0.788	0.05
Constipation	6.7 ± 3.5	6.1 ± 3.6	−2.4 ± 3.8	−1.6 ± 4.2	−0.8	−2.3 to 0.8	0.323	0.20
Diarrhoea	2.6 ± 3.5	4.6 ± 3.9	−1.8 ± 3.8	−3.1 ± 4.7	1.3	−0.4 to 2.9	0.131	0.30
Nausea	3.3 ± 3.2	3.3 ± 3.3	−2.4 ± 3.4	−1.9 ± 4.0	−0.5	−2.0 to 0.9	0.468	0.14
Vomiting	0.7 ± 1.8	0.8 ± 2.3	−0.5 ± 1.5	−0.6 ± 1.9	0.2	−0.5 to 0.8	0.645	0.09
Belching	4.2 ± 3.2	4.1 ± 3.5	−0.6 ± 3.3	−1.1 ± 2.8	0.4	−0.8 to 1.6	0.487	0.14
Dyspepsia	6.2 ± 3.0	6.5 ± 2.9	−2.7 ± 3.8	−3.2 ± 3.5	0.5	−0.9 to 1.9	0.510	0.13

CI, confidence interval; ETD, estimated treatment difference (positive figures favour VSL#3); ITT, intention-to-treat; FMS, fibromyalgia syndrome; LOCF, last observation carried forward; SD, standard deviation.

Table 3. Comparison of the impact of VSL#3® and placebo on gastrointestinal symptoms (complete case analysis).

Gastrointestinal Symptom	Baseline Mean ± SD		Mean Change (±SD) from Baseline to Week 12			Treatment Difference (Placebo Minus VSL#3)			
	Placebo N = 56	VSL#3® N = 54	Placebo N = 53	VSL#3® N = 53	ETD	95%CI	p-Value	Cohen's d
Primary outcome: composite score of Pain + Bloating + Meteorism	20.9 ± 5.6	20.7 ± 5.0	−7.6 ± 6.1	−7.5 ± 8.4	−0.09	−3.7 to 3.5	0.959	0.01
Abdominal pain	6.2 ± 2.5	6.1 ± 2.5	−2.5 ± 2.9	−2.9 ± 3.4	0.4	−1.2 to 2.0	0.620	0.13
Abdominal bloating	7.8 ± 2.2	7.4 ± 2.1	−3.2 ± 2.9	−2.5 ± 3.3	−0.7	−2.3 to 0.9	0.373	0.23
Meteorism	6.9 ± 2.8	7.2 ± 2.5	−2.0 ± 3.0	−2.2 ± 3.3	0.2	−1.4 to 1.8	0.789	0.07
Flatulence	6.5 ± 2.9	6.0 ± 2.3	−1.5 ± 3.3	−1.8 ± 5.0	0.3	−1.5 to 2.1	0.759	0.08

Table 3. Cont.

Gastrointestinal Symptom	Baseline Mean ± SD		Mean Change (±SD) from Baseline to Week 12			Treatment Difference (Placebo Minus VSL#3)		
	Placebo N = 56	VSL#3® N = 54	Placebo N = 53	VSL#3® N = 53	ETD	95%CI	p-Value	Cohen's d
Constipation	6.7 ± 3.5	6.1 ± 3.6	−3.2 ± 3.6	−2.6 ± 4.1	−0.6	−2.6 to 1.3	0.522	0.17
Diarrhoea	2.6 ± 3.5	4.6 ± 3.9	−1.2 ± 3.3	−2.5 ± 4.5	1.3	−0.8 to 3.4	0.213	0.34
Nausea	3.3 ± 3.2	3.3 ± 3.3	−2.8 ± 3.1	−2.6 ± 2.7	−0.2	−1.7 to 1.3	0.787	0.07
Vomiting	0.7 ± 1.8	0.8 ± 2.3	−0.2 ± 1.0	−0.5 ± 1.3	0.4	−0.2 to 1.0	0.231	0.31
Belching	4.2 ± 3.2	4.1 ± 3.5	−1.3 ± 2.9	−1.6 ± 2.4	0.3	−1.1 to 1.7	0.678	0.11
Dyspepsia	6.2 ± 3.0	6.5 ± 2.9	−3.2 ± 3.4	−3.8 ± 3.2	0.7	−1.0 to 2.3	0.444	0.20

CI, confidence interval; ETD, estimated treatment difference (positive figures favour VSL#3); FMS, fibromyalgia syndrome; SD, standard deviation.

Table 4. Comparison of the impact of VSL#3® and placebo on fibromyalgia, sleep, depression and quality of life.

Outcome	Baseline (Mean ± SD)		Mean Change (±SD) from Baseline to Week 12			Treatment Difference (Placebo Minus VSL#3)		
	Placebo N = 56	VSL#3® N = 54	Placebo N = 35	VSL#3® N = 28	ETD	95% CI	p-Value	Cohen's d
FIQR-total	75.5 ± 12.3	70.0 ± 17.8	−12.5 ± 14.1	−7.2 ± 12.5	−5.2	−12.0 to 1.6	0.128	0.40
FIQR-pain	8.0 ± 1.6	7.8 ± 1.6	−0.7 ± 2.0	−0.9 ± 2.3	0.3	−0.8 to 1.3	0.611	0.13
FIQR-energy	7.9 ± 2.4	7.6 ± 2.4	−0.6 ± 3.2	−1.0 ± 2.9	0.4	−1.2 to 1.9	0.635	0.12
FIQR-stiffness	8.1 ± 2.1	7.3 ± 2.5	−1.7 ± 2.9	−0.3 ± 2.3	−1.5	−2.8 to 0.1	0.034	0.56
ISI total	19.9 ± 4.6	17.3 ± 7.0	−1.2 ± 4.0	−1.7 ± 5.9	0.5	−2.0 to 3.0	0.702	0.10
PHQ-9	17.4 ± 5.6	16.3 ± 6.3	−2.5 ± 4.2	−2.2 ± 7.2	−0.3	−3.4 to 2.8	0.846	0.05
SF-36 PCS *	28.4 ± 7.0	27.9 ± 6.3	2.2 ± 6.3	4.5 ± 8.0	−2.3	−5.9 to 1.3	0.211	0.33
SF-36 MCS *	32.1 ± 11.8	32.6 ± 12.8	1.9 ± 12.2	0.8 ± 12.4	1.1	−5.3 to 7.4	0.740	0.09

* The number of observed cases at week 12 was N = 35 and N = 27 for placebo and VSL#3, respectively. CI, confidence interval; ETD, estimated treatment difference (positive figures favour VSL#3); FIQR, Revised Fibromyalgia Impact Questionnaire; ISI, Insomnia Severity Inventory; MCS, Mental Component Score; PHQ-9, 9-item Patient Health Questionnaire; PCS, Physical Component Score; SD, standard deviation; SF-36, Short-Form Health-Survey.

2.4. Tolerability

One-third of the patients in each study group reported at least one adverse event. Seven (13.0%) patients in the VSL#3® group and six (10.7%) in the placebo group discontinued the treatment due to adverse events. The vast majority of the adverse events were gastrointestinal related, with some differences between the two study groups in the adverse event profile. Abdominal distension was more frequent among VSL#3®-treated patients, whereas upper abdominal pain was more frequent among placebo-treated patients; however, none of the differences was statistically significant (Table 5).

Table 5. Safety and tolerability profiles of VSL#3® and placebo.

Outcome [N (%)]	Placebo N = 56	VSL#3® N = 54	p-Value
At least one adverse event	19 (33.9)	20 (37.0)	0.733
Treatment discontinuation due to adverse events	6 (10.7)	7 (13.0)	0.714
Serious adverse events	0 (0.0)	0 (0.0)	NA
Most frequent adverse events [a] (incidence ≥ 3%)			
Abdominal distension	1 (1.8)	5 (9.3)	0.110
Flatulence	3 (5.4)	5 (9.3)	0.490
Abdominal pain	3 (5.4)	3 (5.6)	1.000
Constipation	4 (7.1)	3 (5.6)	1.000
Diarrhoea	0 (0.0)	2 (3.7)	0.240
Vomiting	0 (0.0)	2 (3.7)	0.240
Nausea	3 (5.4)	2 (3.7)	1.000
Disease worsening	0 (0.0)	2 (3.7)	0.240
Dyspepsia	3 (5.4)	0 (0.0)	0.240
Headache	2 (3.6)	0 (0.0)	0.490
Upper abdominal pain	4 (7.1)	0 (0.0)	0.120
Swelling	2 (3.6)	0 (0.0)	0.490
Influenza	2 (3.6)	0 (0.0)	0.490

[a] Adverse events were coded with the Medical Dictionary for Regulatory Activities (MedRA) and are presented as preferred terms. NA = not applicable as the data did not fulfil the criteria required to perform a Fisher's test.

3. Discussion

Overall, our data could not demonstrate any beneficial effects of VSL#3® either on the composite score of severity of abdominal pain, bloating and meteorism or in any of the secondary outcome variables. This lack of benefit can be potentially attributed to several factors, including the elevated placebo response, the high proportion of patients who withdrew from the study, and the presence of rather complicated mechanisms underlying the gastrointestinal manifestations in fibromyalgia.

The relevance of the placebo effect in fibromyalgia clinical trials is substantial and has been investigated in several systematic reviews and meta-analyses [20–22]. It has been estimated that the mean placebo effect for pain reduction in patients with fibromyalgia is 30.8% when considering a 30% pain reduction, and 18.8% when considering a 50% pain reduction [20,21]. A recent meta-analysis found that, in relation to patients that received no treatment, fibromyalgia patients receiving placebo experienced significant improvement not only in pain, but also in fatigue, sleep quality, physical function and FIQ total score [22]. In our study, the proportion of placebo responders for the main outcome variable was 50.9%. Similar placebo effect rates have been described in clinical trials evaluating probiotics in patients with IBS. In their review, Rogers and Mousa indicated the presence of a high placebo effect among patients with IBS ranging between 30% and 50%. Several mediators of the placebo effect, particularly in patients with functional somatic disorders, have been suggested, including Pavlovian conditioning, belief outcomes, and patient expectations, among other factors [23].

The dropout rate was also disproportionately high. Nocebo effect is also very relevant in fibromyalgia clinical trials, and it has been estimated to represent between 9% and 11% of patient dropouts [21,24]. Consistent with these estimations, the percentage of placebo-treated patients in our study that withdrew due to tolerability issues was 10.7% of the sample, slightly less than the dropout rate in the VSL#3® group, which was of 12%. However, 17 (31.5%) patients in the VSL#3®-treated group and 15 (26.8%) in the placebo-treated group withdrew due to reasons unrelated to tolerability and/or efficacy issues, mainly loss of follow up; the percentage of withdrawals was similar across participating centres.

The effects of probiotics on human health seem to be related to different effects, such as a decrease in inflammation, decrease in intestinal permeability, modification of the intestinal microbiota, and metabolism modulation. These effects are mediated by multiple mechanisms of action, including the colonization and normalization of perturbed intestinal microbial communities, competitive exclusion of pathogens, modulation of enzymatic activities and production of volatile fatty acids. Nevertheless, it is important to highlight that the mechanisms underlying the exacerbation of gastrointestinal manifestations in fibromyalgia appear to be far more complex and extend beyond the possible small intestinal bacterial overgrowth, gut microbiota alterations or symbiosis [3]. Therefore, this may provide another possible explanation for the lack of benefit of VSL#3 on the primary efficacy outcome. More research is needed to further understand the specific patient characteristics that may predict a favourable response to VSL#3®.

Interestingly, VSL#3-treated patients who were considered as responders to treatment according to the primary outcome variable maintained the degree of improvement obtained after the treatment period during the follow-up period, whereas in placebo-treated patients who were considered as responders, the improvement decreased during the follow-up period. This suggests that at least a subgroup of patients obtained a benefit from VSL#3® treatment. Unfortunately, we were not able to identify any characteristic that could differentiate placebo- from VSL#3®-responders.

In the last five years, the efficacy of probiotics in the treatment of IBS has been evaluated in several systematic reviews and meta-analyses [17,25–27]. These reviews reached a common conclusion that probiotics seem to be beneficial for IBS symptoms and that their tolerability is generally good, although more information is needed in relation to probiotic type, probiotic dosage and treatment length. With one exception [27], they also agree in considering that multi-strain probiotics seem to be preferable over single-strain probiotics.

The use of probiotics in the management of IBS has been recently revised by the American Gastroenterological Association in a technical review that found that, although data concerning the potential efficacy of probiotics on the management of IBS are substantial, no single strain or combination has been studied in a sufficiently rigorous manner [28]. For this reason, the American Gastroenterological Association advocates the use of probiotics for the treatment of IBS only in the context of a clinical trial [29].

VSL#3® has been the object of two meta-analyses in the treatment of IBS. The first one, published in 2018, evaluated the efficacy and tolerability of VSL3#3® for the treatment of IBS [18]; the authors concluded that, although a trend for global overall improvement was observed, no significant differences with placebo were found for specific symptoms such as abdominal pain, bloating or stool consistency. Probiotic-associated side effects were detailed only in one of the five clinical trials included in the meta-analysis and reported a more frequent worsening of the gastrointestinal symptoms in VSL#3®-treated patients than in placebo-treated patients. In our study, almost all side-effects reported by patients who received VSL#3® were also related to the worsening of the previous gastrointestinal symptoms (Table 5). We would like to note that some authors have reported that the formulation of VSL#3 used in the studies conducted prior to 2016 is not the same as the one used here; thus, the results reported in this meta-analysis could be referred to that formulation and not the one we used in our study [30]. The second meta-analysis was based on the tolerability of VSL#3® in any clinical condition, which included IBS, obesity, ulcerative colitis, and early menopause, concluding that the safety profile of VSL#3® was not significantly different from the placebo, and was similar to that of other probiotics [19]. However, there are uncertainties about this meta-analysis because the actual number of patients examined was too small and the pathologies and the probiotic dosages too heterogeneous.

To the best of our knowledge, only one study has been published evaluating the use of probiotics in the treatment of fibromyalgia [31]. The objective of this randomised, placebo-controlled trial, which also used a multi-strain probiotic, was to investigate the potential efficacy of the probiotic on the cognition, emotional symptoms and functional state of the patients. Thus, we cannot establish any comparison in relation to our primary objective, which was to assess the gastrointestinal symptomatology of the patients. However, the authors assessed other variables that we also evaluated, such as depression, anxiety, fibromyalgia pain and impact and health-related quality of life, As in our case, no significant differences were found between the probiotic and placebo in relation to any of these outcomes.

Our study has some limitations. The high dropout rate and its impact on the study estimates because of the missing data as well as the placebo effect in our study were relatively high, prompting cautious interpretation of the study findings. Although we performed a secondary analysis using a complete case approach in order to limit the influence of the imputation method to handle missing data, it is important to bear in mind that complete case analysis is appropriate only when the participants in the analysis can be regarded as a random sample of the study population (i.e., when the missing mechanism is missing completely at random) [32], which cannot be assumed to be the case in our study; in addition, complete case analysis tends to overestimate treatment effects. Therefore, complete case analysis can only be considered as a sensitivity analysis. In addition, due to the lack of a validated scale for measuring our primary outcome, we had to use an ad hoc instrument to assess the severity of gastrointestinal symptoms. Additionally, the lack of sample size calculation due to the absence of published data on the primary outcome measure may have prevented us from adequately controlling the power in the current study. Finally, we did not investigate the composition of patients' microbiota either at the beginning or the end of the trial; this would have been a worthwhile approach, since different experimental and clinical studies have shown that multi-train probiotics can improve health by modifying the gut microbiota composition [33–36].

4. Materials and Methods

4.1. Study Design

In this study, a randomised double-blind placebo-controlled trial evaluating the efficacy and tolerability of VSL#3® in the treatment of patients with fibromyalgia and associated gastrointestinal symptomatology was conducted. VSL#3® (manufactured for Actial Farmaceutica Srl) is a high-concentration multi-strain probiotic mix, commercially available in 450 billion CFU/sachet, containing the following: (i) one strain of *Streptococcus thermophilus BT01*; (ii) three strains of Bifidobacteria: *B. breve BB02*, *B. animalis subsp. lactis BL03* (previously identified as *B. longum BL03*) and *B. animalis subsp. lactis BI04* (previously identified as *B. infantis BI04*); and (iii) four strains of Lactobacilli: *L. acidophilus BA05*, *L. plantarum BP06*, *L. paracasei BP07* and *L. helveticus BD08* (previously identified as *L. delbrueckii subsp. bulgaricus BD08*) [37]. The composition of the placebo was maltose, cornstarch and silicon dioxide

The treatment was administered during a 12-week period, and the participants were followed for an additional 12-week period in order to follow evolution after treatment. The trial protocol was approved both by the Biomedical Research Ethics Committee of the province of Granada (Granada, Spain) and by the Ethics Committee of the Catholic University of Murcia (Murcia, Spain), the two cities where the trial was carried out. Written informed consent was obtained from every subject before inclusion in the study. The trial was registered at ClinicalTrials.gov with the identifier NCT04256785.

4.2. Participants

Patients were recruited from several fibromyalgia associations who regularly attended the two outpatient clinics where the trial was performed.

The inclusion criteria were the following: (a) diagnosis with fibromyalgia, confirmed at the screening of patients using the ACR 2016 criteria [38]; (b) 18 years of age or older; (c) agreement to voluntarily participate in the study by signing informed consent; (d) willingness to, with no need under medical criteria, maintain the treatment previously received for fibromyalgia, both of pharmacological and non-pharmacological types, with no change in life habits especially regarding habitual diet during the trial's duration; and (e) regular suffering (two or more times per week) from three or more of the following symptoms: abdominal pain, abdominal bloating, meteorism, flatulence, nausea, dyspepsia, eructation, constipation and/or diarrhoea.

The exclusion criteria were as follows: (a) suffering from severe mental illness other than major depression; (b) suffering from severe renal, hepatic or cardiovascular organic disease that, at the discretion of the investigator, could have interfered with participation in the study; (c) suffering from any chronic gastrointestinal disease other than IBS, such as inflammatory bowel disease, active gastroduodenal ulcer or colorectal carcinoma; and (d) pregnancy or breastfeeding. All of the mentioned diseases were required to have been diagnosed by a physician.

4.3. Study Assessments

The severity of the following types of gastrointestinal symptoms was evaluated using a 10-point Visual Analogue Scale (VAS): abdominal pain, abdominal bloating, meteorism, flatulence, constipation, diarrhoea, nausea, eructation and dyspepsia.

Secondary assessments were the following:

(a) The Revised Fibromyalgia Impact Questionnaire (FIQR) [39]: This instrument was created to assess the overall symptoms related to fibromyalgia. The total score of the FIQR ranges from 0 to 100, and the higher the score, the greater the severity of fibromyalgia. The validated Spanish version was used [40].
(b) The 9-item Patient Health Questionnaire (PHQ-9): The objective of this questionnaire is to evaluate depressive symptoms. Its total score ranges from 0 to 27 points; the higher the score, the greater the severity of the depression. Since depression is also a symptom frequently associated with fibromyalgia, it was used to check whether an eventual improvement in gastrointestinal symptoms is reflected in an improvement in depressive symptomatology. A validated Spanish version of the questionnaire was used [41].
(c) The Insomnia Severity Inventory (ISI): This is a brief questionnaire which assesses the severity of insomnia. Its total score ranges from 0 to 28 points; the higher the score, the greater the severity of insomnia. The validated Spanish version of the questionnaire was used [42].
(d) The Short-Form Health-Survey SF-36: This multi-item generic health survey aims to evaluate general health concepts not specific to any age, disease or treatment group and measures eight health domains: physical functioning, physical role limitations, bodily pain, general health perceptions, vitality, social functioning, emotional limitations and mental health. These domains yield two summary measures: the

Physical Component Summary (PCS) and the Mental Component Summary (MCS). The validated Spanish version was applied [43].

(e) A seven-point, Likert-type scale, the Patient Global Improvement Scale, was used to assess the relief of patients' general symptomatology.

4.4. Procedure

At the time of screening, demographic and clinical data from each patient were collected, and the fibromyalgia diagnosis was confirmed. Then, each patient was allocated either to VSL#3® or the matching placebo; the treatment was administered as two sachets of study products twice a day for twelve consecutive weeks. Each sachet of VSL#3® contained 450 billion CFU of live freeze-dried bacteria in powder form (Lot. No. 709002, 709003, 802112, 802113). Patients were randomised in a 1:1 ratio to one of the two treatment groups using a random number generator.

On the day of initiation of treatment, the following questionnaires were administered: VAS of abdominal pain, abdominal bloating, meteorism, flatulence, constipation, diarrhoea, nausea, eructation and dyspepsia; FIQR; ISI; PHQ-9; PGI; and SF-36.

Visual analogue scales of gastrointestinal symptomatology were filled in weekly by the patients during the first 4 weeks of the trial and every 2 weeks between weeks 4 and 12 of the trial. At week 12, FIQR, ISI, PHQ-9 and SF-36 were also completed; PGI was filled in on weeks 4, 8 and 12.

At the end of the treatment period, patients entered into a follow-up period and were monitored at 4, 12 and 24 weeks thereafter; in these visits, the VAS of gastrointestinal symptoms, FIQR, PGI and SF-36 were completed.

Adverse effects potentially associated with treatment were collected at each visit through an open-ended question system. During the 12 weeks of treatment, the medication packages were collected to control therapeutic compliance.

4.5. Statistical Analysis

Given the absence of previous intervention studies in this area and, in general, limited information on this aspect of fibromyalgia, this was considered a pilot study. Thus, the calculation of the sample size was based on the feasibility of recruiting them. The recruitment of 110 patients was estimated as a reasonably attainable goal considering the volume of patients attending each one of the two participating centres.

The primary outcome variable was the mean change from baseline to endpoint in the composite score of the three main gastrointestinal symptoms reported by patients with fibromyalgia, i.e., abdominal pain, abdominal bloating and meteorism, as evaluated with the 10-point VAS. We selected the primary outcome variable considering the most frequent gastrointestinal symptoms previously observed in patients with fibromyalgia [3], which are also the most common ones in IBS. Secondary outcomes were the mean changes from baseline to endpoint in the scores of the FIQR, ISI, PHQ-9 and SF-36. In addition, the proportion of responders regarding gastrointestinal symptoms was calculated in two ways: the proportion of patients with a reduction equal to or greater than 30% in the composite score of abdominal pain, bloating and meteorism, and the proportion of patients who were highly or very highly improved (i.e., a score of 1 or 2) according to the PGI.

All patients who had a postbaseline evaluation were included in the efficacy analyses, and missing data were imputed using the LOCF approach. A complete case analysis was also performed for the analysis of the mean changes in the scores of the gastrointestinal symptoms. The results were analysed by applying Student's t-test to independent samples in order to compare the data between the subjects who received the placebo and those who received the active product, as well as to compare the data in the subgroups of patients treated with the placebo and with VSL#3®. The proportion of responders and other categorical variables were compared using the χ^2 test or Fisher's exact test, as appropriate. Values lower than 0.05 were considered significant. Effect sizes were calculated using Cohen's d and interpreted as trivial if they were <0.2, small if they were between 0.2 and

<0.5, medium if they were between 0.5 and <0.8 and large if they were ≥0.8. All analyses were performed using SPSS version 22.

5. Conclusions

In summary, although VSL#3® displayed favourable safety and tolerability profiles in patients with fibromyalgia, it did not improve their gastrointestinal or fibromyalgia symptomatology compared to the placebo. However, the maintenance of the benefit among VSL#3® responders and not among placebo responders suggests that some patients could benefit from treatment with this probiotic. More research is still needed to further elucidate the specific factors that may predict a favourable response to treatment with VSL#3® in patients with fibromyalgia.

Author Contributions: E.P.C. was responsible for the study design and the writing of the first draft of the manuscript; F.R.-V. was responsible for the interpretation of the data and contributed to the writing and editing of the manuscript; J.M.G.-L. was responsible for the management and distribution of the study products; J.H.-T., R.M.-B., C.M.-H. and M.D.C.-I. were responsible for patient recruitment, treatment and follow up; M.S. contributed to the writing and editing of the manuscript. All authors have read and agreed to the published version of the manuscript.

Funding: Actial Farmaceutica Srl (Rome, Italy) provided the study products and the randomization codes. Ferring SAU (Madrid, Spain) partially funded data management and statistical analysis. Neither Actial Farmaceutica Srl nor Ferring SAU was involved in the study design, data collection, data analysis, data interpretation, writing of the manuscript or decision to submit for publication. Actial Farmaceutica Srl reviewed a final draft of this manuscript and provided non-binding comments to the authors.

Institutional Review Board Statement: The study was conducted according to the guidelines of the Declaration of Helsinki, and approved by both the Biomedical Research Ethics Committee of the province of Granada (Granada, Spain) (protocol code: not available; date of approval: 23 February 2018) and by the Ethics Committee of the Catholic University of Murcia (Murcia, Spain) (protocol code: CE041804; date of approval: 27 April 2018).

Informed Consent Statement: Informed consent was obtained from all subjects involved in the study.

Data Availability Statement: The clinical trial data are available from the corresponding author upon reasonable request.

Acknowledgments: The authors thank Oscar Salamanca Gutierrez, Paula Muñoz Romero and Susana Vara (Apices, Madrid, Spain) for the statistical analysis.

Conflicts of Interest: E.P.C., J.M.G.-L., J.H.-T., R.M.-B., C.M.H. and M.D.C.-I. declare no conflict of interest; F.R.V. received consultancy fees from Ferring SAU; M.S. is an employee of Evidera, which provides consulting and other research services to pharmaceutical, medical device and related organizations.

References

1. Clauw, D.J. Fibromyalgia and related conditions. *Mayo Clin. Proc.* **2015**, *90*, 680–692. [CrossRef]
2. Yunus, M.B. Central Sensitivity Syndromes: An Overview. *J. Musculoskelet. Pain* **2009**, *17*, 400–408. [CrossRef]
3. Slim, M.; Calandre, E.P.; Rico-Villademoros, F. An insight into the gastrointestinal component of fibromyalgia: Clinical manifestations and potential underlying mechanisms. *Rheumatol. Int.* **2015**, *35*, 433–444. [CrossRef] [PubMed]
4. Erdrich, S.; Hawrelak, J.A.; Myers, S.P.; Harnett, J.E. A systematic review of the association between fibromyalgia and functional gastrointestinal disorders. *Ther. Adv. Gastroenterol.* **2020**, *13*, 1756284820977402. [CrossRef] [PubMed]
5. Pimentel, M.; Chow, E.J.; Hallegua, D.; Wallace, D.; Lin, H.C. Small Intestinal Bacterial Overgrowth: A Possible Association with Fibromyalgia. *J. Musculoskelet. Pain* **2001**, *9*, 105–113. [CrossRef]
6. Pimentel, M.; Wallace, D.; Hallegua, D.; Chow, E.; Kong, Y.; Park, S.; Lin, H.C. A link between irritable bowel syndrome and fibromyalgia may be related to findings on lactulose breath testing. *Ann. Rheum. Dis.* **2004**, *63*, 450–452. [CrossRef] [PubMed]
7. Goebel, A.; Buhner, S.; Schedel, R.; Lochs, H.; Sprotte, G. Altered intestinal permeability in patients with primary fibromyalgia and in patients with complex regional pain syndrome. *Rheumatology* **2008**, *47*, 1223–1227. [CrossRef]

8. Nagy-Szakal, D.; Williams, B.L.; Mishra, N.; Che, X.; Lee, B.; Bateman, L.; Klimas, N.G.; Komaroff, A.L.; Levine, S.; Montoya, J.G.; et al. Fecal metagenomic profiles in subgroups of patients with myalgic encephalomyelitis/chronic fatigue syndrome. *Microbiome* **2017**, *5*, 44. [CrossRef]
9. Clos-Garcia, M.; Andres-Marin, N.; Fernandez-Eulate, G.; Abecia, L.; Lavin, J.L.; van Liempd, S.; Cabrera, D.; Royo, F.; Valero, A.; Errazquin, N.; et al. Gut microbiome and serum metabolome analyses identify molecular biomarkers and altered glutamate metabolism in fibromyalgia. *EBioMedicine* **2019**, *46*, 499–511. [CrossRef]
10. Minerbi, A.; Gonzalez, E.; Brereton, N.J.B.; Anjarkouchian, A.; Dewar, K.; Fitzcharles, M.A.; Chevalier, S.; Shir, Y. Altered microbiome composition in individuals with fibromyalgia. *Pain* **2019**, *160*, 2589–2602. [CrossRef]
11. Pamuk, O.N.; Umit, H.; Harmandar, O. Increased frequency of gastrointestinal symptoms in patients with fibromyalgia and associated factors: A comparative study. *J. Rheumatol.* **2009**, *36*, 1720–1724. [CrossRef]
12. Arranz, L.I.; Canela, M.A.; Rafecas, M. Dietary aspects in fibromyalgia patients: Results of a survey on food awareness, allergies, and nutritional supplementation. *Rheumatol. Int.* **2012**, *32*, 2615–2621. [CrossRef]
13. Lopez-Rodriguez, M.M.; Granero Molina, J.; Fernandez Medina, I.M.; Fernandez Sola, C.; Ruiz Muelle, A. Patterns of food avoidance and eating behavior in women with fibromyalgia. *Endocrinol. Diabetes Nutr.* **2017**, *64*, 480–490. [CrossRef] [PubMed]
14. Rico-Villademoros, F.; Postigo-Martin, P.; Garcia-Leiva, J.M.; Ordonez-Carrasco, J.L.; Calandre, E.P. Patterns of pharmacologic and non-pharmacologic treatment, treatment satisfaction and perceived tolerability in patients with fibromyalgia: A patients' survey. *Clin. Exp. Rheumatol.* **2020**, *38* (Suppl. 123), 72–78. [PubMed]
15. Bull, M.J.; Plummer, N.T. Part 2: Treatments for Chronic Gastrointestinal Disease and Gut Dysbiosis. *Integr. Med.* **2015**, *14*, 25–33.
16. Yusof, N.; Hamid, N.; Ma, Z.F.; Lawenko, R.M.; Wan Mohammad, W.M.Z.; Collins, D.A.; Liong, M.T.; Odamaki, T.; Xiao, J.; Lee, Y.Y. Exposure to environmental microbiota explains persistent abdominal pain and irritable bowel syndrome after a major flood. *Gut Pathog.* **2017**, *9*, 75. [CrossRef] [PubMed]
17. Ford, A.C.; Harris, L.A.; Lacy, B.E.; Quigley, E.M.M.; Moayyedi, P. Systematic review with meta-analysis: The efficacy of prebiotics, probiotics, synbiotics and antibiotics in irritable bowel syndrome. *Aliment. Pharmacol. Ther.* **2018**, *48*, 1044–1060. [CrossRef] [PubMed]
18. Connell, M.; Shin, A.; James-Stevenson, T.; Xu, H.; Imperiale, T.F.; Herron, J. Systematic review and meta-analysis: Efficacy of patented probiotic, VSL#3, in irritable bowel syndrome. *Neurogastroenterol. Motil.* **2018**, *30*, e13427. [CrossRef] [PubMed]
19. Panetta, V.; Bacchieri, A.; Papetti, S.; De Stefani, E.; Navarra, P. The safety profile of probiotic VSL#3(R). A meta-analysis of safety data from double-blind, randomized, placebo-controlled clinical trials. *Eur. Rev. Med. Pharmacol. Sci.* **2020**, *24*, 963–973. [CrossRef]
20. Hauser, W.; Bartram-Wunn, E.; Bartram, C.; Tolle, T.R. Placebo responders in randomized controlled drug trials of fibromyalgia syndrome: Systematic review and meta-analysis. *Schmerz* **2011**, *25*, 619–631. [CrossRef]
21. Hauser, W.; Sarzi-Puttini, P.; Tolle, T.R.; Wolfe, F. Placebo and nocebo responses in randomised controlled trials of drugs applying for approval for fibromyalgia syndrome treatment: Systematic review and meta-analysis. *Clin. Exp. Rheumatol.* **2012**, *30*, 78–87.
22. Chen, X.; Zou, K.; Abdullah, N.; Whiteside, N.; Sarmanova, A.; Doherty, M.; Zhang, W. The placebo effect and its determinants in fibromyalgia: Meta-analysis of randomised controlled trials. *Clin. Rheumatol.* **2017**, *36*, 1623–1630. [CrossRef]
23. Musial, F.; Klosterhalfen, S.; Enck, P. Placebo responses in patients with gastrointestinal disorders. *World J. Gastroenterol.* **2007**, *13*, 3425–3429. [CrossRef]
24. Mitsikostas, D.D.; Chalarakis, N.G.; Mantonakis, L.I.; Delicha, E.M.; Sfikakis, P.P. Nocebo in fibromyalgia: Meta-analysis of placebo-controlled clinical trials and implications for practice. *Eur. J. Neurol.* **2012**, *19*, 672–680. [CrossRef]
25. Dale, H.F.; Rasmussen, S.H.; Asiller, O.O.; Lied, G.A. Probiotics in Irritable Bowel Syndrome: An Up-to-Date Systematic Review. *Nutrients* **2019**, *11*, 2048. [CrossRef]
26. Niu, H.L.; Xiao, J.Y. The efficacy and safety of probiotics in patients with irritable bowel syndrome: Evidence based on 35 randomized controlled trials. *Int. J. Surg.* **2020**, *75*, 116–127. [CrossRef]
27. Li, B.; Liang, L.; Deng, H.; Guo, J.; Shu, H.; Zhang, L. Efficacy and Safety of Probiotics in Irritable Bowel Syndrome: A Systematic Review and Meta-Analysis. *Front. Pharmacol.* **2020**, *11*, 332. [CrossRef]
28. Preidis, G.A.; Weizman, A.V.; Kashyap, P.C.; Morgan, R.L. AGA Technical Review on the Role of Probiotics in the Management of Gastrointestinal Disorders. *Gastroenterology* **2020**, *159*, 708–738.e704. [CrossRef] [PubMed]
29. Su, G.L.; Ko, C.W.; Bercik, P.; Falck-Ytter, Y.; Sultan, S.; Weizman, A.V.; Morgan, R.L. AGA Clinical Practice Guidelines on the Role of Probiotics in the Management of Gastrointestinal Disorders. *Gastroenterology* **2020**, *159*, 697–705. [CrossRef] [PubMed]
30. De Simone, C. Comment on: "Search and Selection of Probiotics that Improve Mucositis Symptoms in Oncologic Patients: A Systematic Review. *Nutrients* **2020**, *12*, 399. [CrossRef] [PubMed]
31. Roman, P.; Estevez, A.F.; Miras, A.; Sanchez-Labraca, N.; Canadas, F.; Vivas, A.B.; Cardona, D. A Pilot Randomized Controlled Trial to Explore Cognitive and Emotional Effects of Probiotics in Fibromyalgia. *Sci Rep.* **2018**, *8*, 10965. [CrossRef] [PubMed]
32. Hughes, R.A.; Heron, J.; Sterne, J.A.C.; Tilling, K. Accounting for missing data in statistical analyses: Multiple imputation is not always the answer. *Int. J. Epidemiol.* **2019**, *48*, 1294–1304. [CrossRef] [PubMed]
33. Wang, Y.; Wu, Y.; Sailike, J.; Sun, X.; Abuduwaili, N.; Tuoliuhan, H.; Yusufu, M.; Nabi, X.H. Fourteen composite probiotics alleviate type 2 diabetes through modulating gut microbiota and modifying M1/M2 phenotype macrophage in db/db mice. *Pharmacol Res.* **2020**, *161*, 105150. [CrossRef] [PubMed]

34. Wu, Y.; Wang, L.; Luo, R.; Chen, H.; Nie, C.; Niu, J.; Chen, C.; Xu, Y.; Li, X.; Zhang, W. Effect of a Multispecies Probiotic Mixture on the Growth and Incidence of Diarrhea, Immune Function, and Fecal Microbiota of Pre-weaning Dairy Calves. *Front. Microbiol.* **2021**, *12*, 681014. [CrossRef]
35. Qin, Q.; Liu, H.; Yang, Y.; Wang, Y.; Xia, C.; Tian, P.; Wei, J.; Li, S.; Chen, T. Probiotic Supplement Preparation Relieves Test Anxiety by Regulating Intestinal Microbiota in College Students. *Dis. Markers* **2021**, *2021*, 5597401. [CrossRef]
36. Kim, C.S.; Cha, L.; Sim, M.; Jung, S.; Chun, W.Y.; Baik, H.W.; Shin, D.M. Probiotic Supplementation Improves Cognitive Function and Mood with Changes in Gut Microbiota in Community-Dwelling Older Adults: A Randomized, Double-Blind, Placebo-Controlled, Multicenter Trial. *J. Gerontol. A Biol. Sci. Med. Sci.* **2021**, *76*, 32–40. [CrossRef]
37. Mora, D.; Filardi, R.; Arioli, S.; Boeren, S.; Aalvink, S.; de Vos, W.M. Development of omics-based protocols for the microbiological characterization of multi-strain formulations marketed as probiotics: The case of VSL#3. *Microb. Biotechnol.* **2019**, *12*, 1371–1386. [CrossRef]
38. Wolfe, F.; Clauw, D.J.; Fitzcharles, M.A.; Goldenberg, D.L.; Hauser, W.; Katz, R.L.; Mease, P.J.; Russell, A.S.; Russell, I.J.; Walitt, B. 2016 Revisions to the 2010/2011 fibromyalgia diagnostic criteria. *Semin. Arthritis Rheum.* **2016**, *46*, 319–329. [CrossRef]
39. Bennett, R.M.; Friend, R.; Jones, K.D.; Ward, R.; Han, B.K.; Ross, R.L. The Revised Fibromyalgia Impact Questionnaire (FIQR): Validation and psychometric properties. *Arthritis Res. Ther.* **2009**, *11*, R120. [CrossRef]
40. Salgueiro, M.; Garcia-Leiva, J.M.; Ballesteros, J.; Hidalgo, J.; Molina, R.; Calandre, E.P. Validation of a Spanish version of the Revised Fibromyalgia Impact Questionnaire (FIQR). *Health Qual. Life Outcomes.* **2013**, *11*, 132. [CrossRef]
41. Baader, M.T.; Molina, F.J.L.; Venezian, B.S.; Rojas, C.C.; Farías, S.R.; Fierro-Freixenet, C.; Backenstrass, M.; Mundt, C. Validación y utilidad de la encuesta PHQ-9 (Patient Health Questionnaire) en el diagnóstico de depresión en pacientes usuarios de atención primaria en Chile. *Rev. Chil. De Neuro-Psiquiatr.* **2012**, *50*, 10–22. (In Spanish) [CrossRef]
42. Fernandez-Mendoza, J.; Rodriguez-Munoz, A.; Vela-Bueno, A.; Olavarrieta-Bernardino, S.; Calhoun, S.L.; Bixler, E.O.; Vgontzas, A.N. The Spanish version of the Insomnia Severity Index: A confirmatory factor analysis. *Sleep Med.* **2012**, *13*, 207–210. [CrossRef] [PubMed]
43. Alonso, J.; Prieto, L.; Anto, J.M. The Spanish version of the SF-36 Health Survey (the SF-36 health questionnaire): An instrument for measuring clinical results. *Med. Clin.* **1995**, *104*, 771–776.

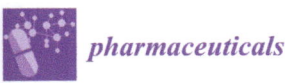

Article

Treatment with an Anti-CX3CL1 Antibody Suppresses M1 Macrophage Infiltration in Interstitial Lung Disease in SKG Mice

Satoshi Mizutani [1], Junko Nishio [1,2], Kanoh Kondo [1], Kaori Motomura [1], Zento Yamada [1], Shotaro Masuoka [1], Soichi Yamada [1], Sei Muraoka [1], Naoto Ishii [3], Yoshikazu Kuboi [3], Sho Sendo [4], Tetuo Mikami [5], Toshio Imai [3] and Toshihiro Nanki [1,*]

[1] Department of Internal Medicine, Division of Rheumatology, Toho University School of Medicine, Ota-ku, Tokyo 143-8541, Japan; satoshi.mizutani@med.toho-u.ac.jp (S.M.); junko.nishio@med.toho-u.ac.jp (J.N.); kano.kondo@med.toho-u.ac.jp (K.K.); kaori.motomura@med.toho-u.ac.jp (K.M.); zento.yamada@med.toho-u.ac.jp (Z.Y.); shoutarou.masuoka@med.toho-u.ac.jp (S.M.); soichi.yamada@med.toho-u.ac.jp (S.Y.); seimuraoka@med.toho-u.ac.jp (S.M.)

[2] Department of Immunopathology and Immunoregulation, Toho University School of Medicine, Ota-ku, Tokyo 143-8540, Japan

[3] KAN Research Institute, Inc., Chuo-ku, Kobe-shi, Hyogo 650-0047, Japan; n-ishii@kan.eisai.co.jp (N.I.); y-kuboi@kan.eisai.co.jp (Y.K.); t-imai@kan.eisai.co.jp (T.I.)

[4] Department of Internal Medicine, Division of Rheumatology and Clinical Immunology, Kobe University Graduate School of Medicine, Chuo-ku, Kobe-shi, Hyogo 650-0017, Japan; sho1000d@med.kobe-u.ac.jp

[5] Department of Pathology, Toho University School of Medicine, Ota-ku, Tokyo 143-8540, Japan; tetsuo.mikami@med.toho-u.ac.jp

* Correspondence: toshihiro.nanki@med.toho-u.ac.jp; Tel.: +81-3-3762-4151 (ext. 6591)

Abstract: CX3C Motif Chemokine Ligand 1 (CX3CL1; fractalkine) has been implicated in the pathogenesis of rheumatoid arthritis (RA) and its inhibition was found to attenuate arthritis in mice as well as in a clinical trial. Therefore, we investigated the effects of an anti-CX3CL1 monoclonal antibody (mAb) on immune-mediated interstitial lung disease (ILD) in SKG mice, which exhibit similar pathological and clinical features to human RA-ILD. CX3CL1 and CX3C chemokine receptor 1 (CX3CR1), the receptor for CX3CL1, were both expressed in the fibroblastic foci of lung tissue and the number of bronchoalveolar fluid (BALF) cells was elevated in ILD in SKG mice. No significant changes were observed in lung fibrosis or the number of BALF cells by the treatment with anti-CX3CL1 mAb. However, significantly greater reductions were observed in the number of M1 macrophages than in M2 macrophages in the BALF of treated mice. Furthermore, CX3CR1 expression levels were significantly higher in M1 macrophages than in M2 macrophages. These results suggest the stronger inhibitory effects of the anti-CX3CL1 mAb treatment against the alveolar infiltration of M1 macrophages than M2 macrophages in ILD in SKG mice. Thus, the CX3CL1-CX3CR1 axis may be involved in the infiltration of inflammatory M1 macrophages in RA-ILD.

Keywords: rheumatoid arthritis; interstitial lung diseases; CX3CL1/fractalkine; CX3CR1; M1 macrophage; M2 macrophage; SKG mice

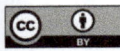

1. Introduction

Rheumatoid arthritis (RA) is a systemic inflammatory disease that is characterized by synovitis, progressive bone erosion, and cartilage destruction [1]. Interstitial lung disease (ILD) develops in 10% of patients with RA, with alveolar septal fibrosis occurring through unknown mechanisms and resulting in more impaired pulmonary gas exchange and shorter life expectancy than in RA patients without ILD [2,3]. Limited information is currently available on the pathogenesis of RA-ILD and its exacerbating factors and an effective therapy has not yet been established [4].

ILD is characterized by abnormal tissue repair after lung tissue damage by chronic inflammation regardless of the cause. Macrophages, which are the most abundant immune cell in the lungs, play a key role in the development of ILD. Activated macrophages are polarized into classically activated M1 macrophages and alternatively activated M2 macrophages [5,6]. In the early inflammatory phase, M1 macrophages produce proinflammatory factors, such as tumor necrosis factor (TNF)-α, interleukin (IL)-1β, and inducible nitric oxide synthase [7–11]. In contrast, M2 macrophages contribute to tissue fibrosis by secreting profibrotic cytokines, including IL-4, IL-10, and transforming growth factor-β [12–15]. Lung macrophages are also classified into alveolar and interstitial macrophages depending on their locations, both of which are involved in the pathogenesis of ILD [16,17]. Although embryonic alveolar macrophages dominant in the steady state, the infiltration of alveolar macrophages derived from circulating monocytes also occurs in murine bleomycin-induced ILD (BLM-ILD) [17]. Monocyte-derived alveolar macrophages, but not embryo-derived resident alveolar macrophages, express profibrotic genes in BLM-ILD [16], suggesting that these migrated monocyte-derived alveolar macrophages are responsible for ILD.

The sole member of the CX3C-type chemokine family, chemokine (C-X3-C motif) ligand 1 (CX3CL1; fractalkine) is a membrane-bound chemokine that is expressed on a number of cells, including endothelial cells, fibroblast-like synoviocytes, osteoblasts, neurons, adipocytes, and intestinal epithelial cells. [18]. The extracellular domain of CX3CL1 is constitutively cleaved and functions as a soluble chemokine [19,20]. In the steady state, circulating monocytes expressing CX3C chemokine receptor 1 (CX3CR1), the receptor for CX3CL1, adhere to endothelial cells through the CX3CL1-CX3CR1 interaction in order to monitor vascular abnormalities [19]. Membrane-bound CX3CL1 is more strongly expressed on endothelial cells under inflammatory conditions, leading to the firm adherence and activation of CX3CR1$^+$ monocytes that initiate local inflammation. The cleavage of membrane CX3CL1 is also promoted by TNF-α, IL-1, and interferon-γ. The recruitment of CX3CR1-expressing inflammatory cells, including monocytes, NK cells, cytotoxic T cells, type 1 helper T cells, and γδ T cells, has been shown to exacerbate local inflammation [21].

Proliferative fibroblast-like synoviocytes express CX3CL1 and inflammatory cells, such as macrophages and T cells, express CX3CR1 in RA joints [22–25]. We previously demonstrated that the blockade of CX3CL1 efficiently suppressed collagen-induced arthritis in mice [25]. A clinical trial on a humanized anti-CX3CL1 monoclonal antibody (mAb) for RA reported clinical efficacy for active RA [26,27]. These findings indicate that the CX3CL1-CX3CR1 axis contributes to the progression of RA through the CX3CL1-dependent migration of activated macrophages into the synovium.

Limited information is currently available on the role of the CX3CL1-CX3CR1 axis in RA-ILD. CX3CL1 is expressed on alveolar and bronchial epithelial cells and vascular endothelial cells in the normal lungs of humans and mice [28,29]. In idiopathic pulmonary fibrosis (IPF) and ILD in polymyositis or dermatomyositis (PM/DM), CX3CL1 is expressed on fibroblasts, inflammatory cells, and alveolar macrophages in addition to the epithelia and vessels [28,29]. Serum CX3CL1 levels were found to correlate with the alveolar-arterial oxygen pressure difference in patients with ILD with PM/DM [30]. On the other hand, CX3CR1$^+$ mononuclear cells infiltrated ILD in patients with systemic sclerosis [31] and PM/DM [30] as well as murine BLM-ILD [32,33]. In BLM-ILD, the depletion of CX3CR1-expressing cells suppressed lung fibrosis and this was accompanied by a decrease in infiltrated macrophages [32]. These findings implicate the CX3CL1-CX3CR1 axis in lung fibrosis.

SKG mice develop RA-like chronic polyarthritis and ILD following an injection of zymosan A [34,35]. Since the point mutation of zeta-chain-associated protein kinase 70 (ZAP-70) in SKG mice promotes autoreactive T-cell development in the thymus, these articular and lung manifestations are considered to develop through autoimmune mechanisms. While arthritis develops in the early stages (4–5 weeks) after the administration of zymosan A, lung inflammation manifests later and fibrosis becomes evident after approximately 12 weeks [34,36]. Therefore, ILD in SKG mice (SKG-ILD) is considered to more closely reflect RA-ILD than other ILD models.

In the present study, we investigated the involvement of CX3CL1 and its inhibition in ILD in SKG mice. A treatment with anti-CX3CL1 mAb suppressed the infiltration of M1 macrophages, but not M2 macrophages, into the alveolar space, but did not attenuate lung fibrosis, suggesting the potential of CX3CL1 to regulate macrophage infiltration in SKG-ILD.

2. Results

2.1. Histopathological Findings of SKG-ILD

SKG mice spontaneously develop ILD at approximately 6 months of age under conventional conditions [34], but not under specific-pathogen-free (SPF) conditions [36]. Therefore, we induced ILD in SKG mice under SPF conditions at 8 weeks of age using the intraperitoneal administration of zymosan A. We confirmed that lung tissues collected 12 weeks after the administration of zymosan A exhibited multiple fibroblastic foci that were fibrotic areas with mononuclear cell infiltration and a consequently altered alveolar structure, while those from mice administered saline showed no signs of inflammation (Figure 1A,B). Masson's trichrome (MT) stain showed collagen deposition colocalized with infiltrating cells in fibroblastic foci (Figure 1B), which confirmed that SKG mice administered zymosan A developed robust ILD in our SPF mouse facility.

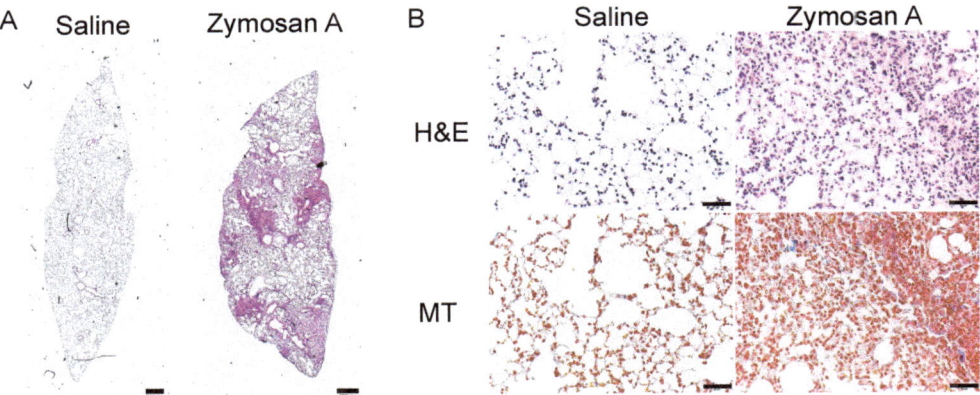

Figure 1. Interstitial lung disease (ILD) induced in SKG/jcl (SKG) mice. ILD was induced in male SKG mice by an intraperitoneal injection of 7.5 mg zymosan A or saline as the control at 8–9 weeks of age. Lung tissue was isolated 12 weeks after the administration of saline or zymosan A and stained with hematoxylin and eosin (H&E) and Masson's trichrome (MT). (**A**) A representative image of whole area of longitudinal H&E section of the lung from SKG mice administered saline or zymosan A at × 40 magnification. Scale bars indicate 500 μm. (**B**) Images of H&E (upper panels) or MT (lower panels) staining at × 200 magnification. Scale bars indicate 50 μm.

2.2. Expression of CX3CL1 and CX3CR1 in Lungs with ILD in SKG Mice

To examine the involvement of CX3CL1 in the pathogenesis of ILD in SKG mice, an immunohistochemical analysis of the expression of CX3CL1 and CX3CR1 in lungs with ILD was performed (Figure 2). While CX3CL1 was expressed on alveolar epithelial cells and macrophages in lungs from both saline-(control) and zymosan A-administered mice, CX3CL1 appeared to accumulate in the fibroblastic foci of lungs in zymosan A-administered mice (Figure 2A, the 3,3′-diaminobenzidine (DAB) staining intensities in control and zymosan A-administered mice, 0.015 vs. 11.136). CX3CR1 was only expressed on alveolar macrophages, the number of which was small, in control mice, whereas CX3CR1-expressing cells massively infiltrated fibroblastic foci in zymosan A-administered mice (Figure 2B, the DAB staining intensities in control and zymosan A-administered mice, 0.094 vs. 5.552). Although alveolar macrophages appeared to be present in the fibrotic foci of lungs with ILD, the destruction of the alveolar structure made them less distinct. These results suggested the involvement of the CX3CL1-CX3CR1 axis in the infiltration of alveolar macrophages and interstitial macrophages in SKG-ILD.

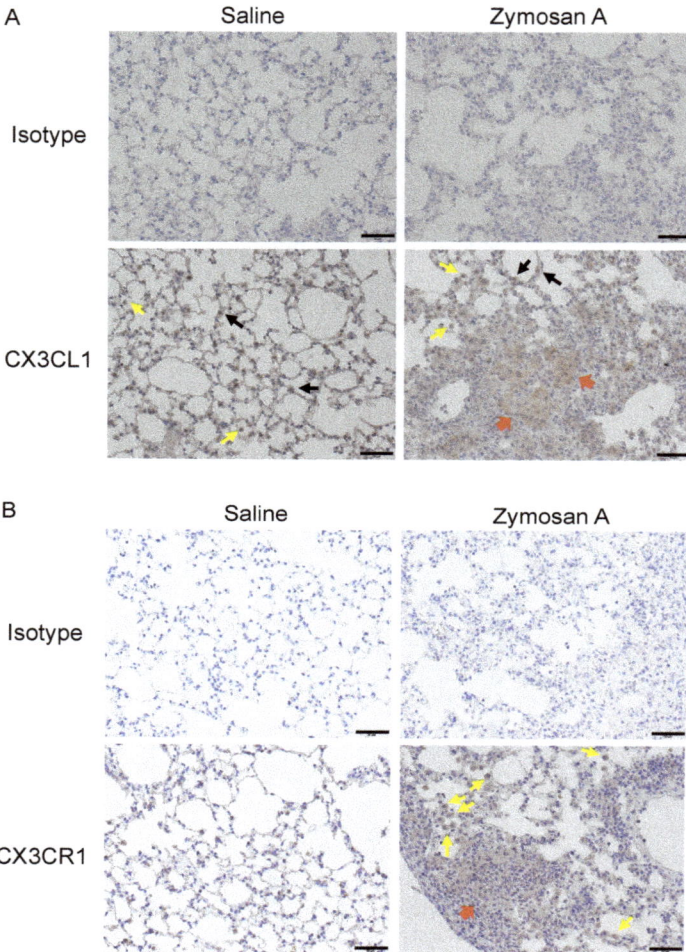

Figure 2. Immunohistochemical (IHC) analysis of CX3CL1 and CX3CR1 in lung tissue from SKG-ILD mice. Lung tissue was obtained as described in Figure 1. Representative images of the IHC analysis of CX3CL1 or CX3CR1 are shown. (**A**) Images of IHC for CX3CL1. Arrows indicate CX3CL1-positive alveolar epithelial cells (black arrows), alveolar macrophages (yellow arrows), or CX3CL1-stained areas in fibroblastic foci (red arrows). (**B**) Images of IHC for CXC3R1. Arrows indicate CX3CR1-positive alveolar macrophages (yellow arrows) or CX3CR1$^+$ cell-infiltrating areas in fibroblastic foci (red arrows). Original magnification of ×200. Scale bars indicate 50 µm.

2.3. Minimal Effects of the Blockade of CX3CL1 in the Lung Pathology of SKG-ILD

Based on the results showing that CX3CR1$^+$ cell numbers increased in the lung tissue of SKG-ILD, we hypothesized that the migration of CX3CR1-positive cells contributes to lung inflammation and fibrosis. To address this hypothesis, we treated SKG-ILD mice with neutralizing anti-CX3CL1 mAb or a control antibody (Ab) and assessed the lung histology of ILD. Anti-CX3CL1 mAb was administered twice a week from the day of the administration of zymosan A until mice were euthanized. Lung tissue from control Ab- and anti-CX3CL1 mAb-treated mice both showed fibroblastic foci with massive cell infiltration and an altered alveolar structure (Figure 3A). The accumulation of collagen bundles was also similarly observed in lungs from control Ab-treated mice and anti-CX3XCL1 mAb-treated mice with MT staining (Figure 3A). No significant differences were noted in Ashcroft scores [37] or collagen-deposited areas between control Ab-treated mice and anti-CX3CL1 mAb-treated mice (Figure 3B,C). These results indicated that the inhibition of CX3CL1 had minimal effects on fibrotic changes in the lungs of SKG-ILD.

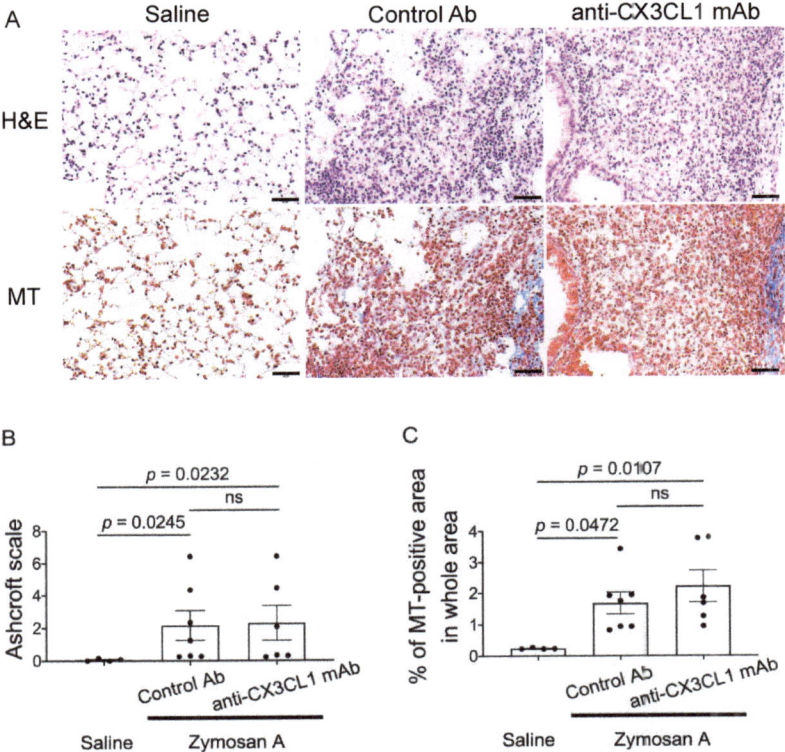

Figure 3. No significant changes in lung fibrosis by the anti-CX3CL1 mAb treatment in SKG-ILD. SKG mice were treated with an intraperitoneal injection of control Ab (hamster immunoglobulin) ($n = 7$) or anti-CX3CL1 mAb ($n = 6$) twice a week for 12 weeks immediately after the administration of zymosan A until euthanization. (**A**) Representative images of lung tissues stained with H&E (upper panels) or MT (lower panels). Original magnification × 200. Scale bars indicate 50 µm. (**B**) The Ashcroft scale was used to assess H&E-stained lung tissues. (**C**) The percentage of MT-positive (blue color-stained) areas in the whole area. The black points indicate each sample value. Data are expressed as means ± standard error of the mean (SEM). ns, not significant. The Kruskal–Wallis test was used with Dunn's test as a post hoc test.

2.4. Flow Cytometric Analysis of Bronchoalveolar Fluid (BALF) Cells in SKG-ILD

Although the inhibition of CX3CL1 only negligibly affected lung fibrosis, marked changes were observed in $CX3CR1^+$ cells that had abundantly infiltrated the alveolar space. We performed a flow cytometric analysis of BALF cells in SKG-ILD to investigate changes in alveolar cell populations following the treatment with anti-CX3CL1 mAb. The numbers of all cells, leukocytes, and T lymphocytes in BALF were significantly higher in SKG-ILD mice than in control saline-injected SKG mice. Furthermore, the number of CD68$^+$ macrophages was markedly higher in SKG-ILD mice than in control SKG mice. No changes were observed in BALF B lymphocytes following the induction of ILD. However, the administration of anti-CX3CL1 mAb did not significantly alter the numbers of these cell populations (Figure 4).

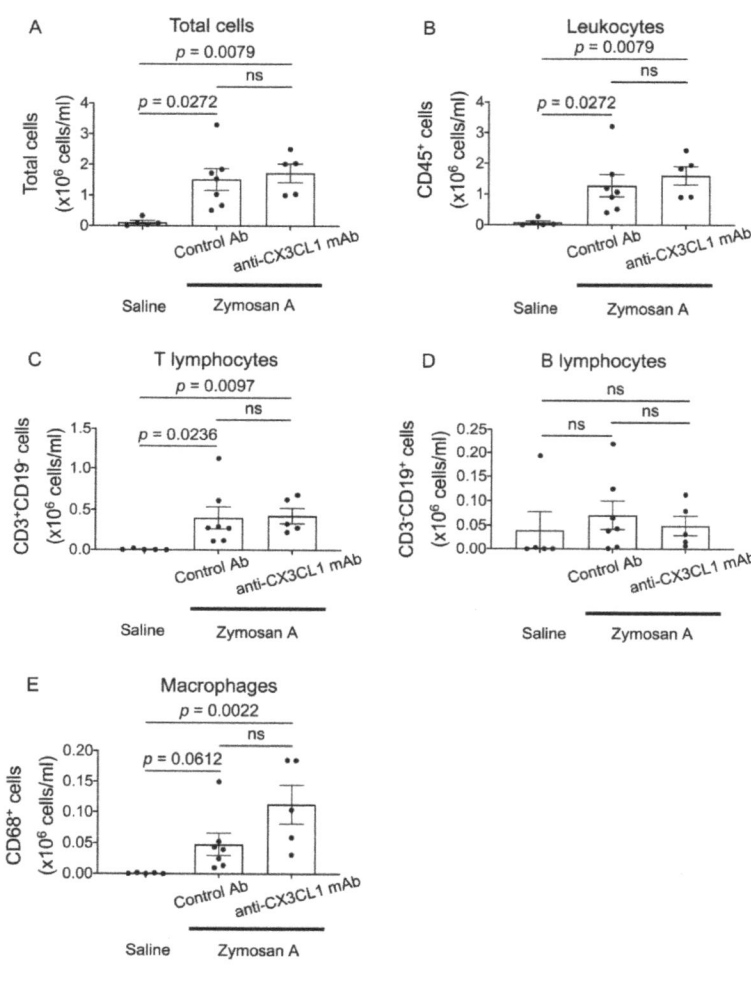

Figure 4. No significant changes in numbers of individual immune cell populations in BALF from SKG-ILD mice treated with anti-CX3CL1 mAb. BALF cells were isolated from saline-administered SKG mice ($n = 5$) or zymosan A-administered SKG mice treated with control Ab ($n = 7$) or anti-CX3CL1 mAb ($n = 5$). The numbers of all cells (**A**), CD45$^+$ cells (**B**), T lymphocytes (**C**), B lymphocytes (**D**), and macrophages (**E**) are shown. Since 4 mL of saline was used to obtain BALF, total cell numbers of individual populations are estimated by multiplying the concentration (cells/mL) by 4 mL. Data are expressed as means ± SEM. The Kruskal–Wallis test was used with Dunn's test as a post hoc test.

2.5. Effects of the Blockade of CX3CL1 on Alveolar Macrophages in SKG-ILD

Since macrophages play a critical role in ILD, we examined M1 (CD86$^+$CD206$^-$) and M2 (CD206$^+$CD86$^-$) macrophages in BALF. The number of M2 macrophages was similar between control Ab-treated mice and anti-CX3CL1 mAb-treated mice (Figure 5A,C), which is consistent with the lack of an effect of the anti-CX3CL1 treatment on fibrosis. In contrast, the number of M1 macrophages significantly decreased following the anti-CX3CL1 mAb treatment (Figure 5B), and consequently the M1/M2 ratio significantly decreased (Figure 5D), suggesting skewed polarization toward M2 macrophages. However, the level of IL-1β in BALF was not altered and IL-6 in BALF rather increased following the anti-CX3CL1 mAb treatment (Figure 5E,F). Thus, these results indicate that anti-CX3CL1 mAb inhibited M1 macrophage infiltration and skewed polarization toward M2 macrophages, consistently with little anti-fibrotic effects of the blockade of CX3CL1.

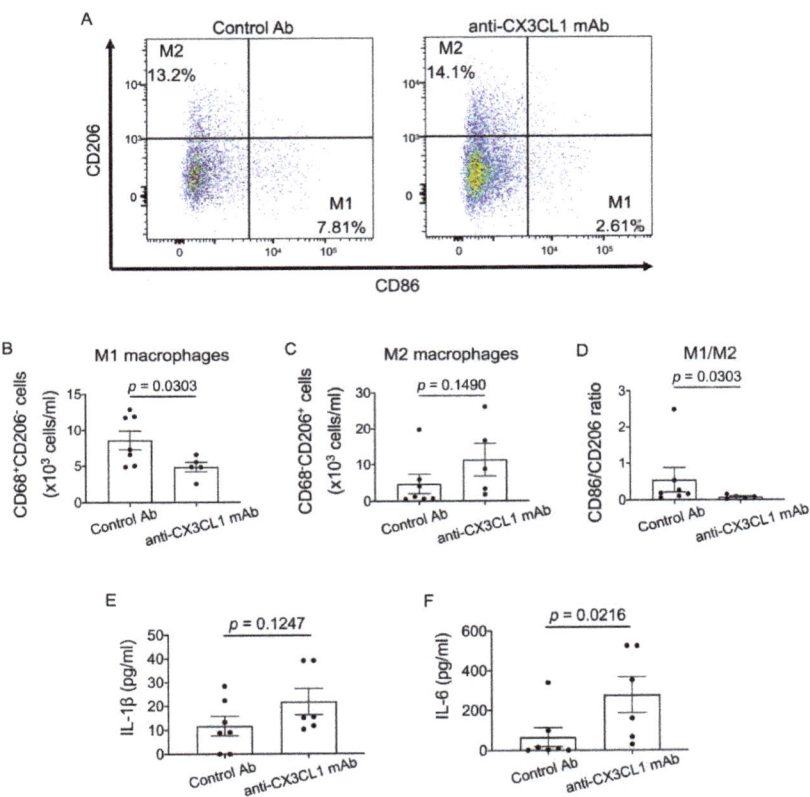

Figure 5. Alterations in M1 and M2 macrophage numbers in BALF following the treatment with anti-CX3CL1 mAb. BALF cells obtained in Figure 4 were analyzed for M1 and M2 macrophages. (**A**) Representative flow cytometry scatter plots for the expression of CD86 and CD206 in $CD68^+$ macrophages. (**B–D**) The numbers of M1 macrophages ($CD86^+CD206^-$ cells; (**B**) and M2 macrophages ($CD206^+CD86^-$ cells; (**C**) and the M1/M2 ratio (**D**) are shown. (**E,F**) Levels of interleukin (IL)-1β (**E**) and IL-6 (**F**) in BALF. Data are expressed as means ± SEM. The Mann–Whitney U test was performed.

2.6. High Expression Levels of CX3CR1 in Alveolar M1 Macrophages

We examined CX3CR1 expression levels on BALF M1 and M2 macrophages in SKG-ILD mice. Although M1 and M2 macrophages both expressed CX3CR1, its expression levels were significantly higher in M1 macrophages than in M2 macrophages (mean fluorescent intensity; M1, 2994 ± 551.6, M2, 767.8 ± 117.9, Figure 6). This result suggested that the higher expression level of CX3CR1 more strongly inhibited the alveolar infiltration of M1 macrophages by anti-CX3CR1 mAb than that of M2 macrophages.

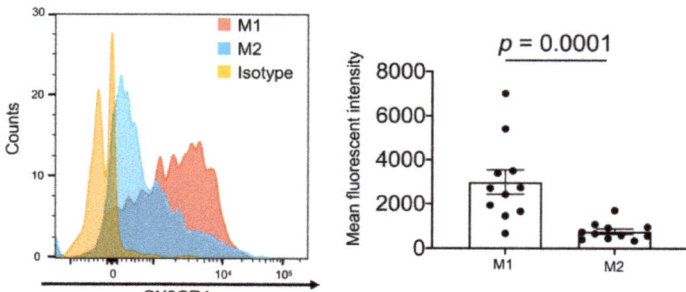

Figure 6. Expression of CX3CR1 on M1 or M2 macrophages. BALF cells obtained from SKG-ILD mice were analyzed for the expression of CX3CR1 on M1 and M2 macrophages. (**A**) Representative histogram of CX3CR1 expression on $CD45^+CD68^+CD86^+CD206^-$-gated cells (M1) or $CD45^+CD68^+CD86^-CD206^+$-gated cells (M2). (**B**) Pooled data on the mean fluorescent intensity of CX3CR1 expression on M1 or M2 macrophages ($n = 11$). Data are expressed as means ± SEM. The Mann–Whitney U test was conducted.

3. Discussion

In the present study, we administered a treatment with anti-CX3CL1 neutralizing mAb to SKG mice with immune-mediated ILD. The results obtained demonstrated that $CX3CL1^+$ and $CX3CR1^+$ cells localized to fibroblastic foci in SKG-ILD and that the anti-CX3CL1 mAb treatment reduced the number of M1 macrophages in BALF. However, the treatment did not significantly alter the number of BALF M2 macrophages or fibrosis in SKG-ILD. We also found that CX3CR1 expression levels in BALF were higher in M1 macrophages than in M2 macrophages in SKG-ILD, suggesting that anti-CX3CL1 mAb more strongly inhibited the migration of M1 macrophages than M2 macrophages.

Although the contribution of the CX3CL1-CX3CR1 axis to the pathogenesis of ILD has already been demonstrated using a murine BLM-ILD model, its involvement in immune-mediated ILD remains unclear. The present study is the first to examine the role of the CX3CL1-CX3CR1 axis in immune-mediated ILD using SKG mice. The expression of CX3CL1 and CX3CR1 in lung fibroblastic foci was observed in SKG-ILD mice, similar to the murine BLM-ILD model [29,32,33]. $CX3CR1^+$ macrophages that localize to fibrotic loci have been shown to promote fibroblast migration or proliferation through the production of platelet-derived growth factor-AA in BLM-ILD [32]. CX3CL1 and CX3CR1 are abundantly expressed in ILD in patients with RA (unpublished data). These findings indicate that the CX3CL1-CX3CR1 axis is involved in the pathogenesis of RA-ILD, similar to the murine model of ILD.

Anti-CX3CL1 mAb therapy reduced the number of BALF M1 macrophages, but not M2 macrophages, in SKG-ILD, and only negligibly attenuated lung fibrosis in SKG-ILD. Based on the result showing that BALF M1 macrophages expressed a significantly higher level of CX3CR1 than BALF M2 macrophages in SKG-ILD, we speculated that anti-CX3CL1 mAb efficiently suppressed the migration of M1 macrophages, but not M2 macrophages.

The minimal effects of anti-CX3CL1 mAb on SKG-ILD is consistent with our recent findings showing the negligible effects of anti-CX3CL1 mAb therapy on the number of infiltrated BALF M2 macrophages in a BLM-ILD model [29]. In contrast, previous studies reported that genetically CX3CR1-depleted mice were resistant to BLM-ILD regardless of whether they were congenic or inducible-deficient mice [32,33]. Therefore, the use of CX3CL1-blocking antibodies may have different outcomes from the complete genetic absence of the CX3CL1-CX3CR1 signal.

ILD is characterized by abnormal tissue repair during chronic inflammation. Although M2 macrophages are considered to play a pivotal role in the process of fibrosis, M1 macrophages are also necessary for inflammation eliciting abnormal tissue repair. In the present study, anti-CX3CL1 mAb successfully inhibited the migration of M1 macrophages, but failed to suppress the migration and/or polarization of M2 macrophages; therefore, it did not exert therapeutic effects against lung fibrosis with CX3CL1 blockade alone. Moreover, the levels of IL-1β and IL-6 in BALF did not decrease following the anti-CX3CL1 mAb treatment. These imply that anti-CX3CL1 mAb treatment could not dampen IL-1β and IL-6 production even though it reduced M1 macrophages in BALF. This is probably partially because these cytokines were also produced by activated fibroblasts and/or the other macrophages in uncontrolled lung fibrosis.

The present study had several limitations that need to be addressed. Although we observed a decrease in BALF M1 macrophages in SKG-ILD following the treatment with anti-CX3CL1 mAb, the number of BALF cells reflects, but may not directly contribute to, inflammation and/or fibrosis in the lung. Therefore, the effects of anti-CX3CL1 mAb on lung-infiltrating cells remain unclear. Another limitation is that anti-CX3CL1 mAb was administered at the same time as the zymosan A injection. In SKG mice, lung fibrosis becomes evident several weeks after an injection of zymosan A. A different treatment outcome may have been observed if anti-CX3CL1 mAb had been administered once lung fibrosis was established.

In summary, our study demonstrated that the CX3CL1-CX3CR1 axis contributed to the pathogenesis of ILD through the migration of CX3CR1[+] cells into inflammatory lung tissue expressing CX3CL1 in SKG mice, a model of RA-ILD. Although anti-CX3CL1 mAb therapy did not attenuate lung fibrosis in SKG-ILD, the infiltration of BALF M1 macrophages strongly expressing CX3CR1 into the lungs was efficiently suppressed. Although anti-CX3CL1 mAb alone did not exert therapeutic effects against lung fibrosis, its combination therapy with anti-fibrotic drugs, such as nintedanib or pirfenidone, may be expected to have a therapeutic effect on ILD.

4. Materials and Methods

4.1. SKG Mice

Male SKG/jcl mice were purchased from CLEA Japan Inc (Tokyo, Japan). SKG/jcl mice aged 8–9 weeks ($n = 11$) were intraperitoneally administered 7.5 mg of zymosan A (Alfa Aesar, Lancashire, UK) dissolved in 0.5 mL of physiological saline. Control mice ($n = 5$) were administered 0.5 mL of saline. Mice were euthanized 12 weeks after the administration of zymosan A to assess pulmonary fibrosis. Regarding the treatment with anti-CX3CL1 mAb, 500 µg of anti-CX3CL1 mAb (5H8-4) [25,38] was intraperitoneally injected twice a week for 12 weeks from the day of the zymosan A administration. Hamster Ig [39] was used as the control Ab for the control group of mice. All experimental procedures were performed in the SPF animal facility of Toho University. Animal experiments were performed according to the animal experiment guidelines approved by Toho University Animal Care and User Committee (approved number: #18-51-398, approved date: 24 May 2018).

4.2. Histopathological Investigation

Mice were euthanized with an overdose of injectable anesthetics 12 weeks after the administration of zymosan A. Left lung tissue was fixed with 10% neutral formalin solution and embedded in paraffin. Three-micrometer-thick sections were used for hematoxylin and eosin (H&E) staining, the MT stain for collagen deposition, and an immunohistochemical analysis. In the immunohistochemical analysis, sections were stained with rabbit immunoglobulin as the isotype control (Dako X0903, Santa Clara, CA, USA), rabbit anti-CX3CL1 polyclonal Ab (pAb, Boster PA1401, Pleasanton, CA, USA), or anti-CX3CR1 (Abcam ab8021, Cambridge, UK,) after blocking endogenous peroxidase and consequent blocking with 2.5% goat serum. An incubation with the primary Ab was conducted at room temperature for 3 h for anti-CX3CL1 pAb or for 30 min for anti-CX3CR1 pAb. The

ImmPRESS polymer kit (Vector MP-7451-15, Burlingame, CA, USA) was used to detect Ab staining, and counterstaining with hematoxylin was performed. All histological images were captured using a BX-63 microscope (Olympus, Tokyo, Japan).

To assess lung fibrosis, ten fields under the ×40 view were randomly selected from each H&E section, scored using the Ashcroft scale [37], and the average score of each section was calculated [37]. Regarding collagen quantification, MT-stained areas and the total cross-section area were quantified by ImageJ software (National Institute of Health) and the percentage of MT areas in the total area was calculated. To assess the intensity of CX3CL1 or CX3CR1 staining in IHC images, the mean value of DAB staining per pixel in the lung interstitial area after thresholding was calculated by ImageJ.

4.3. Flow Cytometric Analysis of BALF

BALF was obtained as previously described [29]. Briefly, 1 mL of saline with 100 μM EDTA was intratracheally injected and aspirated by a 24-G catheter with a 1 mL syringe. This procedure was repeated 4 times and recovered BALF was pooled.

After Fc blocking with 20 μg/mL of rat anti-mouse CD16/CD32 mAb (2.4G2, BD, Franklin Lakes, NJ, USA), BALF cells were stained with PE-conjugated rat anti-mouse CD68 mAb (FA-11, BioLegend, San Diego, CA, USA), BV421-conjugated rat anti mouse CD86 mAb (GL-1, BioLegend), APC-conjugated rat anti mouse CD206 mAb (C068C2, BioLegend), BV510-conjugated rat anti-mouse CD3 mAb (17A2, BioLegend), FITC-conjugated rat anti-mouse CD19 mAb (1D3/CD19, BioLegend), APC/Cy7-conjugated rat anti-mouse CD45 mAb (30-F11, BioLegend), and PE/Cy7-conjugated rat anti-mouse CX3CR1 mAb (SA011F11, BioLegend). A flow cytometric analysis was performed using BD LSRFortessaTM (BD Biosciences, San Jose, CA, USA) and data were analyzed using FlowJo software ver. 10.7.1 (BD Biosciences).

4.4. Enzyme-Linked Immunosorbent Assay (ELISA) for BALF

Supernatant of BALF were collected and stored at −80 °C until subjected to the assay. ELISA was performed to measure the levels of IL-1β and IL-6 using mouse IL-1β ELISA kit (Proteintech KE10003, Rosemont, IL, USA) and mouse IL-6 quantikine ELISA kit (R&D systems 6000B, Minneapolis, MN, USA), respectively by following manufactural protocols.

4.5. Statistical Analysis

Statistical analyses were performed using Graph Pad Prism ver. 8.3.1 (Graph Pad Software, San Diego, CA, USA). The Kruskal–Wallis test was used to compare three groups. Dunn's test was employed as a post hoc test. The Mann–Whitney U test was conducted to compare two groups. A p-value less than 0.05 was considered to be significant. Results were shown as the mean ± SEM.

5. Conclusions

Our study suggests that the CX3CL1-CX3CR1 axis contributes to the pathogenesis of RA-ILD through the migration of CX3CR1+ cells. Anti-CX3CL1 mAb therapy efficiently suppressed the infiltration of BALF M1 macrophages in the mouse model of RA-ILD, and therefore, this therapy combined with anti-fibrotic drugs may have a more robust therapeutic effect on lung fibrosis.

Author Contributions: Conceptualization, S.M. (Satoshi Mizutani) and T.N.; methodology, S.M. (Satoshi Mizutani), J.N. and T.N.; validation, S.M. (Satoshi Mizutani), J.N. and T.N.; formal analysis, S.M. (Satoshi Mizutani); investigation, S.M. (Satoshi Mizutani), J.N., K.K., K.M., Z.Y., S.M. (Shotaro Masuoka), S.Y., S.M. (Sei Muraoka), T.I., Y.K., S.S., T.M., N.I. and T.N.; writing—original draft preparation, S.M. (Satoshi Mizutani); writing—review and editing, S.M. (Satoshi Mizutani), J.N., K.K., K.M., Z.Y., S.M. (Shotaro Masuoka), S.Y., S.M. (Sei Muraoka), T.I., Y.K., S.S., T.M., N.I and T.N.; visualization, S.M. (Satoshi Mizutani) and J.N.; supervision, T.N.; project administration, J.N.; funding acquisition, S.M. (Sei Muraoka), J.N. and T.N. All authors have read and agreed to the published version of the manuscript.

Funding: This study was partly supported by a Research Promotion Grant from the Toho University Graduate School of Medicine (No. 17-01, 20-01) to T.N., the Program for the Strategic Research Foundation for Private Universities (S1411015) from the Ministry of Education, Culture, Sports, Science, and Technology, Japan to T.N., the Private University Research Branding Project from the Ministry of Education, Culture, Sports, Science, and Technology, Japan to T.N., and Grants-in-Aid for Scientific Research (C) (18K07166) to J.N. and for Early-Career Scientists (19K17897) to S.M. (Sei Muraoka) from the Ministry of Education, Culture, Sports, Science, and Technology, Japan.

Institutional Review Board Statement: The study was conducted according to the guidelines of the Declaration of Helsinki and approved by Toho University Animal Care and User Committee (approved number: #18-51-398, approved date: 24 May 2018).

Informed Consent Statement: Not applicable.

Data Availability Statement: The data presented in this study are available on request from the corresponding author.

Acknowledgments: We thank Yasunari Miyazaki, Takashi Yamana, and Masaru Ejima at the Department of Respiratory Medicine, Tokyo Medical and Dental University for their technical advice on removing, treating, and scoring lung tissue. We also thank Motonari Kondo, Yuriko Tanaka, and Marii Ise at the Department of Molecular Immunology, Toho University for their assistance with the flow cytometric analysis.

Conflicts of Interest: S.M. (Sei Muraoka) has received speaker fee from Eisai Co., Ltd. T.I. reports personal fees from KAN Research institute, Inc., during the conduct of the study; in addition, T.I. has a patent COMPOSITIONS AND METHODS FOR TREATING INFLAMMATORY DISORDERS issued. Y.K. reports personal fees from KAN Research institute, Inc., during the conduct of the study; in addition, Y.K. has a patent COMPOSITIONS AND METHODS FOR TREATING INFLAMMATORY DISORDERS issued. N.I. reports personal fees from KAN Research institute, Inc., during the conduct of the study. T.N. received research grants, consulting fees and/or speaking fees from Eisai Co., Ltd. S.M. (Satoshi Mizutani), J.N., K.K., K.M., Z.Y., S.M. (Shotaro Masuoka), S.Y., S.S. and T.M. have declared no conflicts of interest.

References

1. Smolen, J.S.; Aletaha, D.; McInnes, I.B. Rheumatoid arthritis. *Lancet* **2016**, *388*, 2023–2038. [CrossRef]
2. Redente, E.F.; Aguilar, M.A.; Black, B.P.; Edelman, B.L.; Bahadur, A.N.; Humphries, S.M.; Lynch, D.A.; Wollin, L.; Riches, D.W.H. Nintedanib reduces pulmonary fibrosis in a model of rheumatoid arthritis-associated interstitial lung disease. *Am. J. Physiol. Lung Cell Mol. Physiol.* **2018**, *314*, L998–L1009. [CrossRef] [PubMed]
3. Olson, A.L.; Swigris, J.J.; Sprunger, D.B.; Fischer, A.; Fernandez-Perez, E.R.; Solomon, J.; Murphy, J.; Cohen, M.; Raghu, G.; Brown, K.K. Rheumatoid arthritis-interstitial lung disease-associated mortality. *Am. J. Respir Crit. Care Med.* **2011**, *183*, 372–378. [CrossRef] [PubMed]
4. Doyle, T.J.; Dellaripa, P.F.; Batra, K.; Frits, M.L.; Iannaccone, C.K.; Hatabu, H.; Nishino, M.; Weinblatt, M.E.; Ascherman, D.P.; Washko, G.R.; et al. Functional impact of a spectrum of interstitial lung abnormalities in rheumatoid arthritis. *Chest* **2014**, *146*, 41–50. [CrossRef]
5. Mantovani, A.; Biswas, S.K.; Galdiero, M.R.; Sica, A.; Locati, M. Macrophage plasticity and polarization in tissue repair and remodelling. *J. Pathol.* **2013**, *229*, 176–185. [CrossRef]
6. Wynn, T.A.; Vannella, K.M. Macrophages in Tissue Repair, Regeneration, and Fibrosis. *Immunity* **2016**, *44*, 450–462. [CrossRef]
7. Robbe, P.; Draijer, C.; Borg, T.R.; Luinge, M.; Timens, W.; Wouters, I.M.; Melgert, B.N.; Hylkema, M.N. Distinct macrophage phenotypes in allergic and nonallergic lung inflammation. *Am. J. Physiol. Lung Cell Mol. Physiol.* **2015**, *308*, L358–L367. [CrossRef]
8. Sierra-Filardi, E.; Nieto, C.; Dominguez-Soto, A.; Barroso, R.; Sanchez-Mateos, P.; Puig-Kroger, A.; Lopez-Bravo, M.; Joven, J.; Ardavin, C.; Rodriguez-Fernandez, J.L.; et al. CCL2 shapes macrophage polarization by GM-CSF and M-CSF: Identification of CCL2/CCR2-dependent gene expression profile. *J. Immunol.* **2014**, *192*, 3858–3867. [CrossRef]
9. Sierra-Filardi, E.; Vega, M.A.; Sanchez-Mateos, P.; Corbi, A.L.; Puig-Kroger, A. Heme Oxygenase-1 expression in M-CSF-polarized M2 macrophages contributes to LPS-induced IL-10 release. *Immunobiology* **2010**, *215*, 788–795. [CrossRef]
10. Lu, H.L.; Huang, X.Y.; Luo, Y.F.; Tan, W.P.; Chen, P.F.; Guo, Y.B. Activation of M1 macrophages plays a critical role in the initiation of acute lung injury. *Biosci. Rep.* **2018**, *38*. [CrossRef]
11. Xie, N.; Cui, H.; Ge, J.; Banerjee, S.; Guo, S.; Dubey, S.; Abraham, E.; Liu, R.M.; Liu, G. Metabolic characterization and RNA profiling reveal glycolytic dependence of profibrotic phenotype of alveolar macrophages in lung fibrosis. *Am. J. Physiol. Lung Cell Mol. Physiol.* **2017**, *313*, L834–L844. [CrossRef]

12. Yao, Y.; Wang, Y.; Zhang, Z.; He, L.; Zhu, J.; Zhang, M.; He, X.; Cheng, Z.; Ao, Q.; Cao, Y.; et al. Chop Deficiency Protects Mice Against Bleomycin-induced Pulmonary Fibrosis by Attenuating M2 Macrophage Production. *Mol. Ther.* **2016**, *24*, 915–925. [CrossRef]
13. Florez-Sampedro, L.; Song, S.; Melgert, B.N. The diversity of myeloid immune cells shaping wound repair and fibrosis in the lung. *Regeneration* **2018**, *5*, 3–25. [CrossRef]
14. Moore, B.B.; Kolodsick, J.E.; Thannickal, V.J.; Cooke, K.; Moore, T.A.; Hogaboam, C.; Wilke, C.A.; Toews, G.B. CCR2-mediated recruitment of fibrocytes to the alveolar space after fibrotic injury. *Am. J. Pathol.* **2005**, *166*, 675–684. [CrossRef]
15. Sun, L.; Louie, M.C.; Vannella, K.M.; Wilke, C.A.; LeVine, A.M.; Moore, B.B.; Shanley, T.P. New concepts of IL-10-induced lung fibrosis: Fibrocyte recruitment and M2 activation in a CCL2/CCR2 axis. *Am. J. Physiol. Lung Cell Mol. Physiol.* **2011**, *300*, L341–L353. [CrossRef]
16. Misharin, A.V.; Morales-Nebreda, L.; Reyfman, P.A.; Cuda, C.M.; Walter, J.M.; McQuattie-Pimentel, A.C.; Chen, C.I.; Anekalla, K.R.; Joshi, N.; Williams, K.J.N.; et al. Monocyte-derived alveolar macrophages drive lung fibrosis and persist in the lung over the life span. *J. Exp. Med.* **2017**, *214*, 2387–2404. [CrossRef]
17. McCubbrey, A.L.; Barthel, L.; Mohning, M.P.; Redente, E.F.; Mould, K.J.; Thomas, S.M.; Leach, S.M.; Danhorn, T.; Gibbings, S.L.; Jakubzick, C.V.; et al. Deletion of c-FLIP from CD11b(hi) Macrophages Prevents Development of Bleomycin-induced Lung Fibrosis. *Am. J. Respir. Cell Mol. Biol.* **2018**, *58*, 66–78. [CrossRef]
18. Kim, K.W.; Vallon-Eberhard, A.; Zigmond, E.; Farache, J.; Shezen, E.; Shakhar, G.; Ludwig, A.; Lira, S.A.; Jung, S. In vivo structure/function and expression analysis of the CX3C chemokine fractalkine. *Blood* **2011**, *118*, e156–e167. [CrossRef]
19. Garton, K.J.; Gough, P.J.; Blobel, C.P.; Murphy, G.; Greaves, D.R.; Dempsey, P.J.; Raines, E.W. Tumor necrosis factor-alpha-converting enzyme (ADAM17) mediates the cleavage and shedding of fractalkine (CX3CL1). *J. Biol. Chem.* **2001**, *276*, 37993–38001. [CrossRef]
20. Tsou, C.L.; Haskell, C.A.; Charo, I.F. Tumor necrosis factor-alpha-converting enzyme mediates the inducible cleavage of fractalkine. *J. Biol. Chem.* **2001**, *276*, 44622–44626. [CrossRef]
21. Nishimura, M.; Umehara, H.; Nakayama, T.; Yoneda, O.; Hieshima, K.; Kakizaki, M.; Dohmae, N.; Yoshie, O.; Imai, T. Dual functions of fractalkine/CX3C ligand 1 in trafficking of perforin+/granzyme B+ cytotoxic effector lymphocytes that are defined by CX3CR1 expression. *J. Immunol.* **2002**, *168*, 6173–6180. [CrossRef] [PubMed]
22. Ruth, J.H.; Volin, M.V.; Haines, G.K., 3rd; Woodruff, D.C.; Katschke, K.J., Jr.; Woods, J.M.; Park, C.C.; Morel, J.C.; Koch, A.E. Fractalkine, a novel chemokine in rheumatoid arthritis and in rat adjuvant-induced arthritis. *Arthritis Rheum.* **2001**, *44*, 1568–1581. [CrossRef]
23. Koizumi, K.; Saitoh, Y.; Minami, T.; Takeno, N.; Tsuneyama, K.; Miyahara, T.; Nakayama, T.; Sakurai, H.; Takano, Y.; Nishimura, M.; et al. Role of CX3CL1/fractalkine in osteoclast differentiation and bone resorption. *J. Immunol.* **2009**, *183*, 7825–7831. [CrossRef] [PubMed]
24. Blaschke, S.; Koziolek, M.; Schwarz, A.; Benohr, P.; Middel, P.; Schwarz, G.; Hummel, K.M.; Muller, G.A. Proinflammatory role of fractalkine (CX3CL1) in rheumatoid arthritis. *J. Rheumatol.* **2003**, *30*, 1918–1927.
25. Nanki, T.; Urasaki, Y.; Imai, T.; Nishimura, M.; Muramoto, K.; Kubota, T.; Miyasaka, N. Inhibition of fractalkine ameliorates murine collagen-induced arthritis. *J. Immunol.* **2004**, *173*, 7010–7016. [CrossRef]
26. Tanaka, Y.; Takeuchi, T.; Yamanaka, H.; Nanki, T.; Umehara, H.; Yasuda, N.; Tago, F.; Kitahara, Y.; Kawakubo, M.; Torii, K.; et al. Efficacy and Safety of E6011, an Anti-Fractalkine Monoclonal Antibody, in Patients With Active Rheumatoid Arthritis With Inadequate Response to Methotrexate: Results of a Randomized, Double-Blind, Placebo-Controlled Phase II Study. *Arthritis Rheumatol.* **2020**. [CrossRef]
27. Tanaka, Y.; Takeuchi, T.; Umehara, H.; Nanki, T.; Yasuda, N.; Tago, F.; Kawakubo, M.; Kitahara, Y.; Hojo, S.; Kawano, T.; et al. Safety, pharmacokinetics, and efficacy of E6011, an antifractalkine monoclonal antibody, in a first-in-patient phase 1/2 study on rheumatoid arthritis. *Mod. Rheumatol.* **2018**, *28*, 58–65. [CrossRef]
28. Rivas-Fuentes, S.; Herrera, I.; Salgado-Aguayo, A.; Buendia-Roldan, I.; Becerril, C.; Cisneros, J. CX3CL1 and CX3CR1 could be a relevant molecular axis in the pathophysiology of idiopathic pulmonary fibrosis. *Int. J. Med. Sci.* **2020**, *17*, 2357–2361. [CrossRef]
29. Yamada, S.; Miyoshi, S.; Nishio, J.; Mizutani, S.; Yamada, Z.; Kusunoki, N.; Sato, H.; Kuboi, Y.; Hoshino-Negishi, K.; Ishii, N.; et al. Effects of CX3CL1 inhibition on murine bleomycin-induced interstitial pneumonia. *Eur. J. Inflamm.* **2020**, *18*. [CrossRef]
30. Suzuki, F.; Kubota, T.; Miyazaki, Y.; Ishikawa, K.; Ebisawa, M.; Hirohata, S.; Ogura, T.; Mizusawa, H.; Imai, T.; Miyasaka, N.; et al. Serum level of soluble CX3CL1/fractalkine is elevated in patients with polymyositis and dermatomyositis, which is correlated with disease activity. *Arthritis Res. Ther.* **2012**, *14*, R48. [CrossRef]
31. Hoffmann-Vold, A.M.; Weigt, S.S.; Palchevskiy, V.; Volkmann, E.; Saggar, R.; Li, N.; Midtvedt, O.; Lund, M.B.; Garen, T.; Fishbein, M.C.; et al. Augmented concentrations of CX3CL1 are associated with interstitial lung disease in systemic sclerosis. *PLoS ONE* **2018**, *13*, e0206545. [CrossRef]
32. Aran, D.; Looney, A.P.; Liu, L.; Wu, E.; Fong, V.; Hsu, A.; Chak, S.; Naikawadi, R.P.; Wolters, P.J.; Abate, A.R.; et al. Reference-based analysis of lung single-cell sequencing reveals a transitional profibrotic macrophage. *Nat. Immunol.* **2019**, *20*, 163–172. [CrossRef]
33. Ishida, Y.; Kimura, A.; Nosaka, M.; Kuninaka, Y.; Hemmi, H.; Sasaki, I.; Kaisho, T.; Mukaida, N.; Kondo, T. Essential involvement of the CX3CL1-CX3CR1 axis in bleomycin-induced pulmonary fibrosis via regulation of fibrocyte and M2 macrophage migration. *Sci. Rep.* **2017**, *7*, 16833. [CrossRef]

34. Sakaguchi, N.; Takahashi, T.; Hata, H.; Nomura, T.; Tagami, T.; Yamazaki, S.; Sakihama, T.; Matsutani, T.; Negishi, I.; Nakatsuru, S.; et al. Altered thymic T-cell selection due to a mutation of the ZAP-70 gene causes autoimmune arthritis in mice. *Nature* **2003**, *426*, 454–460. [CrossRef]
35. Sakaguchi, S.; Sakaguchi, N.; Yoshitomi, H.; Hata, H.; Takahashi, T.; Nomura, T. Spontaneous development of autoimmune arthritis due to genetic anomaly of T cell signal transduction: Part 1. In *Seminars in Immunology*; Academic Press: Cambridge, MA, USA, 2006; Volume 18, pp. 199–206.
36. Shiomi, A.; Usui, T.; Ishikawa, Y.; Shimizu, M.; Murakami, K.; Mimori, T. GM-CSF but not IL-17 is critical for the development of severe interstitial lung disease in SKG mice. *J. Immunol.* **2014**, *193*, 849–859. [CrossRef]
37. Ashcroft, T.; Simpson, J.M.; Timbrell, V. Simple method of estimating severity of pulmonary fibrosis on a numerical scale. *J. Clin. Pathol.* **1988**, *41*, 467–470. [CrossRef]
38. Suzuki, F.; Nanki, T.; Imai, T.; Kikuchi, H.; Hirohata, S.; Kohsaka, H.; Miyasaka, N. Inhibition of CX3CL1 (fractalkine) improves experimental autoimmune myositis in SJL/J mice. *J. Immunol.* **2005**, *175*, 6987–6996. [CrossRef]
39. Hoshino-Negishi, K.; Ohkuro, M.; Nakatani, T.; Kuboi, Y.; Nishimura, M.; Ida, Y.; Kakuta, J.; Hamaguchi, A.; Kumai, M.; Kamisako, T.; et al. Role of Anti-Fractalkine Antibody in Suppression of Joint Destruction by Inhibiting Migration of Osteoclast Precursors to the Synovium in Experimental Arthritis. *Arthritis Rheumatol.* **2019**, *71*, 222–231. [CrossRef]

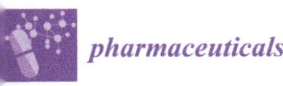

Article

Higher Ventricular-Arterial Coupling Derived from Three-Dimensional Echocardiography Is Associated with a Worse Clinical Outcome in Systemic Sclerosis

Francesco Tona [1,*,†], Elisabetta Zanatta [2,†], Roberta Montisci [3], Denisa Muraru [1], Elena Beccegato [1], Elena De Zorzi [2], Francesco Benvenuti [2], Giovanni Civieri [1], Franco Cozzi [2], Sabino Iliceto [1] and Andrea Doria [2]

[1] Department of Cardiac, Thoracic, Vascular Sciences and Public Health, 35128 Padova, Italy; denisa.muraru@unipd.it (D.M.); elena.beccegato@unipd.it (E.B.); giovanni.civieri@yahoo.it (G.C.); sabino.iliceto@unipd.it (S.I.)

[2] Department of Medicine, Padova University Hospital, 35128 Padova, Italy; elisabettazanatta86@gmail.com (E.Z.); elena.dezorzi@gmail.com (E.D.Z.); fran.benvenuti@gmail.com (F.B.); franco.cozzi@unipd.it (F.C.); andrea.doria@unipd.it (A.D.)

[3] Clinical Cardiology, AOU Cagliari, Department of Medical Science and Public Health, University of Cagliari, 09042 Cagliari, Italy; rmontisc@gmail.com

* Correspondence: francesco.tona@unipd.it; Tel.: +39-0498211844

† These two authors contributed equally to the article.

Abstract: Primary myocardial involvement is common in systemic sclerosis (SSc). Ventricular-arterial coupling (VAC) reflecting the interplay between ventricular performance and arterial load, is a key determinant of cardiovascular (CV) performance. We aimed to investigate VAC, VAC-derived indices, and the potential association between altered VAC and survival free from death/hospitalization for major adverse CV events (MACE) in scleroderma. Only SSc patients without any anamnestic and echocardiographic evidence of primary myocardial involvement who underwent three-dimensional echocardiography (3DE) were included in this cross-sectional study and compared with healthy matched controls. 3DE was used for noninvasive measurements of end-systolic elastance (E_{es}), arterial elastance (E_a), VAC (E_a/E_{es}) and end-diastolic elastance (E_{ed}); the occurrence of death/hospitalization for MACE was recorded during follow-up. Sixty-five SSc patients (54 female; aged 56 ± 14 years) were included. E_{es} ($p = 0.04$), E_a ($p = 0.04$) and E_{ed} ($p = 0.01$) were higher in patients vs. controls. Thus, VAC was similar in both groups. E_{es} was lower and VAC was higher in patients with diffuse cutaneous form (dcSSc) vs. patients with limited form (lcSSc) ($p = 0.001$ and $p = 0.02$, respectively). Over a median follow-up of 4 years, four patients died for heart failure and 34 were hospitalized for CV events. In patients with VAC > 0.63 the risk of MACE was higher (HR 2.5; 95% CI 1.13–5.7; $p = 0.01$) and survival free from death/hospitalization was lower ($p = 0.005$) than in those with VAC < 0.63. Our study suggests that VAC may be impaired in SSc patients without signs and symptoms of primary myocardial involvement. Moreover, VAC appears to have a prognostic role in SSc.

Keywords: heart failure; 3D-echocardiography; ventricular function; outcome; systemic sclerosis; ventricular-arterial coupling

Citation: Tona, F.; Zanatta, E.; Montisci, R.; Muraru, D.; Beccegato, E.; De Zorzi, E.; Benvenuti, F.; Civieri, G.; Cozzi, F.; Iliceto, S.; et al. Higher Ventricular-Arterial Coupling Derived from Three-Dimensional Echocardiography Is Associated with a Worse Clinical Outcome in Systemic Sclerosis. *Pharmaceuticals* **2021**, *14*, 646. https://doi.org/10.3390/ph14070646

Academic Editors: Francesco Salton, Barbara Ruaro and Paola Confalonieri

Received: 2 March 2021
Accepted: 2 July 2021
Published: 5 July 2021

Publisher's Note: MDPI stays neutral with regard to jurisdictional claims in published maps and institutional affiliations.

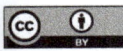

Copyright: © 2021 by the authors. Licensee MDPI, Basel, Switzerland. This article is an open access article distributed under the terms and conditions of the Creative Commons Attribution (CC BY) license (https://creativecommons.org/licenses/by/4.0/).

1. Introduction

Systemic sclerosis (SSc) is a chronic systemic autoimmune disease characterized by widespread vascular lesions and fibrosis of skin and internal organs [1]. Although often clinically silent [2,3], primary cardiac involvement is one of the main causes of death in SSc [4,5]. Thus, a yearly transthoracic echocardiography is recommended in patients with SSc to assess systolic pulmonary artery pressure as well as diastolic and systolic function of the left ventricle (LV) [6]. In this regard, some measurements such as end-diastolic diameter, fractional shortening, or LV ejection fraction (LVEF) are routinely used in clinical practice. However, these indices are load-dependent and do not systematically reflect the contractile state of the myocardium [7]. The interplay between cardiac function and arterial system—commonly defined as ventricular-arterial coupling (VAC)—is a major determinant of ventricular performance as it reflects global cardiovascular (CV) efficiency [8], and can be mathematically expressed as the ratio between arterial elastance (Ea) and end-systolic elastance (Ees) of the LV. VAC has been recently recognized as a key determinant of cardiovascular performance, and in fact, ventricular-arterial uncoupling which occurs in various clinical conditions, may predict morbidity and mortality [9–11].

The advantages of three-dimensional echocardiography (3DE) vs. 2-dimensional echocardiography (2DE) lie in its better accuracy, precision, and reproducibility for volume measurements [12], and consequently for VAC assessment [13].

We aimed to investigate VAC by 3DE in SSc patients, as well as potential differences in VAC values and VAC-derived indices by comparing patients with a limited and diffuse cutaneous form of SSc (lcSSc and dcSSc, respectively). Moreover, we set out to evaluate a potential association between altered VAC and survival-free from major adverse cardiovascular events (MACEs) in SSc.

2. Results

2.1. Echocardiography and Pressure-Volume Curve Parameters in SSc Patients and Controls

Baseline characteristics of the 65 patients enrolled in the study are shown in Table 1. LV diastolic dimension, wall thickness, and mass index were comparable in patients and in controls. Regional contractility was normal in all patients and controls. Left ventricular end-systolic volume (LVESV), LV end-diastolic volume (LVEDV), stroke volume (SV), and LVEF were similar in both groups. Systolic and diastolic blood pressure were comparable in patients and controls. E/e' was higher in patients vs. controls (10.02 ± 4.3 vs. 6.5 ± 2.2, $p < 0.0001$). Ees and Ea were higher in patients vs. controls (3.95 ± 1.8 vs. 2.99 ± 0.7 mmHg/mL, $p = 0.002$; 2.28 ± 0.11 vs. 1.73 ± 0.07 mmHg/mL, $p = 0.001$, respectively), whereas VAC was comparable in both groups (0.60 ± 0.1 vs. 0.62 ± 0.2, $p = 0.59$). Diastolic elastance (Eed) was higher in patients (0.23 ± 0.01 vs. 0.16 ± 0.03 mmHg/mL, $p = 0.001$). Stroke work (SW), potential energy (PE), pressure-voulme area (PVA) and LV efficiency indicating mechanical energy exerted by the left ventricle were similar in both groups.

Table 1. Clinical and Echocardiographic Features in SSc Patients with and without VAC > 0.63.

	All Patients (n = 65)	VAC ≤ 0.63 (n = 34)	VAC > 0.63 (n = 31)	p Value
Age, years	56 ± 14	58 ± 13	53 ± 16	0.12
Female, n (%)	54 (83)	29 (85)	25 (81)	0.61
Body weight, Kg	60 ± 11	62 ± 9	59 ± 10	0.81
BMI, Kg/m^2	25 ± 2	26 ± 3	25 ± 1	0.80
Systolic blood pressure, mmHg	126 ± 21	127 ± 20	125 ± 22	0.55
Diastolic blood pressure, mmHg	74 ± 10	70 ± 9	79 ± 6	0.69
Hemoglobin, g/dL	14 ± 0.8	15 ± 0.6	13 ± 0.2	0.71
Creatinine, mg/dL	0.98 ± 0.02	0.95 ± 0.01	1.02 ± 0.02	0.81
Clinical Features				
Disease duration, years	19 ± 11	16 ± 9	22 ± 12	0.03
Diffuse cutaneous form, n (%)	27 (41)	10 (29)	17 (55)	0.03
PAH, n (%)	22 (34)	6 (17)	16 (47)	0.57
ILD on HRCT, n (%)	37 (57)	20 (59)	17 (55)	0.86
Digital ulcers, n (%)	39 (60)	20 (58)	19 (61)	0.66

Table 1. Cont.

	All Patients (n = 65)	VAC ≤ 0.63 (n = 34)	VAC > 0.63 (n = 31)	p Value
Treatment, n (%)				
Prostanoid ev	12 (18)	4 (12)	8 (26)	0.40
ET-1 inhibitors	22 (34)	14 (41)	8 (26)	0.33
Immunosuppressants	30 (46)	18 (53)	12 (39)	0.28
Echocardiographic Measurements				
LVEDD, mm	44.9 ± 0.5	45.1 ± 0.6	44.7 ± 0.5	0.94
IVS thickness, mm	11.4 ± 1.2	9.9 ± 1.9	13.6 ± 1.6	0.28
PW thickness, mm	11.5 ± 1.3	9.6 ± 1.9	13.2 ± 1.6	0.21
LV mass, g	155 ± 59	151 ± 63	161 ± 53	0.33
LVEDV, mL	88 ± 26	85 ± 29	91 ± 24	0.24
LVESV, mL	33 ± 11	28 ± 10	38 ± 11	<0.0001
SV, mL	55 ± 17	57 ± 19	52 ± 14	0.41
LVEF (%)	62 ± 5	67 ± 3	57 ± 2	<0.0001
Aorta, mm	30 ± 0.3	30 ± 0.3	30 ± 0.4	0.69
Left atrium, mm	49.8 ± 9	47.7 ± 8	51.9 ± 9	0.12
RVEDD, cm^2	19 ± 5	18.2 ± 5	20 ± 5	0.08
TAPSE, cm	2.25 ± 0.5	2.31 ± 0.5	2.19 ± 0.5	0.24
Peak E velocity, m/s	0.86 ± 0.2	0.85 ± 0.1	0.88 ± 0.2	0.58
Peak A velocity, m/s	0.79 ± 0.2	0.84 ± 0.2	0.75 ± 0.2	0.13
DT, ms	199 ± 60	219 ± 62	179 ± 52	0.08
E/A ratio	1.14 ± 0.3	1.07 ± 0.3	1.21 ± 0.3	0.16
E/e' ratio	10.2 ± 4.3	10.9 ± 4.7	9.3 ± 3.6	0.23
PAP, mmHg	34 ± 19	32 ± 16	37 ± 21	0.42
Pressure-Volume Curve Relationships				
End-diastolic elastance, mmHg/mL	0.21 (0.17–0.28)	0.23 (0.17–0.29)	0.21 (0.16–0.24)	0.42
Arterial elastance, mmHg/mL	2.10 (1.82–2.80)	2.10 (1.78–3.01)	2.10 (1.87–2.80)	0.69
End-systolic elastance, mmHg/mL	3.79 (2.87–5.30)	4.43 (3.3–6.3)	2.94 (2.53–4.12)	<0.0001
Ventricular-arterial coupling	0.57 (0.49–0.72)	0.51 (0.45–0.53)	0.73 (0.68–0.75)	<0.0001
Stroke work, mmHg·mL	6021 (4275–8424)	6351 (4325–8991)	5346 (4252–7695)	0.38
Potential energy, mmHg·mL	1566 (1258–2413)	1532 (1194–2103)	1935 (1521–3087)	0.001
Pressure-volume area, mmHg·mL	7659 (5798–11,102)	8008 (5550–11,274)	7281 (5798–10,410)	0.86
LV efficiency, %	78 (73–80)	79 (78–81)	73 (72–74)	<0.0001

BMI, body mass index; DT, E-wave deceleration time; ET-1, endothelin 1; E/A, ratio of early transmitral diastolic flow velocity (E) and flow velocity during atrial contraction (A); HRCT, high resolution computed tomography; ILD, interstitial lung disease; IVS, interventricular septum; LV, left ventricle; LVEDD, left ventricular end-diastolic diameter; LVEDV, left ventricular end-diastolic volume; LVEF, left ventricular ejection fraction; LVESV, left ventricular end-systolic volume; PAH, pulmonary arterial hypertension; PAP, pulmonary arterial pressure; PW, posterior wall; RP, Raynaud phenomenon; RVEDD, right ventricular end-diastolic dimension; SSc, systemic sclerosis; SV, stroke volume; TAPSE, tricuspid annular plane excursion. Values are mean ± SD or median (IQR).

2.2. Echocardiography and Pressure-Volume Curve Parameters According to VAC Value

Patients in the higher VAC group (>0.63) had significantly higher LVESV ($p < 0.0001$) with reduced LVEF ($p < 0.0001$) than those with lower VAC (≤0.63). Ees was lower in patients with VAC > 0.63 ($p < 0.0001$) whereas Ea was similar in both groups (Table 1). Disease duration was longer ($p = 0.03$) and the prevalence of diffuse cutaneous SSc (dcSSc) was higher ($p = 0.03$) in patients with VAC > 0.63. Ongoing medications were comparable between the two groups.

2.3. Echocardiography and Pressure-Volume Curve Parameters in dcSSc and lcSSc Patients

Table 2 shows the differences between patients with dcSSc vs. lcSSc. In particular, LVEDV ($p = 0.004$), LVESV ($p = 0.001$), and SV ($p = 0.03$) were higher in dcSSc patients and LVEF was lower, albeit within the normal range ($p = 0.01$). Ea ($p = 0.01$) and Ees ($p = 0.001$) were lower in dcSSc patients. VAC was significantly higher in dcSSc patients ($p = 0.02$). PE was higher in dcSSc ($p = 0.01$) and LV efficiency was lower ($p = 0.02$) (Table 2). Ees correlated with Ea ($\rho = 0.851$, $p < 0.0001$). However, in dcSSc the correlation line is shifted upward and to the left. For the same Ea value, patients with dcSSc presented a lower Ees, indicative of inadequate contractility (Figure 1).

Table 2. Clinical and Echocardiographic Features in dcSSc Patients versus lcSSc Patients.

	dcSSc (n = 27)	lcSSc (n = 38)	*p* Value
Age, years	51 ± 14	59 ± 14	0.02
Female, n (%)	19 (70)	35 (92)	0.01
Body weight, Kg	60 ± 5	57 ± 2	0.52
BMI, Kg/m^2	26 ± 2	25 ± 2	0.61
Systolic blood pressure, mmHg	124 ± 22	128 ± 21	0.44
Diastolic blood pressure, mmHg	77 ± 8	72 ± 7	0.62
Hemoglobin, g/dL	13 ± 0.3	15 ± 0.1	0.58
Creatinine, mg/dL	0.98 ± 0.01	0.93 ± 0.03	0.34
Clinical features			
Disease duration, years	14 ± 7	22 ± 12	0.005
PAH, n (%)	10 (37)	12 (31)	0.25
ILD on HRCT, n (%)	12 (44)	25 (66)	0.01
Digital ulcers, n (%)	17 (62)	22 (58)	0.83
Treatment, n (%)			
Prostanoid ev	7 (26)	5 (13)	0.21
ET-1 inibithors	9 (33)	13 (34)	0.44
Immunosuppressants	8 (29)	22 (58)	0.008
Echocardiographic measurements			
LVEDD, mm	46 ± 0.6	44 ± 0.5	0.07
IVS thickness, mm	10 ± 0.2	12 ± 0.2	0.46
PW thickness, mm	10 ± 0.2	12 ± 0.3	0.83
LV mass, g	148 ± 51	166 ± 71	0.54
LVEDV, mL	101 ± 29	82 ± 21	0.004
LVESV, mL	39 ± 12	29 ± 9	0.001
SV, mL	62 ± 20	52 ± 13	0.03

Table 2. *Cont.*

	dcSSc (n = 27)	lcSSc (n = 38)	*p* Value
LVEF (%)	60 ± 6	64 ± 5	0.01
Aorta, mm	29 ± 0.4	30 ± 0.3	0.12
Left atrium, mm	48 ± 0.8	50 ± 0.9	0.50
RVEDD, cm^2	19.9 ± 5	18.3 ± 5	0.32
TAPSE, cm	2.24 ± 0.5	2.30 ± 0.5	0.65
Peak E velocity, cm/s	0.90 ± 0.2	0.84 ± 0.2	0.53
Peak A velocity, cm/s	0.81 ± 0.2	0.78 ± 0.2	0.53
DT, ms	180 ± 54	211 ± 61	0.38
E/A ratio	1.19 ± 0.3	1.11 ± 0.2	0.44
E/e' ratio	8.6 ± 2	10.7 ± 4	0.07
PAP, mmHg	32 ± 3	34 ± 3	0.75
Pressure-volume curve relationships			
End-diastolic elastance, mmHg/mL	0.17 (0.13–0.22)	0.23 (0.19–0.28)	0.03
Arterial elastance, mmHg/mL	1.83 (1.53–2.20)	2.21 (1.88–2.73)	0.01
End-systolic elastance, mmHg/mL	2.90 (2.22–3.56)	4.06 (3.12–5.49)	0.001
Ventricular-arterial coupling	0.69 (0.52–0.74)	0.52 (0.45–0.65)	0.02
Stroke work, mmHg·mL	6284 (4045–8748)	5805 (4680–8748)	0.25
Potential energy, mmHg·mL	1863 (1493–2973)	1552 (1215–2268)	0.01
Pressure-volume area, mmHg·mL	8008 (5487–11,522)	7357 (6138–11,016)	0.12
LV efficiency, %	74 (72–78)	79 (76–81)	0.02

Abbreviations as in Table 1. Values are mean ± SD or median (IQR).

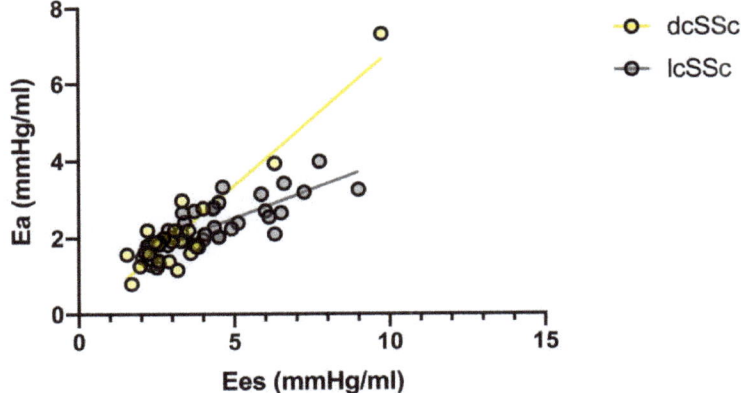

Figure 1. Scatterplot of the relationship between Ea and Ees in patients with lcSSc and patients with dcSSc. Ees correlates with Ea both in lcSSc ($\rho = 0.779$, $p < 0.0001$) and, albeit more weakly, in dcSSc ($\rho = 0.599$, $p = 0.002$).

2.4. Correlations of Pressure-Volume Curve Parameters

Unlike Ees and VAC ($\rho = -0.456$, $p < 0.0001$ and $\rho = 0.336$, $p = 0.008$, respectively), Ea did not correlate with time elapsed from SSc diagnosis ($\rho = 0.035$, $p = 0.78$). Ea positively correlated with Eed ($\rho = 0.857$, $p < 0.0001$) and systolic pulmonary arterial pressure ($\rho = 0.401$, $p = 0.002$), and inversely with TAPSE ($\rho = -0.434$, $p = 0.007$). Ees positively correlated with Eed (ρ = 0.811, $p < 0.0001$). Eed inversely correlated with TAPSE (ρ = −0.447, $p = 0.001$).

2.5. Association between VAC and Other Clinical Variables

At univariate linear regression analysis, diagnosis of dcSSc ($p = 0.009$), therapy with prostanoid ($p = 0.03$), disease duration ($p = 0.01$) and age at diagnosis ($p = 0.02$) were determinants of VAC. To further investigate the potential factors involved in VAC alterations, we performed a multivariable linear regression (stepwise) including significant factors at univariate linear regression analysis which revealed that only diagnosis of dcSSc had an independent influence on VAC (Table 3).

Table 3. Independent Effects of Clinical Variables on VAC.

	b	95% CI	p Value
dcSSc	0.342	0.020–0.184	0.01
Prostanoid ev	0.247	(−0.008)–0.154	0.07
Disease duration	0.133	(−0.002)–0.005	0.39
Age at SSc diagnosis	−0.077	(−0.004)–0.002	0.63
Corrected R^2			0.008

Note: Using multivariable linear regression analysis with stepwise method.

2.6. Factors Associated with VAC > 0.63

In univariable logistic regression VAC > 0.63 was associated with time elapsed from diagnosis ($p = 0.01$), age at SSc onset ($p = 0.04$), diagnosis of dcSSc ($p = 0.03$), and LVESV ($p = 0.002$). In multivariable logistic regression, adjusted for age and sex, VAC > 0.63 was associated with LVESV (OR 1.076; 95% CI 1.012–1.144; $p = 0.02$) and time elapsed from diagnosis (OR 1.057; 95% CI 1.008–1.127; $p = 0.04$).

2.7. Major Adverse Cardiac Events

During a 4-year median follow-up (IQR, 2–10 years), 38 patients (58.5%) developed major adverse cardiac events (MACEs). Four patients (6%) died from heart failure, 16 (24%) were hospitalized for heart failure and 18 (28%) for angina (n = 12, 67%; nine without coronary epicardial stenosis and three with epicardial coronary stenosis), or myocardial infarction (n = 6, 33%). Twelve out of 16 (75%) of the heart failure episodes were with low ejection fraction (HFrEF). No heart failure episode was of right-sided origin. There were non-cardiovascular death or events during the follow-up period.

Differences between patients with and without MACEs are shown in Table 4. Time from SSc diagnosis was longer and LVEF was lower in patients with MACEs ($p = 0.03$ and $p = 0.01$, respectively). LVESV tended to be greater in patients with MACEs ($p = 0.06$). Ea was similar in patients with and without MACEs ($p = 0.52$). Ees was lower ($p = 0.01$) and VAC was higher ($p = 0.008$) in patients with MACEs. LV efficiency was lower in patients with MACEs ($p = 0.01$). VAC was >0.63 in 23/38 (60%) patients with MACEs and in 8/27 (29%) patients without MACEs ($p = 0.01$). Figure 2 shows the cumulative survival free from MACEs according to VAC value.

Table 4. Clinical and Echocardiographic Features in Patients with and without MACEs.

	No MACEs (n = 27)	MACEs (n = 38)	p Value
Age, years	55 ± 11	56 ± 16	0.66
Female, n (%)	22 (81)	32 (84)	0.77
Body weight, Kg	58 ± 3	59 ± 2	0.81
BMI, Kg/m^2	25 ± 1	26 ± 2	0.89
Systolic blood pressure, mmHg	133 ± 19	122 ± 22	0.04
Diastolic blood pressure, mmHg	75 ± 6	73 ± 7	0.49
Hemoglobin, g/dL	14 ± 0.3	15 ± 0.4	0.68
Creatinine, mg/dL	0.95 ± 0.04	0.96 ± 0.01	0.89
Clinical features			
Disease duration, years	10 ± 1	16 ± 1	0.03
dcSSc, n (%)	9 (33)	16 (42)	0.43
PAH, n (%)	8 (30)	14 (36)	0.69
ILD on HRCT, n (%)	10 (37)	27 (71)	0.03
Digital ulcers, n (%)	16 (59)	23 (60)	0.75
Treatment, n (%)			
Prostanoid ev	6 (22)	6 (15)	0.64
ET-1 inibithors	9 (33)	13 (34)	0.44
Immunosuppressants	6 (22)	24 (63)	0.007
Echocardiographic measurements			
LVEDD, mm	43 ± 0.5	45 ± 0.5	0.13
IVS thickness, mm	10 ± 0.2	13 ± 0.2	0.18
PW thickness, mm	9 ± 0.2	12 ± 0.3	0.22
LV mass, g	143 ± 50	168 ± 66	0.17
LVEDV, mL	85 ± 24	91 ± 28	0.36
LVESV, mL	30 ± 10	35 ± 12	0.06
SV, mL	54 ± 15	55 ± 18	0.84
LVEF (%)	64 ± 5	60 ± 5	0.01
Aorta, mm	30 ± 0.3	29 ± 0.3	0.46
Left atrium, mm	52 ± 0.9	48 ± 0.8	0.13
RVEDD, cm^2	17.7 ± 3	20 ± 6	0.12
TAPSE, cm	2.35 ± 0.5	2.15 ± 0.5	0.23
Peak E velocity, cm/s	0.92 ± 0.2	0.82 ± 0.3	0.50
Peak A velocity, cm/s	0.80 ± 0.2	0.73 ± 0.2	0.41
DT, ms	189 ± 50	200 ± 55	0.36
E/A ratio	1.17 ± 0.3	1.13 ± 0.2	0.71
E/e' ratio	11 ± 4	9.2 ± 4	0.24
PAPs, mmHg	29 ± 9	37 ± 23	0.14
Pressure-volume curve relationships			
End-diastolic elastance, mmHg/mL	0.23 (0.18–0.27)	0.19 (0.16–0.24)	0.68
Arterial elastance, mmHg/mL	1.25 (1.96–2.84)	1.95 (1.69–2.45)	0.52
End-systolic elastance, mmHg/mL	4.50 (3.08–6.08)	3.30 (2.70–3.89)	0.01

Table 4. Cont.

	No MACEs (n = 27)	MACEs (n = 38)	p Value
Ventricular-arterial coupling	0.51 (0.45–0.64)	0.63 (0.53–0.72)	0.008
Stroke work, mmHg·mL	6588 (4781–8910)	5400 (4230–6705)	0.44
Potential energy, mmHg·mL	1521 (1257–2322)	1748 (1527–2252)	0.52
Pressure-volume area, mmHg·mL	8100 (6169–11,381)	7380 (5620–9459)	0.67
LV efficiency, %	79 (75–81)	75 (73–78)	0.01

Abbreviations as in Table 1. Values are mean ± SD or median (IQR).

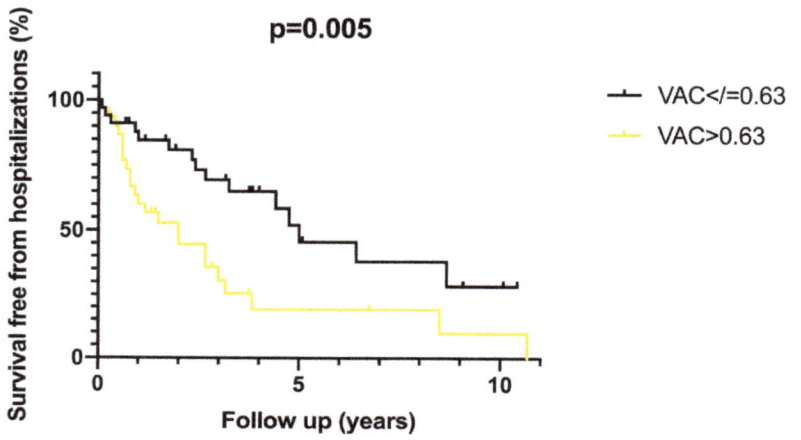

Figure 2. Kaplan Meier estimate of survival free from hospitalizations of patients with VAC ≤ 0.63 (in black), and patients with VAC > 0.63 (in yellow).

2.8. Risk Factors for MACEs in the Study Cohort

In univariable Cox regression analysis, MACEs were associated with VAC > 0.63 ($p = 0.008$), LVEF < 62% ($p = 0.02$), LV efficiency < 76% ($p = 0.02$) and disease duration ($p = 0.01$). In the final multivariable regression model, also adjusted for age, sex, pulmonary hypertension, dcSSc and interstitial lung disease, VAC > 0.63 was independently associated with MACEs (HR 2.5; 95% CI 1.13–5.7; $p = 0.01$) (Table 5). The C statistic for multivariable model increased from 0.82 to 0.92 when adding VAC > 0.63 ($p = 0.001$) (Figure 3).

Table 5. Univariate and Multivariable Predictors of MACEs.

	Univariate		Multivariable Model	
	HR (95% CI)	p Value	HR (95% CI)	p Value
Age > 60 years	1.5 (1.2–2.9)	0.20		
Female	2.0 (1.2–5.2)	0.15		
Disease duration, years	1.03 (1.006–1.06)	0.01		
Diffuse cutaneous form	1.7 (1.1–3.3)	0.13		
PAH	1.0 (0.3–3.4)	0.94		
ILD on HRCT	1.2 (0.5–2.6)	0.54		
Immunosuppressants	1.7 (0.8–3.8)	0.13		

Table 5. Cont.

	Univariate		Multivariable Model	
	HR (95% CI)	p Value	HR (95% CI)	p Value
Echocardiographic measurements				
LVEDV > 85 mL	1.0 (0.5–1.9)	0.97		
LVESV > 34 mL	1.1 (0.6–2.2)	0.61		
SV < 53 mL	1.3 (0.7–2.6)	0.31		
LVEF < 62%	2.1 (1.0–4.1)	0.02		
TAPSE < 2.1 cm	1.6 (0.6–4.3)	0.29		
E/e' ratio > 9	2.1 (0.6–6.8)	0.21		
PAP > 30 mmHg	0.8 (0.4–1.6)	0.56		
Pressure-volume curve relationships				
End-diastolic elastance > 0.21 mmHg/mL	1.0 (0.3–3.2)	0.86		
Arterial elastance > 2 mmHg/mL	0.8 (0.4–1.5)	0.56		
End-systolic elastance < 3.4 mmHg/mL	1.4 (0.7–2.8)	0.24		
Ventricular-arterial coupling > 0.63	2.4 (1.2–4.8)	0.008	2.5 (1.13–5.7)	0.01
Stroke work < 5671 mmHg·mL	1.5 (0.8–2.9)	0.19		
Potential energy > 1621 mmHg·mL	1.1 (0.6–2.2)	0.62		
Pressure-volume area < 7498 mmHg·mL	0.9 (0.4–1.7)	0.75		
LV efficiency < 76%	2.1 (1.09–4.1)	0.02		

CI. confidence interval; HR, hazard ratio; HRCT, high resolution computed tomography; ILD, interstitial lung disease; LVEDV, left ventricular end-diastolic volume; LVEF, left ventricular ejection fraction; LVESV, left ventricular end-systolic volume; MACE, major adverse cardiac events; PAH, pulmonary arterial hypertension; PAP, pulmonary arterial pressure; SV, stroke volume; TAPSE, tricuspid annular plane excursion.

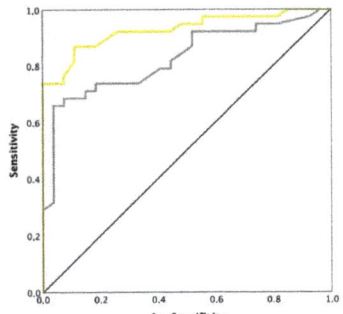

	C-statistic	CI 95%	p value*
Model 1	0.825	0.72-0.92	
Model 2 (+ VAC)	0.927	0.86-0.99	0.001

Figure 3. Receiving operating curves in model 1 and model 2 (including VAC > 0.63) for MACEs. C-statistic improves adding VAC > 0.63 in the multivariable model * p value is derived from comparison of model 1 to model 1 plus VAC > 0.63 (model 2).

2.9. Incremental Value of VAC for Predicting Adverse Cardiac Events

To assess the incremental prognostic value of VAC, global chi-square scores were calculated (Figure 4). The addition of VAC > 0.63 (global chi-square: 13.1) significantly increased the global chi-square score (19.2; $p = 0.02$).

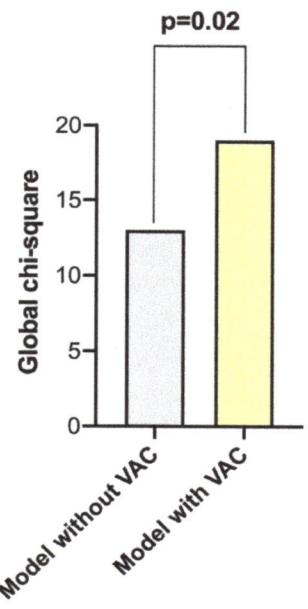

Figure 4. Incremental prognostic value of VAC > 0.63 when added to LVEF, LV efficiency, disease duration, age, sex, pulmonary hypertension, dcSSc and interstitial lung disease (Model 1).

2.10. Intra and Interobserver Reproducibility of VAC by 3D

Intraobserver reproducibility was high (r = 0.98, SEE = 0.12); the mean difference was −0.02 and the upper and lower limits of agreement between the measurements were +0.14 (95% CI, +0.08 to +0.2) and −0.19 (95% CI, −0.26 to −0.13), respectively; intraclass correlation coefficient was 0.986. Interobserver reproducibility was also high (r = 0.96, SEE =0.18); the mean difference was 0.01 and the upper and lower limits of agreement between the 2 measurements were +0.36 (95% CI, +0.26 to +0.45) and −0.33 (95% CI, −0.43 to −0.23), respectively; intraclass correlation coefficient was 0.966.

2.11. Ventricular-Arterial Coupling by 2D and 3D Echo Modalities

Table 6 presents the comparison between 2D and 3D parameters. Although Ea and VAC were similar between 2D and 3D echocardiography, Ees was lower by 3D echocardiography.

Table 6. Arterial elastance, End-systolic elastance and Ventricular-arterial coupling by 2D and 3D echocardiography (*n* = 65).

	2D Echo	3D Echo	*p* Value
Arterial elastance, mmHg/mL	2.29 (1.93–2.70)	2.04 (1.77–2.66)	0.23
End-systolic elastance, mmHg/mL	4.17 (3.38–4.97)	3.41 (2.57–4.50)	0.02
Ventricular-arterial coupling	0.57 (0.44–0.66)	0.62 (0.48–0.71)	0.15

Figure 5 presents a linear regression plot (left panel) and Bland–Altman analysis (right panel) for VAC computed by 2D- and 3D-echocardiography.

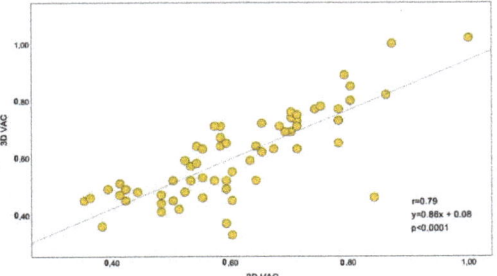 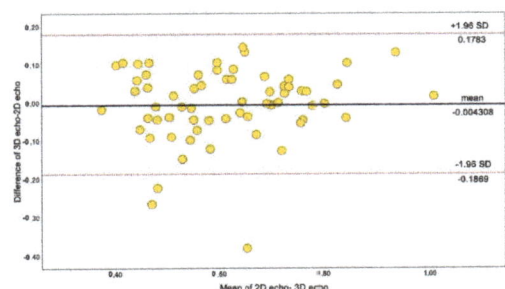

Figure 5. Linear regression (**left**) and Bland-Altman analysis (**right**) for VAC between 2D and 3D-echocardiography. Scattergram (**left** panel) showing the correrelation plot between VAC obtained by 2D- and 3D echocardiography. Plot of the difference (**right** panel) between the VAC measurements against their mean is shown. Medial line represents bias while the upper and lower red dotted lines the levels of agreement Dotted lines represent boundaries of means ± 2 SD, from −1.96 to +1.96. Relative mean error was calculated by the ratio of absolute difference of two values over their average.

3. Discussion

Standard transthoracic measurements derived from echocardiography such as end-diastolic diameter, fractional shortening, or LVEF are routinely used in clinical practice. However, these indices are load-dependent and do not systematically reflect the contractile state of the myocardium.

Our main findings indicate that: (1) VAC by 3DE may be significantly higher in dcSSc patients than in lcSSc patients, despite normal LVEF and worsen in relation to disease duration; (2) VAC by 3DE may predict major cardiovascular events in SSc.

As LV and arterial system are anatomically continuous, their interaction is a crucial determinant of cardiovascular function [14,15]. Notably, and to the best of our knowledge, this is the first study to assess LV pressure-volume relationship and VAC by 3DE in SSc. 3DE allows for a more precise evaluation of LV volumes than 2D echocardiography [12] and this is paramount for a correct assessment of VAC. Comparison with two-dimensional measurements was beyond the scope of our study. Nevertheless, in our 65 patients we found a Pearson correlation r = 0.87 between 2D and 3D echocardiography ($p = 0.0001$) (data not shown).

In our study, the traditional indices of the LV (i.e., LVEDV, LVESV and LVEF) in SSc patients were similar to that observed in controls and SV tended to be lower ($p = 0.07$) in the former. However, Ea was higher and Ees was significantly higher in SSc patients. Thus, VAC was similar in SSc patients and controls. Eed was higher in patients, indicating high filling pressure. This hemodynamic arrangement is peculiar to heart failure with preserved ejection fraction (HFpEF) [11,14], one of the typical and prognostically negative clinical manifestations of cardiac involvement in SSc. We corroborated previous reports indicating high frequencies of impaired diastolic function in SSc. A recent study conducted on a large and unselected SSc cohort showed more frequent and severe diastolic dysfunction (2016 guidelines definition) during the disease course and a high impact on mortality in SSc [16].

Many studies have reported a low prevalence of systolic dysfunction in SSc patients [3,17,18]. However, we hypothesize that conventional echocardiography may cause LV systolic dysfunction to be underestimated. Although we found no differences in the diastolic function between dcSSc and lcSSc, as previously reported [16], there appears to be significant hemodynamic differences between the two main subgroup of SSc patients with different cutaneous form. In fact, our findings point to a predominant intrinsic LV systolic dysfunction in dcSSc and LV inability to compensate higher afterload, rather than important differences in load. The higher afterload in SSc may be attributable to increased arterial stiffness from deposition of collagen and other matrix components [19]. This is supported by the higher Ea value found in our study and correlates with a worse prognosis. In fact, in the recent consensus on the role of VAC [11] the Authors highlighted that extracellular matrix and cytoskeleton regulation processes are biochemical pathways that concomitantly affect cardiac and arterial structure and function through replacement or reactive fibrosis, which typically occurs in in SSc patients. The same Authors note that the measurement of VAC may be useful for not only SSc patients but also for patients with other cardiovascular diseases [11].

The inability of the contractile function of the myocardium to adapt to the afterload is evident from our results, mostly in patients with dcSSc. Impaired contractility and ventricular-arterial uncoupling may stem from coronary microvascular dysfunction and remodeling [20]. Moreover, VAC may be associated with future risk of coronary events due to microvascular dysfunction rather than coronary epicardial atherosclerotic stenosis. Endothelial-derived nitric oxide, oxidative stress and cytokines are main regulators of myocardial microcirculation, as well as aortic vasoreactivity. Furthermore, the decreased autonomic nervous system activity in SSc individuals may result in significant impairment of LV structure, function and mechanics [21]. Finally, as above mentioned, myocardial fibrosis could also play a prominent role [1]. In this regards, the imbalance between extracellular matrix synthesis and degradation by metalloproteinases has been highlighted as a prominent mechanism underlying impaired VAC.

Pulmonary arterial hypertension (PAH) typically affects the right ventricle, whereas the presence of LV abnormalities due to PAH is very uncommon (less than 1% of patients). In this regards, some studies have demonstrated the occurrence of right ventricular-arterial uncoupling in PAH but, to the best of our knowledge, no study have investigated or demonstrated the presence of high left VAC in PAH, due to the absence of a pathophysiological rationale. Moreover, the values of PAPs in our SSc patients with PAH are quite low (mean 34 mmHg), so the possibility of an impact on the left heart is highly unlikely. In line with this rationale, our study patients with VAC > 0.63 did not shown higher rate of PAH or higher level of pulmonary pressure values. Moreover, PAH was not a determinant of VAC in our linear regression analysis. Considering all this aspects, we did not consider useful to exclude these patients, which would considerably reduce the sample size of the study and its relevance.

VAC has been recently recognized as a key determinant of cardiovascular performance and its prognostic role has been demonstrated in various conditions [11]. For the first time, we provided data on the prognostic role of VAC in SSc, thus contributing to clarify the prognostic significance of subclinical cardiac alterations detected by imaging, one of the main unresolved issues in SSc. Our findings support a possible role for VAC in stratifying SSc patients with a major cardiovascular risk. Further prospective studies on larger cohorts are warranted to corroborate our findings.

While specific therapies for SSc cardiomyopathy are still lacking, vasoactive drugs have proven effective in mitigating myocardial perfusion and function abnormalities using conventional techniques. In addition, even low-dose acetylsalicylic acid has been recently associated with a lower incidence of distinct primary myocardial disease manifestations in SSc [22,23]. In this scenario, VAC evaluation may help identify patients who would most benefit from an early and more aggressive treatment with vasodilators and acetylsalicylic acid, to prevent myocardial dysfunction and reduce future MACEs. In this regards it is worth mentioning that—according to emerging evidences—even subclinical inflammation seems play a role in SSc cardiomyopathy. Given that systemic inflammation has been recognized as another potential pathogenetic mechanisms underlying VAC, its assessment might be useful in the longitudinal evaluation of SSc patients ad it pertains the potential benefit of immunosuppressants on subclinical myocardial dysfunction in SSc, as it has been suggested for rheumatoid arthritis.

As a limitation of the study, we should mention the relatively small sample size and monocentric nature of our study. Although statistically significant differences were observed, we acknowledge that our study may be slightly underpowered. A post-hoc power analysis (assuming $\alpha = 0.05$) estimated that with 34 patients with VAC ≤ 0.63 and

31 patients with VAC > 0.63, with an event incidence of 44% in patients with VAC ≤ 0.63 and 74% in patients with VAC > 0.63, we reject the null hypothesis of equal survival with 75% power. In addition, we were not able to demonstrate the exact mechanisms underlying the subtle changes in myocardial contractility, based on other methods, such as cardiac magnetic resonance imaging. Myocardial fibrosis, which is a potential mechanism of myocardial dysfunction in SSc, was not investigated. Although we did not perform coronary angiography to exclude coronary heart disease, all patients were asymptomatic and the pre-test probability was low based on atherosclerotic risk factors, and there were no significant differences vs. controls. Moreover, we did not measure the global longitudinal strain (GLS) and therefore we do not have data of correlation between GLS and LV elastance. Therefore, because LGS is an early and well proved indicator of LV systolic dysfunction, it would be useful for identification of LV dysfunction in SSc patients.

4. Materials and Methods

4.1. Study Population

We conducted a retrospective cohort study that comprised patients attending the Rheumatology Unit of Padova University Hospital. The study population was retrieved from the database of our Echocardiography Laboratory. Overall, three hundred fifty patients underwent echocardiogram between January 2014 and March 2016 [24].

- Inclusion and Exclusion Criteria

Among the 350 patients, only those patients who were evaluated by 3DE were included (Figure 6). All patients were affected with SSc according to ACR/EULAR classification criteria [24].

Exclusion criteria were as follows: patients undergoing only 2DE (n = 250); patients (n = 35) with evidence of structural heart diseases (cardiomyopathy of any origin, significant valvular heart disease, coronary artery disease or myocardial infarction), atrial fibrillation, diabetes mellitus or systemic arterial hypertension grade II/III according to the European Society of Hypertension/European Society of Cardiology 2018 guidelines [25]; glomerular filtration rate <30 mL min^{-1} per 1.73 m^2, cancer in the past 5 years, end-stage ILD and dyslipidemia.

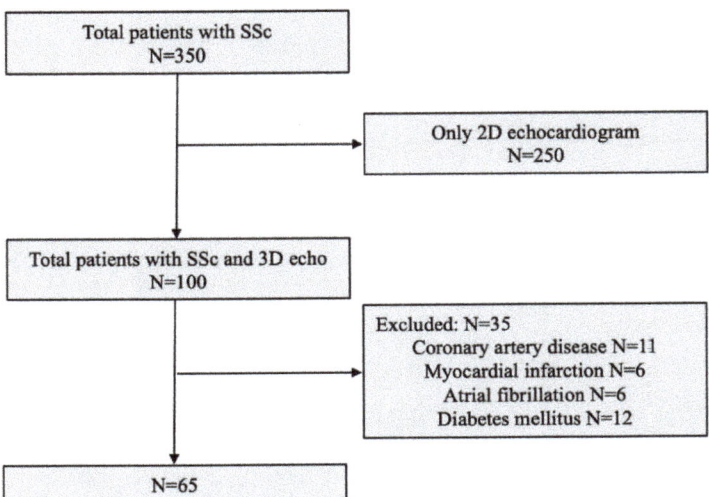

Figure 6. Study flow diagram. SSc, Sytemic Sclerosis.

Ultimately, we enrolled 65 SSc patients (54 female; age 56 ± 14 years) with no signs and symptoms of primary myocardial involvement (Figure 6), according to the available echocardiogram, and to clinical history, physical examination and ECG reported in clinical records within the previous six months.

Baseline evaluation included physical examination, gathering demographic and clinical data, and echocardiographic features (Table 1). Several disease features (e.g., cutaneous form, digital ulcers) and other organ involvement (e.g., interstitial lung disease, ILD) were recorded.

A series of 30 age- and sex-matched subjects satisfying the same exclusion criteria were evaluated by 3DE as controls. Given the retrospective nature of the study the written informed consent had been obtained by all patients at time of 3DE examination: this was a generic consensus to the acquisition of 3D images, beyond 2D standard Echocardiography.

4.2. Echocardiography

Echocardiography was performed using Vivid 7 ultrasound systems (GE Healthcare, Horten, Norway) with a 2.5-MHz transducer by 2 experienced cardiologists (F.T. and D.M.). All participants were examined with conventional 2-dimensional echocardiography and color tissue Doppler (TDI). All echocardiograms were stored on magneto-optical disks and an external FireWire hard drive (LaCie, France) and analyzed off line with commercially available software (EchoPac version 2008; GE Medical, Horten, Norway). Measurements of LV internal dimensions and LV mass index (LVMI) were performed and calculated according to European and American recommendations [26]. LV mass/body surface area ≤ 116 g/m^2 in men and ≤ 104 g/m^2 in women was considered normal. None of the patients suffered from significant valvular disease. In each subject, LVEF was measured and diastolic dysfunction was defined according to the American Society of Echocardiography criteria [27]. We considered abnormal an $E/e' > 14$, and sign of diastolic dysfunction.

Echocardiographic parameters of diastolic function including the ratio between early (E) and late (A) peak velocities of the mitral inflow, E/A, and pulsed-wave tissue Doppler velocities of the mitral annulus in early diastole in the lateral wall (e$'$) were used as surrogates of LV diastolic relaxation and compliance and the deceleration time (DT) as a surrogate of early LV stiffness, and E/e' as surrogate estimate of LV filling pressure [28]. All measures were averaged over 3 heart cycles.

4.2.1. Transthoracic Real-Time 3D Imaging

Three-dimensional echocardiography data set acquisition of the LV was performed by the same examiner at the end of the standard 2DE examination using a 3Volume matrix-array transducer (GE Healthcare). A full-volume scan was acquired using second-harmonic imaging from apical approach, and care was taken to encompass the entire LV cavity in the data set. Consecutive four- to six-beat ECG-gated subvolumes were acquired during an end-expiratory apnoea to generate the full-volume data set. The quality of the acquisition was then verified in each patient by selecting twelve-slice display mode available on the machine to ensure that the entire LV cavity is included in the 3DE full volume, and, if unsatisfactory, the data set was re-acquired. Data sets were stored digitally in raw-data format and exported to a separate workstation equipped with commercially available software for offline analysis of LV volumes and LVEF from 3DE data sets: 4D AutoLVQ™ (EchoPac 202, GE Vingmed, Horten, Norway).

4.2.2. Left Ventricular Volume Measurements

Left ventricular analysis was performed in several steps [29,30]:

(1) Automatic slicing of LV full-volume data set. The end-diastolic frames needed for contour detection were automatically displayed in quad-view: apical four-, two-chamber, long-axis views and LV short-axis plane. Each longitudinal view was color-coded and indicated on the short-axis image at 60° between each plane. Both

reference frames in the end-systole and end-diastole could be also manually selected, if necessary.

(2) Alignment. Rapid manual alignment by pivoting and translating the four-chamber plane was first performed in order that the corresponding intersection line of all planes was placed in the middle of the LV cavity, crossing the LV apex and the center of mitral valve opening in each view. Aligning one plane automatically changed the others. Once LV central longitudinal axis was identified, accurate orientation of LV views was ensured by manual refinement of the angles between the LV planes on the LV short-axis view, in order to correspond to the defining anatomical landmarks of each view.

(3) Left ventricular reference point identification. To subsequently identify a fitting geometric model, the software required manual input of only two single points in any of the three LV apical planes (on points on mitral annulus, and one at the apex) first in end-diastolic frames, and then for corresponding end-systolic frames.

(4) Automated identification of endocardial border. The software automatically detected LV cavity endocardial border in 3D and provided the measured end-diastolic volume (LVEDV). Three additional short-axis views at different levels were displayed in order to facilitate verification of the accuracy of endocardial surface detection both in cross-section and in long-axis by rotating and translating active view plane. At this stage, LV borders could be manually adjusted, if unsatisfactory, by (dis)placing as many additional points as needed (manually corrected AutoLVQ), with secondary immediate automated refinement of boundary detection accordingly. This could be done on each of the six simultaneously displayed LV views, but also possible in between reference planes for LV with distorted shape. After completing steps 1–4 for end-diastolic views, only 3–4 sequence was required for end-systolic frames, since adjustments done in steps 1–2 were automatically carried out subsequently in end-systolic views.

(5) Final quantitative analysis and data display. Using the initial contours in both end-systole and end-diastole, a corresponding dynamic surface-rendered LV cast was derived. Final data panel automatically displayed LVEDV, LVESV, LVEF, SV, cardiac output, and heart rate values. A volume–time plot was also provided.

The intra- and inter-observer reproducibility for systolic function parameters in 20 randomly selected patients were good. Concordance between two raters using the Kappa statistic was 0.95 ($p < 0.0001$).

4.2.3. Variables Derived from Left Ventricular Pressure-Volume Relations

To noninvasively quantify ventricular contractility, we calculated Ees as end-systolic pressure (ESP) divided by LVESV. LVEDV is an index of LV size and quantifies the degree of cardiac remodeling. The end-systolic pressure volume relationship (ESPVR) provides a load-independent measure of contractile function. The ESPVR is typically assumed to be linear and is therefore defined by a slope and an intercept. Although many studies focus on the slope alone, both the slope (end-systolic elastance [Ees]) and the intercept (V_0) are required to describe the contractile state of the left ventricle. Ees quantifies ventricular elastance (stiffness) at end-systole, and V_0 is a measure of ventricular volume at a theoretical end systolic pressure of 0 mm Hg. Because V_0 is an extrapolated value obtained at a non-physiological pressure, the LVESV at a systolic pressure of 100 mm Hg (V_{100}) is also often described. For arterial load, Ea was the ratio of ESP to stroke volume (SV), and VAC was defined as the ratio of Ea to Ees. For these equations, LVESV and SV were obtained from 3DE results. ESP was defined as 0.9 x systolic blood pressure determined by noninvasive blood pressure measurement at the same time as 3DE. As recommended by the ESC guidelines on hypertension, patients were seated comfortably in a quiet environment for 5 min before beginning blood pressure measurements. Three blood pressure measurements were recorded, 1–2 min apart, and additional measurements only if the first two readings differed by >10 mmHg. We used a standard bladder cuff (12–13 cm wide and 35 cm long) for all patients and controls. End-diastolic elastance (Eed) was the ratio of left ventricular end-diastolic pressure (EDP) to LVEDV. We estimated EDP with a formula using the E/e' ratio (11.96 + 0.596 E/e') [31].We estimated mechanical energy including SW, PE, PVA, and LV mechanical efficiency [32]. (Figure 7).

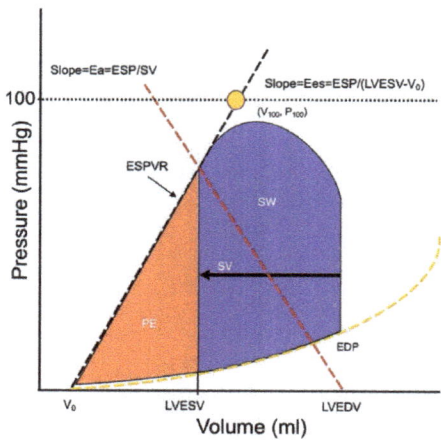

Figure 7. Pressure-volume loops of the left ventricle (**left**). Measurement of parameters derived from a pressure-volume loop of the left ventricle (**right**). End-systolic elastance (Ees) represents the slope of the end-systolic pressure volume relationship (ESPVR) where ESP denotes end-systolic pressure, and Ees represents the noninvasively derived single-beat estimation of this parameter. LVEDV is the end-diastolic volume, and LVESV is the end-systolic volume. V0 is the intercept of the ESPVR at an end-systolic pressure of 0 mm Hg, and V100 is the point on the end-systolic pressure volume line at an end-systolic pressure of 100 mm Hg. Effective arterial elastance (Ea) represents the negative slope joining the end-systolic pressure volume point to the point on the volume axis at end-diastole, where SV represents stroke volume.

4.3. Primary Study Endpoint: Major Adverse Cardiovascular Events (MACEs) during Follow-up

The primary study endpoint was a composite endpoint of MACEs during follow-up. MACEs were defined by the occurrence of death for heart failure or hospitalization from CV causes (i.e., angina, myocardial infarction or heart failure). Angina and myocardial infarctions were defined according to ESC guidelines [33,34]. Two physicians (E.Z. and E.B.) blinded to 3DE findings reviewed all the medical records of included patients, regularly follow-up every 6 months—as per usual protocol at our Rheumatology Unit. In addition, further information were also obtained by evaluating hospital discharge cards and the personal status (i.e., alive/dead) that is recorded in the medical information system of our region.

4.4. Statistical Analysis

Continuous variables with no/mild skew were presented as mean ± SD; skewed measures were represented as median with first and third quartiles (Q1-Q3). Discrete variables were summarized as frequencies and percentages. The distribution of the data was analysed with a 1-sample Kolmogorov-Smirnov test. Categorical variables were compared by the χ^2 test or the Fisher exact test as appropriate. Continuous data were compared using the 2-tailed unpaired t test (for normally distributed data sets) or the Mann-Whitney U test (for skewed variables). Time-dependent receiver operating characteristic curves were used to determine the optimal cutoffs for the primary composite endpoint based on the Youden index. Bivariate correlations were assessed by the Spearman coefficient (ρ). In unadjusted and multivariable-adjusted linear regression analyses, we expressed association between VAC and other clinical variables. Logistic regressions with odds ratios (ORs) and 95% confidence intervals (CIs) were applied to investigate associations between

VAC > 0.63 and clinical characteristics. Event rates are plotted in Kaplan-Meier curves for the primary composite end point and cardiovascular death, and groups were compared using the log-rank test. Univariate and multivariable Cox proportional hazards models were performed to identify the independent determinants of the primary composite end point. Variables with $p < 0.05$ at univariate analysis were included as covariables in multivariable models. Multivariable analyses were performed using a backward-conditional selection procedure on the remaining variables demonstrated a p value < 0.05. Pulmonary hypertension, dcSSc and interstitial lung disease, which have proven important in systemic sclerosis, were forced into the multivariable models, because model's adjustments should take into account factors with well-established clinical relevance. Moreover, VAC was introduced separately in the multivariable analysis to compare incremental value in predicting outcome. To assess the incremental value of VAC in addition to other risk factors for predicting adverse events, we calculated the improvement in global χ^2 value. Multivariable Cox models were discriminated by the C-index (values > 0.7 were deemed acceptable). The agreement between 2D-or 3D-echocardiography was tested by the Bland-Altman method and by the concordance correlation coefficient comparing the mean differences between the two methods of measurements and 95% limits of agreement as the mean difference. Intraobserver and interobserver reproducibilities of VAC were evaluated by linear regression analysis and expressed as correlation of coefficients (r) and standard error of estimates (SEE), and by the intraclass correlation coefficient. Reproducibility is considered satisfactory if the intraclass correlation coefficient is between 0.81 and 1.0. Intraobserver and interobserver reproducibility measurements were calculated in all 65 patients. All tests were two-sided and statistical significance was accepted if the null hypothesis could be rejected at $p < 0.05$. Data were analyzed with SPSS software version 24.0 (SPSS, Inc., Chicago, IL, USA). The study was approved by the institutional ethics committee.

5. Conclusions

In conclusion, our results may help better identify primary cardiac involvement in SSc. We provided the first evidence that VAC may be impaired in SSc and, importantly, that it seems to play a prognostic role in these patients. Our results also suggest that patients with dcSSc present an intrinsic LV systolic dysfunction, which seems to worsen over time and is responsible for the LV inability to compensate higher afterload. Further prospective studies are warranted to ascertain whether early intervention can improve outcomes in patients with "abnormal" VAC.

Author Contributions: Conceptualization, F.T. and E.Z.; data curation, F.T. and R.M.; investigation, D.M., E.B., E.D.Z., F.B., G.C.; resources, F.C.; supervision, S.I. and A.D. All authors have read and agreed to the published version of the manuscript.

Funding: This research received no external funding.

Institutional Review Board Statement: The study was conducted according to the guidelines of the Declaration of Helsinki, and approved by the Institutional Review Board (or Ethics Committee) of AOU of Padova (protocol number 3487/AO/15—13/7/2015 updated number 4895/AT/20—23/7/2020).

Informed Consent Statement: Informed consent was obtained from all subjects involved in the study.

Data Availability Statement: The data sets used and/or analyzed during the current study are available from the corresponding author on reasonable request.

Conflicts of Interest: The authors declare no conflict of interest and have no known competing financial interests or personal relationships that may have influenced the work reported in this paper.

References

1. Denton, C.P.; Khanna, D. Systemic sclerosis. *Lancet* **2017**, *390*, 1685–1699. [CrossRef]
2. Zanatta, E.; Famoso, G.; Boscain, F.; Montisci, R.; Pigatto, E.; Polito, P.; Schiavon, F.; Iliceto, S.; Cozzi, F.; Doria, A.; et al. Nailfold avascular score and coronary microvascular dysfunction in systemic sclerosis: A newsworthy association. *Autoimmun. Rev.* **2019**, *18*, 177–183. [CrossRef]
3. Bissell, L.-A.; Yusof, Y.M.; Buch, M. Primary myocardial disease in scleroderma—A comprehensive review of the literature to inform the UK Systemic Sclerosis Study Group cardiac working group. *Rheumatology* **2016**, *56*, 882–895. [CrossRef] [PubMed]
4. Zanatta, E.; Colombo, C.; D'Amico, G.; D'Humières, T.; Lin, C.D.; Tona, F. Inflammation and Coronary Microvascular Dysfunction in Autoimmune Rheumatic Diseases. *Int. J. Mol. Sci.* **2019**, *20*, 5563. [CrossRef] [PubMed]
5. Rangarajan, V.; Matiasz, R.; Freed, B.H. Cardiac complications of systemic sclerosis and management: Recent progress. *Curr. Opin. Rheumatol.* **2017**, *29*, 574–584. [CrossRef] [PubMed]
6. Zanatta, E.; Polito, P.; Famoso, G.; LaRosa, M.; De Zorzi, E.; Scarpieri, E.; Cozzi, F.; Doria, A. Pulmonary arterial hypertension in connective tissue disorders: Pathophysiology and treatment. *Exp. Biol. Med.* **2019**, *244*, 120–131. [CrossRef] [PubMed]
7. Park, J.J.; Park, J.-B.; Park, J.-H.; Cho, G.-Y. Global Longitudinal Strain to Predict Mortality in Patients with Acute Heart Failure. *J. Am. Coll. Cardiol.* **2018**, *71*, 1947–1957. [CrossRef]
8. Asanoi, H.; Sasayama, S.; Kameyama, T. Ventriculoarterial coupling in normal and failing heart in humans. *Circ. Res.* **1989**, *65*, 483–493. [CrossRef]
9. Ky, B.; French, B.; Khan, A.M.; Plappert, T.; Wang, A.; Chirinos, J.A.; Fang, J.C.; Sweitzer, N.K.; Borlaug, B.A.; Kass, D.A.; et al. Ventricular-Arterial Coupling, Remodeling, and Prognosis in Chronic Heart Failure. *J. Am. Coll. Cardiol.* **2013**, *62*, 1165–1172. [CrossRef]
10. Milewska, A.; Minczykowski, A.; Krauze, T.; Piskorski, J.; Heathers, J.; Szczepanik, A.; Banaszak, A.; Guzik, P.; Wykretowicz, A. Prognosis after acute coronary syndrome in relation with ventricular–arterial coupling and left ventricular strain. *Int. J. Cardiol.* **2016**, *220*, 343–348. [CrossRef]
11. Ikonomidis, I.; Aboyans, V.; Blacher, J.; Brodmann, M.; Brutsaert, D.L.; Chirinos, J.A.; De Carlo, M.; Delgado, V.; Lancellotti, P.; Lekakis, J.; et al. The role of ventricular–arterial coupling in cardiac disease and heart failure: Assessment, clinical implications and therapeutic interventions. A consensus document of the European Society of Cardiology Working Group on Aorta & Peripheral Vascular Diseases, European Association of Cardiovascular Imaging, and Heart Failure Association. *Eur. J. Heart Fail.* **2019**, *21*, 402–424. [CrossRef]
12. Dorosz, J.L.; Lezotte, D.C.; Weitzenkamp, D.A.; Allen, L.A.; Salcedo, E.E. Performance of 3-Dimensional Echocardiography in Measuring Left Ventricular Volumes and Ejection Fraction: A systematic review and meta-analysis. *J. Am. Coll. Cardiol.* **2012**, *59*, 1799–1808. [CrossRef] [PubMed]
13. Gayat, E.; Mor-Avi, V.; Weinert, L.; Yodwut, C.; Lang, R.M. Noninvasive quantification of left ventricular elastance and ventricular-arterial coupling using three-dimensional echocardiography and arterial tonometry. *Am. J. Physiol. Heart Circ. Physiol.* **2011**, *301*, H1916–H1923. [CrossRef] [PubMed]
14. Chirinos, J.A. Ventricular–arterial coupling: Invasive and non-invasive assessment. *Artery Res.* **2013**, *7*, 2–14. [CrossRef]
15. Sunagawa, K.; Maughan, W.L.; Burkhoff, D. Left ventricular interaction with arterial load studied in isolated canine ventricle. *Am. J. Physiol.* **1983**, *245 Pt 1*, H773–H780. [CrossRef]
16. Tennøe, A.H.; Murbræch, K.; Andreassen, J.C.; Fretheim, H.; Garen, T.; Gude, E.; Andreassen, A.; Aakhus, S.; Molberg, Ø; Hoffmann-Vold, A.-M. Left Ventricular Diastolic Dysfunction Predicts Mortality in Patients With Systemic Sclerosis. *J. Am. Coll. Cardiol.* **2018**, *72*, 1804–1813. [CrossRef]
17. Hinchcliff, M.; Desai, C.S.; Varga, J.; Shah, S.J. Prevalence, prognosis, and factors associated with left ventricular diastolic dysfunction in systemic sclerosis. *Clin. Exp. Rheumatol.* **2012**, *30* (Suppl. 71), S30–S37. [PubMed]
18. Butt, S.A.; Jeppesen, J.L.; Torp-Pedersen, C.; Sam, F.; Gislason, G.; Jacobsen, S.; Andersson, C. Cardiovascular Manifestations of Systemic Sclerosis: A Danish Nationwide Cohort Study. *J. Am. Heart Assoc.* **2019**, *8*, e013405. [CrossRef] [PubMed]
19. Constans, J.; Germain, C.; Gosse, P.; Taillard, J.; Tiev, K.; Delevaux, I.; Mouthon, L.; Schmidt, C.; Granel, F.; Soria, P.; et al. Arterial stiffness predicts severe progression in systemic sclerosis: The ERAMS study. *J. Hypertens.* **2007**, *25*, 1900–1906. [CrossRef] [PubMed]
20. Faccini, A.; Kaski, J.C.; Camici, P.G. Coronary microvascular dysfunction in chronic inflammatory rheumatoid diseases. *Eur. Heart J.* **2016**, *37*, 1799–1806. [CrossRef]
21. Di Franco, M.; Paradiso, M.; Riccieri, V.; Basili, S.; Mammarella, A.; Valesini, G. Autonomic dysfunction and microvascular damage in systemic sclerosis. *Clin. Rheumatol.* **2007**, *26*, 1278–1283. [CrossRef] [PubMed]
22. Valentini, G.; Huscher, D.; Riccardi, A.; Fasano, S.; Irace, R.; Messiniti, V.; Matucci-Cerinic, M.; Guiducci, S.; Distler, O.; Maurer, B.; et al. Vasodilators and low-dose acetylsalicylic acid are associated with a lower incidence of distinct primary myocardial disease manifestations in systemic sclerosis: Results of the DeSScipher inception cohort study. *Ann. Rheum. Dis.* **2019**, *78*, 1576–1582. [CrossRef] [PubMed]
23. Zanatta, E.; Codullo, V.; Avouac, J.; Allanore, Y. Systemic sclerosis: Recent insight in clinical management. *Jt. Bone Spine* **2020**, *87*, 293–299. [CrossRef]

24. Van Den Hoogen, F.; Khanna, D.; Fransen, J.; Johnson, S.R.; Baron, M.; Tyndall, A.; Matucci-Cerinic, M.; Naden, R.P.; Medsger, T.A., Jr.; Carreira, P.E.; et al. 2013 Classification Criteria for Systemic Sclerosis: An American College of Rheumatology/European League Against Rheumatism Collaborative Initiative. *Arthritis Rheum.* **2013**, *65*, 2737–2747. [CrossRef]
25. Williams, B.; Mancia, G.; Spiering, W.; Rosei, E.A.; Azizi, M.; Burnier, M.; Clement, D.; Coca, A.; De Simone, G.; Dominiczak, A.; et al. 2018 Practice Guidelines for the management of arterial hypertension of the European Society of Cardiology and the European Society of Hypertension ESC/ESH Task Force for the Management of Arterial Hypertension. *J. Hypertens.* **2018**, *36*, 2284–2309. [CrossRef]
26. Devereux, R.B.; Alonso, D.R.; Lutas, E.M.; Gottlieb, G.J.; Campo, E.; Sachs, I.; Reichek, N. Echocardiographic assessment of left ventricular hypertrophy: Comparison to necropsy findings. *Am. J. Cardiol.* **1986**, *57*, 450–458. [CrossRef]
27. Galderisi, M.; Cosyns, B.; Edvardsen, T.; Cardim, N.; Delgado, V.; Di Salvo, G.; Donal, E.; Sade, L.E.; Ernande, L.; Garbi, M.; et al. Reviewers: This document was reviewed by members of the 2016–2018 EACVI Scientific Documents Committee. Standardization of adult transthoracic echocardiography reporting in agreement with recent chamber quantification, diastolic function, and heart valve disease recommendations: An expert consensus document of the European Association of Cardiovascular Imaging. *Eur. Heart J. Cardiovasc. Imaging* **2017**, *18*, 1301–1310. [CrossRef]
28. Nagueh, S.F.; Appleton, C.P.; Gillebert, T.; Marino, P.; Oh, J.K.; Smiseth, O.A.; Waggoner, A.D.; Flachskampf, F.A.; Pellikka, P.A.; Evangelisa, A. Recommendations for the Evaluation of Left Ventricular Diastolic Function by Echocardiography. *Eur. Heart J. Cardiovasc. Imaging* **2008**, *10*, 165–193. [CrossRef]
29. Muraru, D.; Badano, L.; Piccoli, G.; Gianfagna, P.; Del Mestre, L.; Ermacora, D.; Proclemer, A. Validation of a novel automated border-detection algorithm for rapid and accurate quantitation of left ventricular volumes based on three-dimensional echocardiography. *Eur. Hear. J. Cardiovasc. Imaging* **2010**, *11*, 359–368. [CrossRef] [PubMed]
30. Muraru, D.; Badano, L.; Peluso, D.; Bianco, L.D.; Casablanca, S.; Kocabay, G.; Zoppellaro, G.; Iliceto, S. Comprehensive Analysis of Left Ventricular Geometry and Function by Three-Dimensional Echocardiography in Healthy Adults. *J. Am. Soc. Echocardiogr.* **2013**, *26*, 618–628. [CrossRef]
31. Ommen, S.R.; Nishimura, R.A.; Appleton, C.P.; Miller, F.A.; Oh, J.K.; Redfield, M.M.; Tajik, A.J. Clinical utility of Doppler echocardi-ography and tissue Doppler imaging in the estimation of left ventricular filling pressures. A comparative simultaneous Doppler-catheterization study. *Circulation* **2000**, *102*, 1788–1794. [CrossRef]
32. Chantler, P.D.; Lakatta, E.; Najjar, S.S. Arterial-ventricular coupling: Mechanistic insights into cardiovascular performance at rest and during exercise. *J. Appl. Physiol.* **2008**, *105*, 1342–1351. [CrossRef]
33. Thygesen, K.; Alpert, J.S.; Jaffe, A.S.; Chaitman, B.R.; Bax, J.J.; Morrow, D.A.; White, H.D.; ESC Scientific Document Group. Fourth universal definition of myocardial infarction. *Eur. Heart J.* **2019**, *40*, 237–269. [CrossRef]
34. Roffi, M.; Patrono, C.; Collet, J.-P.; Mueller, C.; Valgimigli, M.; Andreotti, F.; Bax, J.J.; Borger, M.; Brotons, C.; Chew, D.P.; et al. 2015 ESC Guidelines for the management of acute coronary syndromes in patients presenting without persistent ST-segment elevation. *Eur. Heart J.* **2015**, *37*, 267–315. [CrossRef]

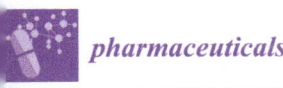

Article

The Effect of Transcutaneous Vagus Nerve Stimulation in Patients with Polymyalgia Rheumatica

Jacob Venborg [1], Anne-Marie Wegeberg [2], Salome Kristensen [3,4], Birgitte Brock [5], Christina Brock [2,3] and Mogens Pfeiffer-Jensen [1,6,7,*]

1. Department of Rheumatology, Aarhus University Hospital, 8200 Aarhus, Denmark; jacob.venborg@clin.au.dk
2. Mech-Sense, Department of Gastroenterology and Hepatology, Aalborg University Hospital, 9000 Aalborg, Denmark; a.wegeberg@rn.dk (A.-M.W.); christina.brock@rn.dk (C.B.)
3. Department of Rheumatology, Aalborg University Hospital, 9000 Aalborg, Denmark; sakr@rn.dk
4. Department of Clinical Medicine, Aalborg University, 9000 Aalborg, Denmark
5. Steno Diabetes Center Copenhagen, 2820 Gentofte, Denmark; birgitte.brock@regionh.dk
6. Department of Clinical Medicine, Faculty of Health Sciences, University of Copenhagen, 2200 Copenhagen, Denmark
7. Copenhagen Center for Arthritis Research (COPECARE), Center for Rheumatology and Spine Diseases, Rigshospitalet, 2600 Glostrup, Denmark
* Correspondence: mogenspfeiffer@dadlnet.dk

Abstract: (1) Polymyalgia rheumatica (PMR) is an inflammatory disease characterised by pain, morning stiffness, and reduced quality of life. Recently, vagus nerve stimulation (VNS) was shown to have anti-inflammatory effects. We aimed to examine the effect of transcutaneous VNS (t-VNS) on PMR. (2) Fifteen treatment-naïve PMR patients completed the study. Patients underwent a 5-day protocol, receiving 2 min of t-VNS stimulation bilaterally on the neck, three times daily. Cardiac vagal tone (CVT) measured on a linear vagal scale (LVS), blood pressure, heart rate, patient-reported outcome, and biochemical changes were assessed. (3) t-VNS induced a 22% increase in CVT at 20 min after initial stimulations compared with baseline (3.4 ± 2.2 LVS vs. 4.1 ± 2.9 LVS, $p = 0.02$) and was accompanied by a 4 BPM reduction in heart rate (73 ± 11 BPM vs. 69 ± 9, $p < 0.01$). No long-term effects were observed. Furthermore, t-VNS induced a 14% reduction in the VAS score for the hips at day 5 compared with the baseline (5.1 ± 2.8 vs. 4.4 ± 2.8, $p = 0.04$). No changes in CRP or proinflammatory analytes were observed. (4) t-VNS modulates the autonomic nervous system in patients with PMR, but further investigation of t-VNS in PMR patients is warranted.

Keywords: polymyalgia rheumatica; vagus nerve stimulation; inflammatory response; PMR; t-vns

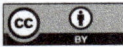

1. Introduction

Polymyalgia rheumatica (PMR) is an inflammatory rheumatic disease of unknown aetiology characterised by muscle pain and morning stiffness in the shoulders, pelvic girdle, and neck. PMR is rarely seen in persons below the age of 50, and can occur independently or alongside giant cell arteritis [1,2]. Typically, PMR will "burn out" after approximately 2 years and it is not associated with increased mortality [3–5]. Nevertheless, ordinary daily activities become immensely difficult and painful to accomplish, consequently, PMR patients often describe a great decline in quality of life. Finally, the disease is associated with increased usage of primary healthcare [6], and thus effective treatment restoring quality of life is of paramount importance to patients with PMR and their families. The first-choice treatment is systemically administered low doses (initially 12.5–25 mg/day) corticosteroids [7]. Although this treatment provides quick and efficient recovery, the adverse effects are typically numerous and severe [8]. Among these, osteoporosis, skin thinning, cushingoid appearance, weight gain, myopathy, and mood disorders are common [9]; as such, effective treatments with less negative and unwanted side effects are warranted. Biological anti-inflammatory drugs are frequently used within rheumatology. Recent studies have demonstrated that PMR patients had increased serum levels of interleukin 6 (IL-6) in comparison with healthy controls, suggesting that IL-6 was part of the pathogenesis of PMR [10,11]. This is supported by the efficient use of monotherapy with IL-6 inhibitors in PMR patients [12–15]. However, treatment with biological drugs is still associated with side effects, such as the increased risk of infection, fever, and rash.

It is generally accepted that the autonomic nervous system regulates neuro-immune communication primarily through the vagal nerve. In vitro studies have shown the inhibition of macrophage cytokine release in lipopolysaccharide-stimulated human macrophage cultures enriched with the cholinergic neurotransmitter acetylcholine [16]. Moreover direct electrical stimulation of the vagus nerve in rats diminished serum levels of tumour necrosis factor-alpha (TNF-α) [17]. Vagal nerve stimulation (VNS) is also believed to diminish levels of pro-inflammatory cytokines, such as IL-1 and IL-6, the latter of which is of great interest in PMR patients [18]. In studies of healthy humans, transcutaneous vagus nerve stimulation (t-VNS) was shown to modulate the inflammatory response by increasing the cardiac vagal tone (CVT) and decreasing the systemic level of TNF-α [16,19]. Finally, t-VNS has reduced disease activity scores in patients with well-controlled psoriatic arthritis (PsA) and rheumatoid arthritis (RA) with no reported adverse effects [20,21]. However, a knowledge gap remains, as no studies have previously investigated the effect of t-VNS as an exclusive treatment in treatment-naïve patients with diseases characterised by high-grade inflammation.

Thus, we aimed to investigate the effect of 5-day t-VNS in treatment-naïve patients with PMR. We hypothesised that t-VNS would increase CVT and consequently reduce the inflammatory response, leading to clinical improvement in patients with PMR. Thus, the aims of this proof-of-concept study were to assess (1) the acute and 5-day CVT response to t-VNS; (2) the effect of 5-day t-VNS on cardiac-derived parameters, such as blood pressure (BP) and heart rate (HR); (3) the effect of t-VNS on inflammatory biomarkers; and (4) patient-reported inflammatory pain.

2. Results

Fifteen of the twenty enrolled patients completed the study. The baseline characteristics of the population are shown in Table 1. The intention-to-treat approach was used, and due to the investigation of various parameters, some datapoints may be missing in a subgroup of patients either because they were extreme values or because the assays were performed incorrectly. Consequently, such values were excluded from further analyses. No adverse events were reported. On average, each patient received 24 stimulations, which means they received fewer than planned (26).

Table 1. Demographic and General Population Characteristics.

Characteristic	PMR Patients (n = 15)
Sex (female)	13 (87)
Age (years)	65 ± 10
Height (cm)	169 ± 6
Weight (kg)	72 ± 12
Body mass index (kg/m^2)	25 ± 4
Currently using NSAIDs (yes)	6 (40.0)
Daily NSAID dose (mg ibuprofen)	833 ± 480
Ethnicity (Caucasian)	15 (100.0)
Smoking, ever (yes)	7 (47)
Smoking (pack-years)	16 ± 12
Daily caffeine intake (yes)	15 (100)
Stimulations pr. patient (mean out of 26)	24 (91)
Amplitude of baseline stimulation	33 ± 6

Data are given as mean ± SD or no. (%) unless stated otherwise.

2.1. Changes in Primary Outcome: Cardiac Vagal Tone

One patient had faulty CVT recordings at all visits; consequently, these measurements were excluded. Another patient showed an extreme value of CVT on day 2; thus, this single measurement was excluded. Only measurements of CVT were excluded; the other parameters were not.

An acute 22% increase in CVT was observed 20 min after the initial t-VNS (3.4 ± 2.2 LVS vs. 4.1 ± 2.9 LVS, $p = 0.02$). However, no changes in CVT were observed on day 2 (3.4 ± 2.2 LVS vs. 3.9 ± 2.7 LVS, $p = 0.50$) nor on day 5 (3.4 ± 2.2 LVS vs. 4.2 ± 2.9, $p = 0.20$). The results are shown in Table 2.

Table 2. Changes in Outcomes.

	Baseline	20 min	24 h	Day 5	p-Value
Cardiac vagal tone (LVS)	3.4 ± 2.2	4.1 ± 2.9	3.9 ± 2.7	4.2 ± 2.9	0.02 *
Systolic blood pressure (mmHG)	139 ± 22	141 ± 22	135 ± 19	137 ± 24	0.38
Diastolic blood pressure (mmHG)	79 ± 10	81 ± 10	77 ± 8	82 ± 15	0.53
Heart rate (BPM)	73 ± 11	69 ± 9	74 ± 11	70 ± 14	0.01 *
MHAQ score	0.9 ± 0.5	-	0.9 ± 0.5	0.8 ± 0.5	0.19
VAS score of PMR-influence	6.7 ± 2.6	-	6.4 ± 2.6	6.1 ± 2.5	0.23
VAS score in hips	5.1 ± 2.8	-	5.0 ± 3.1	4.4 ± 2.8	0.04
Global VAS score	6.2 ± 2.8	-	6.1 ± 2.7	5.9 ± 2.5	0.54
Duration of morning stiffness (minutes)	124 ± 89	-	120 ± 79	108 ± 65	0.19
C-reactive protein (mg/L)	32.3 ± 19.7	-	32.4 ± 19.3	35.9 ± 24.6	0.74
IFN-γ (pg/mL)	5.40 ± 2.67	-	-	6.20 ± 5.94	0.29
IL-2 (pg/mL)	0.06 (0.10)	-	-	0.12 (0.24)	0.06
IL-4 (pg/mL)	0.01 ± 0.01	-	-	0.03 ± 0.03	0.82
IL-6 (ng/L)	4.81 (4.80)	-	-	4.50 (6.25)	0.19
IL-8 (pg/mL)	12.72 ± 6.58	-	-	12.68 ± 6.90	0.37
IL-10 (pg/mL)	0.27 (0.14)	-	-	0.32 (0.12)	0.91
TNF-α (pg/mL)	1.35 ± 0.43	-	-	1.32 ± 0.44	0.67

Data are given as mean $\pm$ SD or median (interquartile range) unless otherwise stated. The p-values are a comparison between baseline and day 5. * Comparison between baseline and 20 min

2.2. Changes in Secondary Outcomes

2.2.1. Changes in Cardiac-Derived Parameters

An acute decrease of 4 BPM in resting HR was observed 20 min after initial t-VNS (73 ± 11 BPM vs. 69 ± 9, $p < 0.01$). No changes in resting HR were observed on day 2 (73 ± 11 BPM vs. 74 ± 11 BPM, $p = 0.77$) or on day 5 (73 ± 11 BPM vs. 70 ± 14, $p = 0.27$). No changes in systolic or diastolic BP were observed 20 min after initial t-VNS, on day 2, or on day 5. The results are shown in Table 2 and Figure 1.

2.2.2. Changes in CRP and Proinflammatory Analytes

Two patients were diagnosed obs. pro PMR but had no concomitant increase in markers of CRP; consequently, they were excluded from the analysis of changes in CRP. Furthermore, a single patient showed extreme values for CRP due to an infection and was excluded for analysis.

No changes in CRP were observed in response to t-VNS on day 2 (32.3 ± 19.7 mg/L vs. 32.4 ± 19.3, $p = 0.94$) or on day 5 (32.3 ± 19.7 mg/L vs. 35.9 ± 24.6 mg/L, $p = 0.33$) in comparison with the baseline. The results are shown in Table 2 and Figure 1. No changes were observed in any of the investigated analytes.

2.2.3. Changes in Patient-Reported Outcome

A 14% reduction in the VAS score for the hips was shown on day 5 in comparison with baseline (5.1 ± 2.8 vs. 4.4 ± 2.8, $p < 0.05$). No significant changes were observed in MHAQ scores, VAS score of PMR influence, global VAS score, or duration of morning stiffness on day 2 or on day 5. The results are shown in Table 2 and Figure 1.

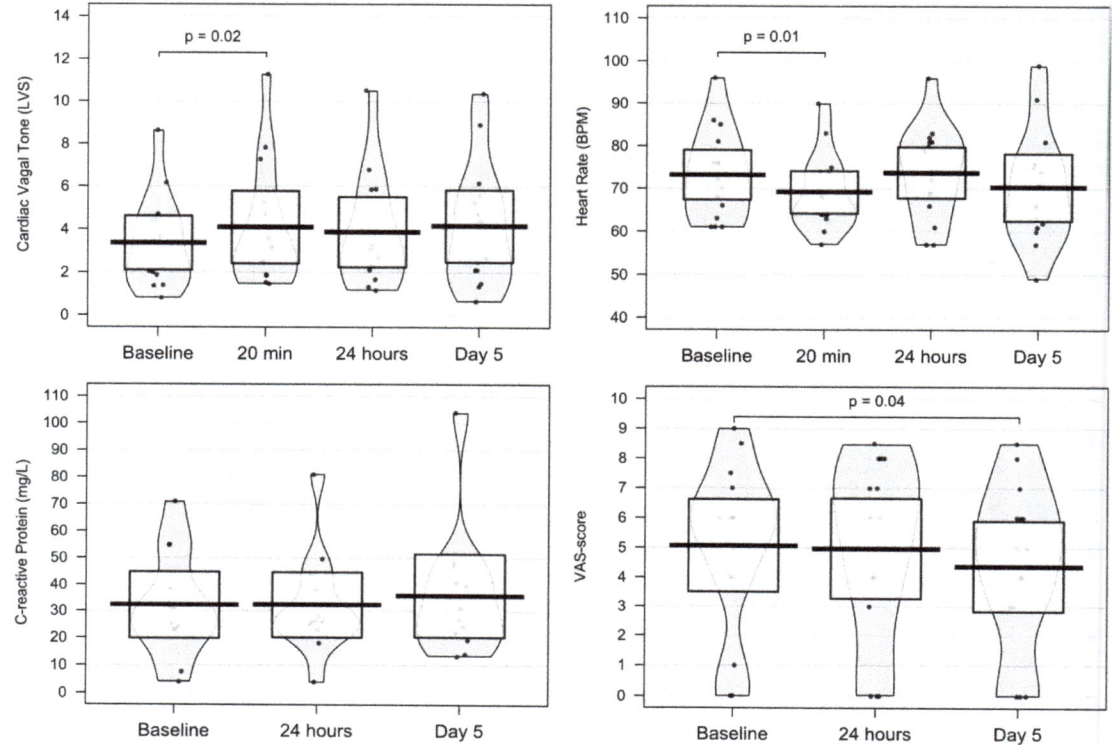

Figure 1. Raw data points, mean, and 95% CI of selected outcomes.

3. Discussion

To our knowledge, this is the first report of response to t-VNS in patients with PMR. We demonstrated that t-VNS caused an acute increase in CVT alongside a decrease in HR in treatment-naïve patients with PMR as a response to bilateral stimulation, indicating that an acute modulation of the autonomic nervous system was obtained. Furthermore, we demonstrated pain relief related to the hips in response to t-VNS.

In this study, we found lower mean values of CVT at baseline and on day 5 when compared with healthy individuals of similar age [22]. However, although this is the first preliminary report on CVT values in patients with PMR, it is consistent with low CVT values in patients with chronic pancreatitis and diabetes mellitus type 1 [23,24]. Furthermore, impaired parasympathetic activity has been demonstrated in patients with Crohn's disease [25]. Thus, our findings seem to support that the autonomic nervous system regulates neuro-immune communication and the activation of the cholinergic anti-inflammatory reflex. A true increase in CVT following 5 days of stimulation may exist; however, this result may subsequently be hampered by the presence of a type 2 error due to low power.

PMR is a clinical diagnosis that may be difficult to establish with certainty due to the heterogeneity of the disease [26]. In 2012, The European League Against Rheumatism (EULAR) in collaboration with the American College of Rheumatology (ACR) developed provisional classification criteria for PMR in order to make the process of diagnosis more consistent [27]. However, these criteria are not meant for diagnostic purposes. Patients were eligible for inclusion if the doctor's putative diagnosis was PMR or obs. pro. PMR, and thus, the diagnoses were not definitive at the point of enrolment.

We observed a 14% decrease in VAS score of the pain related to the hips, and similar trends were shown for the rest of the parameters. This suggests that t-VNS might reduce pain. Furthermore, although PMR is not associated with increased mortality, patients with PMR typically describe an immense loss in quality of life. To evaluate the patient's self-reported function and quality of life, MHAQ score, VAS scores, and duration of morning stiffness were evaluated but were not altered in response to t-VNS.

We did not observe any decrease in the objective biochemical profile, including CRP and IL-6, which are of particular interest in PMR. This contrasts with findings in other inflammatory diseases, such as rheumatoid and psoriatic arthritis, where t-VNS resulted in decreased levels of CRP [21]. These contrasting findings may be due to the high-grade inflammation in PMR patients. Koopman et al. demonstrated inhibited levels of TNF-α and improved disease scores in response to VNS stimulation for 42 days with an implanted device in patients with RA, suggesting the long-term activation of the cholinergic anti-inflammatory reflex [28]. In contrast, we applied stimulation three times per day over 5 days with a handheld, non-invasive device, and the treatment was mostly patient-administered. Thus, this study might underestimate the potential benefit of VNS on pro- and anti-inflammatory cytokines in PMR.

Limitations

This study is the first of its kind to investigate the effect of transcutaneous vagal nerve stimulation in patients with PMR characterised by high-grade inflammation. It is, however, an open-label, proof-of-concept study and thus has inherent limitations. First, as we did not have a sham control group, we cannot make firm conclusions on the observed changes in response to VNS. Second, as the study was open-label, all patients were aware of any beneficial effect and may have influenced subjective outcomes. However, all patients were examined by the same two researchers; thus, instructions on how to use the gammaCore were standardised, which minimised the risk of difference in the quality of the stimulation. Third, the study may be underpowered as we aimed to include 20 patients, but only 15 completed the protocol. Therefore, the sample size was small and vulnerable to inducing error. However, similar explorative pilot studies have been able to show differences in response to t-VNS in patient groups with established rheumatoid diagnoses [20,21]. Fourth, the intervention length of 5 days may have been insufficient for t-VNS to alter the disease activity. However, as these patients were treatment-naïve and suffered from pain, we did not believe it ethical to prolong this explorative treatment. Consequently, all patients in the study went on to be treated with prednisolone. Nonetheless, we cannot rule out the possibility that a longer intervention might have produced pronounced effects. Fifth, it has been questioned whether 5 min CVT was a reliable biomarker of parasympathetic activation, but the measure has been shown to perform better than heart rate variability measures [29]. Lastly, with only three out of the total 26 stimulations being supervised, we could not ensure the quality of each stimulation.

4. Materials and Methods

4.1. Study Design

This study was an open-label, proof-of-concept experimental pilot study investigating the effect of t-VNS in patients with inflammatory diseases. Two centres were used for inclusion: Mech-Sense, Aalborg University Hospital, and Department of Rheumatology, Aarhus University Hospital. A 5-day protocol was used, which was believed to be of adequate length to demonstrate our hypothesis, but did not unnecessarily delay treatment with glucocorticoids.

4.2. Cohort

Forty-two patients did not meet any exclusion criteria and were eligible for screening by a trained doctor to confirm the diagnosis of either (1) a well-established diagnosis of PMR (certain diagnosis) or (2) a putative PMR diagnosis, where no alternative pathology could explain the case better (obs. pro PMR). Exclusion criteria were any corticosteroid treatment within 5 weeks prior to inclusion, age < 18 years, known cardiovascular disease, hypotension (<100 mmHg systolic and <60 mmHg diastolic), pregnancy (positive U-HCG) or current lactation, and non-compliance with the protocol. Inclusion criteria were newly diagnosed, treatment-naïve PMR patients. No drugs were used besides NSAIDs and paracetamol; while the usage of NSAIDs during the protocol was not disallowed, it was recommended that patients did not use it.

If the eligible patients agreed to participate, they signed an informed consent form. Twenty patients were included; however, 5 patients dropped out before completion, leaving 15 patients for analysis. Reasons for drop-out were: non-compliance with the protocol (n = 1), withdrawal of consent (n = 2), and did not show (n = 2).

4.3. Vagus Nerve Stimulation

t-VNS was performed using a non-invasive, handheld gammaCore® device (electroCore, Inc., Basking Ridge, NJ, USA) providing transcutaneous low-voltage electric stimulation on the cervical part of the vagus nerve. The signal consisted of five 5000 Hz sine-wave pulses repeated at a rate of 25 Hz. Patients were given clear instructions to place the two gel-covered conductors on top of the common carotid arteries on the neck. The amplitude of the electric signal, ranging from 0 to 40 on an arbitrary scale, could be adjusted via two control buttons on the device. Each stimulation lasted 2 min, after which the device would stop automatically.

On days 1–4, stimulations were carried out bilaterally three times a day (morning, noon, and evening), while on day 5 only one stimulation was carried out. A total of 26 stimulations were planned for each patient. Compliance was assured by counting the remaining stimulations when the device was returned. The patients were given clear instructions to position the device correctly, and the amplitude was to be slowly increased until a mild contraction of the ipsilateral oral commissure was seen or the pain from the stimulation was unbearable. At the second visit, the patients performed a stimulation under the supervision of the investigator to ensure safe and proper usage.

4.4. Outcomes

4.4.1. Primary Outcome: Resting Cardiac Vagal Tone

The primary outcome was a change in resting CVT between baseline and day 5 (long-term response) and differences between baseline and 20 min after the first stimulation (acute response).

CVT is a non-invasive measure of the efferent parasympathetic cardiac vagal tone, which is computed from a five-minute ECG recording; incoming QRS complexes are compared with a template derived from the initial part of the recording, and changes in R–R intervals are detected via phase shift demodulation [22]. CVT was measured on a linear vagal scale where 0 represents full atropinisation [30]. Resting CVT was assessed via a three-lead ECG (eMotion Faros180° portable cardiac monitoring device, Bittium, Oulu, Finland) using Ambu BlueSensor P ECG-electrodes (Ambu, Copenhagen, Denmark), placed on cleaned and dried skin, and assessments were performed in conformity with international recommendations [31]. The recordings were analysed using ProCVT software (ProBiometrics, London, UK) to derive CVT.

On days 1, 2, and 5, five-minute ECG recordings were conducted. On day 1, two recordings were made to evaluate the acute response; one prior to the first stimulation (baseline) and the second after 20 min. On days 2 and 5, a single CVT recording was performed before stimulation. The successful recordings were manually edited if needed, i.e., changes in HR exceeding 15 beats per minute (BPM) between two consecutive heartbeats were treated as artefacts, e.g., coughing or sudden movements. If artefacts were present in the data, the five heartbeats before and after were discarded by the underlying algorithm.

4.4.2. Secondary Outcomes: Cardiac-Derived Parameters, CRP, Proinflammatory Analytes, and Patient-Reported Outcome

Patient-reported outcomes were assessed on days 1, 2, and 5, with each patient completing two questionnaires. Firstly, the modified health assessment questionnaire (MHAQ), which consists of eight questions measuring the ability to perform common daily life activities, such as dressing, arising, eating, walking, hygiene, reaching, and gripping. Each patient was asked to rate their ability to perform these activities on a scale ranging from 1 to 4: 1 = without difficulty, 2 = with some difficulty, 3 = with much difficulty, and 4 = unable to do the requested task. The second questionnaire consisted of three assessments on a validated continuous (0–100 mm) visual analogue scale (VAS scoring) and an evaluation of the duration of morning joint stiffness. For the VAS score, three domains were assessed: (1) general pain, (2) pain related to the hips, and (3) a general, overall assessment of the negative effect and influences caused by PMR.

Measurement of BP and HR was carried out prior to each ECG recording. Each measurement was performed on the upper left arm using an electronic sphygmomanometer (UA-852; A&D Company, Limited, Tokyo, Japan).

Blood samples were drawn on days 1, 2, and 5 prior to other measurements. Samples for routine clinical biochemistry, alongside EDTA-plasma and serum, were drawn on baseline day and day 5 for analysis of proinflammatory analytes IFN-γ, IL-, 1β, IL-2, IL-4, IL-6, IL-8, IL-10, IL-13, and TNF-α. Analyses of cytokines were performed via Luminex multiplexing technology using the Inflammation 20-Plex Human ProcartaPlex™ Panel (Invitrogen, Thermo Fisher Scientific, Waltham, MA, USA) and a MAGPIX instrument (Luminex, Austin, TX, USA) in accordance with the manufacturer's protocol. For each analyte, extreme outliers, defined as values above $Q3 + 3 \times IQR$ or below $Q1 - 3 \times IQR$, were identified and removed.

4.5. Statistical Methods

Data were presented as mean ± standard deviation (SD) unless otherwise clarified. All data were evaluated for normality using Shapiro–Wilk test for normality or through visual inspection of QQ plots. For statistical comparison between baseline and visit values, paired t-test was used for data of normal distribution, and Wilcoxon signed-rank test was used for data of non-normal distribution. A p-value less than 0.05 was considered significant. All data analyses were performed in STATA version 16.0 (StataCorp, TX, USA) and R version 4.0.3 (The R Foundation for Statistical Computing). Likewise, all graphical outputs were produced using the same version of R.

5. Conclusions

In conclusion, we showed an acute modulation of the autonomic nervous system in patients with PMR as evidenced by increased CVT and decreased HR. Furthermore, we showed alleviation of hip pain in response to a five-day protocol, but this was not reflected in the cytokine profile. Further investigation of t-VNS in PMR patients is warranted, preferably in blinded, randomised, sham-controlled trials, before any firm conclusion is drawn upon the ability to activate the cholinergic anti-inflammatory reflex in this patient group.

Author Contributions: Conceptualization, B.B., C.B., M.P.-J.; Methodology, B.B., M.P.-J.; Validation, A.-M.W., B.B., C.B., M.P.-J.; Formal analysis, J.V., C.B.; Investigation, J.V., A.-M.W., S.K.; Data curation, J.V., A.-M.W., C.B.; Writing—original draft preparation, J.V.; Writing—review and editing, J.V., A.-M.W., S.K., C.B., M.P.-J.; Visualization, J.V., C.B.; Supervision, A.-M.W., M.P.-J.; Project administration, B.B., C.B., M.P.-J.; Funding acquisition, J.V., M.P.-J. All authors have read and agreed to the published version of the manuscript.

Funding: J. Venborg was financially supported by the Danish Rheumatism Association.

Institutional Review Board Statement: The study was conducted in conformity with the Good Clinical Practice Unit (CPMP/ICH/135/95) and approved by the Central Denmark Region Committees on Health Research Ethics (1-10-72-199-16), the Danish Data Protection Agency (1-16-02-442-16), the

Danish Medicines Agency (2016024373), and the European Databank on Medical Devices (CIV-16-03-015125).

Informed Consent Statement: Informed consent was obtained from all subjects involved in the study.

Data Availability Statement: Data is contained within the article.

Acknowledgments: The gammaCore devices used for intervention were supplied by electroCore, Inc. The authors would like to thank the Department of Clinical Biochemistry, Aarhus University Hospital, for carrying out the blood samples analyses. Additionally, a special thank goes out to all participating patients for making the project possible.

Conflicts of Interest: The authors declare no conflict of interest.

References

1. Camellino, D.; Giusti, A.; Girasole, G.; Bianchi, G.; Dejaco, C. Pathogenesis, Diagnosis and Management of Polymyalgia Rheumatica. *Drugs Aging* **2019**. [CrossRef] [PubMed]
2. Salvarani, C.; Cantini, F.; Hunder, G.G. Polymyalgia Rheumatica and Giant-Cell Arteritis. *Lancet* **2008**, *372*, 234–245. [CrossRef]
3. Barraclough, K.; Liddell, W.G.; du Toit, J.; Foy, C.; Dasgupta, B.; Thomas, M.; Hamilton, W. Polymyalgia Rheumatica in Primary Care: A Cohort Study of the Diagnostic Criteria and Outcome. *Fam. Pract.* **2008**, *25*, 328–333. [CrossRef] [PubMed]
4. Myklebust, G.; Wilsgaard, T.; Jacobsen, B.K.; Gran, J.T. Causes of Death in Polymyalgia RheumaticaA Prospective Longitudinal Study of 315 Cases and Matched Population Controls. *Scand. J. Rheumatol.* **2003**, *32*, 38–41. [CrossRef] [PubMed]
5. Schaufelberger, C.; Bengtsson, B.-Å.; Andersson, R. Epidemiology and Mortality in 220 Patients with Polymyalgia Rheumatica. *Rheumatology* **1995**, *34*, 261–264. [CrossRef]
6. Hutchings, A.; Hollywood, J.; Lamping, D.L.; Pease, C.T.; Chakravarty, K.; Silverman, B.; Choy, E.H.S.; Scott, D.G.I.; Hazleman, B.L.; Bourke, B.; et al. Clinical Outcomes, Quality of Life, and Diagnostic Uncertainty in the First Year of Polymyalgia Rheumatica. *Arthritis Care Res.* **2007**, *57*, 803–809. [CrossRef]
7. Dejaco, C.; Singh, Y.P.; Perel, P.; Hutchings, A.; Camellino, D.; Mackie, S.; Abril, A.; Bachta, A.; Balint, P.; Barraclough, K.; et al. 2015 Recommendations for the Management of Polymyalgia Rheumatica: A European League Against Rheumatism/American College of Rheumatology Collaborative Initiative. *Arthritis Rheumatol.* **2015**, *67*, 2569–2580. [CrossRef]
8. Curtis, J.R.; Westfall, A.O.; Allison, J.; Bijlsma, J.W.; Freeman, A.; George, V.; Kovac, S.H.; Spettell, C.M.; Saag, K.G. Population-Based Assessment of Adverse Events Associated with Long-Term Glucocorticoid Use. *Arthritis Care Res.* **2006**, *55*, 420–426. [CrossRef]
9. Gaffo, A.; Saag, K.G.; Curtis, J.R. Treatment of Rheumatoid Arthritis. *Am. J. Health Syst. Pharm.* **2006**, *63*, 2451–2465. [CrossRef] [PubMed]
10. Alvarez-Rodríguez, L.; Lopez-Hoyos, M.; Mata, C.; Marin, M.J.; Calvo-Alen, J.; Blanco, R.; Aurrecoechea, E.; Ruiz-Soto, M.; Martínez-Taboada, V.M. Circulating Cytokines in Active Polymyalgia Rheumatica. *Ann. Rheum. Dis.* **2010**, *69*, 263–269. [CrossRef]
11. Van der Geest, K.S.M.; Abdulahad, W.H.; Rutgers, A.; Horst, G.; Bijzet, J.; Arends, S.; Roffel, M.P.; Boots, A.M.H.; Brouwer, E. Serum Markers Associated with Disease Activity in Giant Cell Arteritis and Polymyalgia Rheumatica. *Rheumatology* **2015**, *54*, 1397–1402. [CrossRef] [PubMed]
12. Macchioni, P.; Boiardi, L.; Catanoso, M.; Pulsatelli, L.; Pipitone, N.; Meliconi, R.; Salvarani, C. Tocilizumab for Polymyalgia Rheumatica: Report of Two Cases and Review of the Literature. *Semin. Arthritis Rheum.* **2013**, *43*, 113–118. [CrossRef] [PubMed]
13. Devauchelle-Pensec, V.; Berthelot, J.M.; Cornec, D.; Renaudineau, Y.; Marhadour, T.; Jousse-Joulin, S.; Querellou, S.; Garrigues, F.; Bandt, M.D.; Gouillou, M.; et al. Efficacy of First-Line Tocilizumab Therapy in Early Polymyalgia Rheumatica: A Prospective Longitudinal Study. *Ann. Rheum. Dis.* **2016**, *75*, 1506–1510. [CrossRef]
14. Camellino, D.; Soldano, S.; Cutolo, M.; Cimmino, M.A. Dissecting the Inflammatory Response in Polymyalgia Rheumatica: The Relative Role of IL-6 and Its Inhibition. *Rheumatol. Int.* **2018**, *38*, 1699–1704. [CrossRef]
15. Chino, K.; Kondo, T.; Sakai, R.; Saito, S.; Okada, Y.; Shibata, A.; Kurasawa, T.; Okuyama, A.; Takei, H.; Amano, K. Tocilizumab Monotherapy for Polymyalgia Rheumatica: A Prospective, Single-Center, Open-Label Study. *Int. J. Rheum. Dis.* **2019**, *22*, 2151–2157. [CrossRef]
16. Borovikova, L.V.; Ivanova, S.; Zhang, M.; Yang, H.; Botchkina, G.I.; Watkins, L.R.; Wang, H.; Abumrad, N.; Eaton, J.W.; Tracey, K.J. Vagus Nerve Stimulation Attenuates the Systemic Inflammatory Response to Endotoxin. *Nature* **2000**, *405*, 458. [CrossRef]
17. Borovikova, L.V.; Ivanova, S.; Nardi, D.; Zhang, M.; Yang, H.; Ombrellino, M.; Tracey, K.J. Role of Vagus Nerve Signaling in CNI-1493-Mediated Suppression of Acute Inflammation. *Auton. Neurosci.* **2000**, *85*, 141–147. [CrossRef]
18. Rasmussen, S.E.; Pfeiffer-Jensen, M.; Drewes, A.M.; Farmer, A.D.; Deleuran, B.W.; Stengaard-Pedersen, K.; Brock, B.; Brock, C. Vagal Influences in Rheumatoid Arthritis. *Scand. J. Rheumatol.* **2018**, *47*, 1–11. [CrossRef] [PubMed]
19. Brock, C.; Brock, B.; Aziz, Q.; Møller, H.J.; Jensen, M.P.; Drewes, A.M.; Farmer, A.D. Transcutaneous Cervical Vagal Nerve Stimulation Modulates Cardiac Vagal Tone and Tumor Necrosis Factor-Alpha. *Neurogastroenterol. Motil.* **2017**, *29*, e12999. [CrossRef]

20. Drewes, A.M.; Brock, C.; Rasmussen, S.E.; Møller, H.J.; Brock, B.; Deleuran, B.W.; Farmer, A.D.; Pfeiffer-Jensen, M. Short-Term Transcutaneous Non-Invasive Vagus Nerve Stimulation May Reduce Disease Activity and pro-Inflammatory Cytokines in Rheumatoid Arthritis: Results of a Pilot Study. *Scand. J. Rheumatol.* **2021**, *50*, 20–27. [CrossRef]
21. Brock, C.; Rasmussen, S.E.; Drewes, A.M.; Møller, H.J.; Brock, B.; Deleuran, B.; Farmer, A.D.; Pfeiffer-Jensen, M. Vagal Nerve Stimulation-Modulation of the Anti-Inflammatory Response and Clinical Outcome in Psoriatic Arthritis or Ankylosing Spondylitis. *Mediat. Inflamm.* **2021**, *2021*, e9933532. [CrossRef] [PubMed]
22. Farmer, A.D.; Coen, S.J.; Kano, M.; Weltens, N.; Ly, H.G.; Botha, C.; Paine, P.A.; Oudenhove, L.V.; Aziz, Q. Normal Values and Reproducibility of the Real-Time Index of Vagal Tone in Healthy Humans: A Multi-Center Study. *Ann. Gastroenterol. Q. Publ. Hell. Soc. Gastroenterol.* **2014**, *27*, 362–368.
23. Juel, J.; Brock, C.; Olesen, S.S.; Madzak, A.; Farmer, A.D.; Aziz, Q.; Frøkjær, J.B.; Drewes, A.M. Acute Physiological and Electrical Accentuation of Vagal Tone Has No Effect on Pain or Gastrointestinal Motility in Chronic Pancreatitis. *J. Pain Res.* **2017**, *10*, 1347–1355. [CrossRef] [PubMed]
24. Brock, C.; Jessen, N.; Brock, B.; Jakobsen, P.E.; Hansen, T.K.; Rantanen, J.M.; Riahi, S.; Dimitrova, Y.K.; Dons-Jensen, A.; Aziz, Q.; et al. Cardiac Vagal Tone, a Non-Invasive Measure of Parasympathetic Tone, Is a Clinically Relevant Tool in Type 1 Diabetes Mellitus. *Diabet. Med.* **2017**, *34*, 1428–1434. [CrossRef]
25. Engel, T.; Ben-Horin, S.; Beer-Gabel, M. Autonomic Dysfunction Correlates with Clinical and Inflammatory Activity in Patients with Crohn's Disease. *Inflamm. Bowel Dis.* **2015**, *21*, 2320–2326. [CrossRef] [PubMed]
26. Dasgupta, B.; Hutchings, A.; Matteson, E.L. Polymyalgia Rheumatica: The Mess We Are Now in and What We Need to Do about It. *Arthritis Care Res.* **2006**, *55*, 518–520. [CrossRef] [PubMed]
27. Dasgupta, B.; Cimmino, M.A.; Kremers, H.M.; Schmidt, W.A.; Schirmer, M.; Salvarani, C.; Bachta, A.; Dejaco, C.; Duftner, C.; Jensen, H.S.; et al. 2012 Provisional Classification Criteria for Polymyalgia Rheumatica: A European League Against Rheumatism/American College of Rheumatology Collaborative Initiative. *Arthritis Rheum.* **2012**, *64*, 943–954. [CrossRef]
28. Koopman, F.A.; Chavan, S.S.; Miljko, S.; Grazio, S.; Sokolovic, S.; Schuurman, P.R.; Mehta, A.D.; Levine, Y.A.; Faltys, M.; Zitnik, R.; et al. Vagus Nerve Stimulation Inhibits Cytokine Production and Attenuates Disease Severity in Rheumatoid Arthritis. *Proc. Natl. Acad. Sci. USA* **2016**, *113*, 8284–8289. [CrossRef]
29. Wegeberg, A.-M.; Lunde, E.D.; Riahi, S.; Ejskjaer, N.; Drewes, A.M.; Brock, B.; Pop-Busui, R.; Brock, C. Cardiac Vagal Tone as a Novel Screening Tool to Recognize Asymptomatic Cardiovascular Autonomic Neuropathy: Aspects of Utility in Type 1 Diabetes. *Diabetes Res. Clin. Pract.* **2020**, *170*, 108517. [CrossRef]
30. Julu, P.O.O. A Linear Scale for Measuring Vagal Tone in Man. *J. Auton. Pharmacol.* **1992**, *12*, 109–115. [CrossRef]
31. Malik, M. Heart Rate Variability. *Ann. Noninvasive Electrocardiol.* **1996**, *1*, 151–181. [CrossRef]

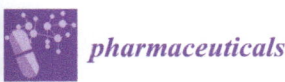

Review

Respiratory Manifestations in Systemic Lupus Erythematosus

Salvatore Di Bartolomeo [1], Alessia Alunno [2] and Francesco Carubbi [3,*]

[1] Department of Medicine, ASL 1 Avezzano-Sulmona-L'Aquila, 67039 Sulmona, Italy; salvatore.dibart@gmail.com
[2] Rheumatology Unit, Department of Medicine, University of Perugia, 06123 Perugia, Italy; alessia.alunno82@gmail.com
[3] Internal Medicine and Nephrology Unit, Department of Life, Health & Environmental Sciences, University of L'Aquila and Department of Medicine, ASL 1 Avezzano-Sulmona-L'Aquila, 67100 L'Aquila, Italy
* Correspondence: francescocarubbi@libero.it; Tel.: +39-086-226-8315

Abstract: Systemic lupus erythematosus (SLE) is a chronic systemic autoimmune disease characterized by a wide spectrum of clinical manifestations. The respiratory system can be involved in up to 50–70% of patients and be the presenting manifestation of the disease in 4–5% of cases. Every part of the respiratory part can be involved, and the severity can vary from mild self-limiting to life threatening forms. Respiratory involvement can be primary (caused by SLE itself) or secondary (e.g., infections or drug toxicity), acute or chronic. The course, treatment and prognosis vary greatly depending on the specific pattern of the disease. This review article aims at providing an overview of respiratory manifestations in SLE along with an update about therapeutic approaches including novel biologic therapies.

Keywords: systemic lupus erythematosus; airway disease; interstitial lung disease; shrinking lung syndrome; diffuse alveolar hemorrhage; pleurisy; infection

---

Citation: Di Bartolomeo, S.; Alunno, A.; Carubbi, F. Respiratory Manifestations in Systemic Lupus Erythematosus. *Pharmaceuticals* **2021**, *14*, 276. https://doi.org/10.3390/ph14030276

Academic Editor: Barbara Ruaro

Received: 28 January 2021
Accepted: 16 March 2021
Published: 18 March 2021

Publisher's Note: MDPI stays neutral with regard to jurisdictional claims in published maps and institutional affiliations.

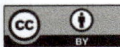

Copyright: © 2021 by the authors. Licensee MDPI, Basel, Switzerland. This article is an open access article distributed under the terms and conditions of the Creative Commons Attribution (CC BY) license (https://creativecommons.org/licenses/by/4.0/).

1. Introduction

Systemic lupus erythematosus (SLE) is a chronic, systemic autoimmune disease with a relapsing–remitting course and characterized by the production of a wide range of autoantibodies. Although people of any age and gender can be involved, females of childbearing age are the most affected, with a female-to-male ratio of about 9:1 [1].

SLE can have a wide range of manifestations, involving virtually every organ or apparatus, and its severity can vary from very mild disease without major organ involvement, to severe life-threatening conditions. Clinical manifestations may include cytopenia, fever, malar and other skin rashes, oral ulcers, polyarthralgia/non erosive arthritis, vasculitis, renal, neurological, cardiac and pleuro-pulmonary involvement [2–4]. Recently, a new set of classification criteria was proposed by American College of Rheumatology/European League Against Rheumatism (ACR/EULAR), designed to increase classification sensitivity and specificity for inclusion in SLE research studies and trials [5]. Furthermore, recommendations on disease management from EULAR were recently updated [6,7].

SLE pathogenesis is multifactorial and not completely understood, and includes an interaction between non-Mendelian genetic predisposition, hormonal and environmental factors, ultimately leading to an alteration in both innate and adaptive immunity. In particular, SLE pathogenesis is characterized by an impaired apoptotic cell clearance by phagocytes, B-cell and T-cell autoreactivity leading to an abnormal production of autoantibodies, and immune complexes (ICs) formation with nuclear and cytosolic antigens. ICs can, in turn, activate the classical pathway of the complement system contributing to inflammation and damage in target organs [4,8].

Although the exact prevalence is unknown, respiratory tract involvement can be present in 50–70% of SLE patients, being the presenting symptom of the disease in 4–5% of cases and more frequent in men [8–10]. Every part of the respiratory tract can be involved:

upper and lower airways, vessels, pleura, lung parenchyma and respiratory muscles (Figure 1). Respiratory manifestations can be acute or chronic, primary (directly caused by the disease) or secondary (due to concomitant complications such as infections). Interestingly, acute manifestations may be associated with generalized lupus disease activity, while chronic complications may progress independently to general disease activity [10].

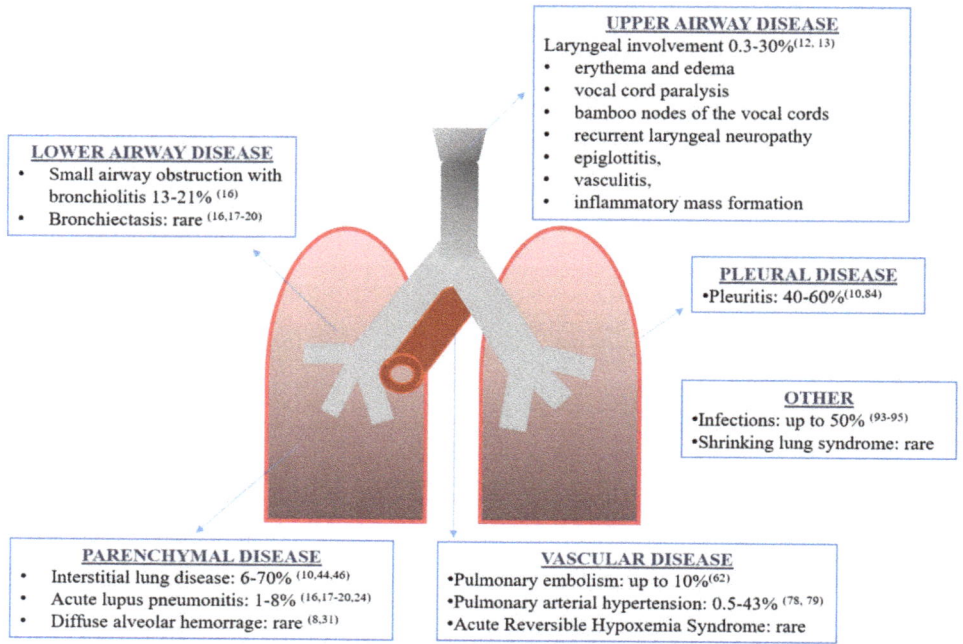

Figure 1. Overview of respiratory manifestations in systemic lupus erythematosus along with the prevalence and corresponding references.

Respiratory manifestations of SLE are associated with a variable mortality rate, depending to the type of involvement, its extension, and the presence of comorbidities. In particular, pulmonary involvement is associated with higher mortality and with negative effect on patient-reported outcomes, patient-performed outcome and quality of life [11]. Unfortunately, clinical and therapeutic trial data specifically focused on respiratory manifestations of SLE are scarce, so treatment options are based on evidence from other organ involvement in SLE, or from respiratory manifestations in other autoimmune diseases, or based on case reports or small cases series.

In this review, we provide an overview of the scientific literature about the respiratory involvement in SLE, and highlight the progress achieved so far in the understanding of pathogenic mechanisms and in the identification of therapeutic strategies needing to be addressed in future studies. In particular, we designed a comprehensive literature search on this topic, by a review of reported published articles in indexed international journals up until 31st October 2019, following proposed guidelines for preparing a biomedical narrative review [12].

2. Airway Disease

Laryngeal involvement can occur in 0.3–30% of SLE patients and range from asymptomatic to severe life-threatening upper airway obstruction [13]. Clinical manifestations are non-specific and include hoarseness, cough, dyspnea, and stridor. Mucosal inflammation with erythema and edema is the major manifestation; other findings include vocal cord paralysis, bamboo nodes of the vocal cords, recurrent laryngeal neuropathy, epiglottitis, rheumatoid nodules [14], vasculitis, inflammatory mass formation and late subglottic stenosis. It usually responds well to corticosteroids (CS) therapy. However, in severe cases of respiratory failure, advanced airway management may be necessary [13,15,16].

Other airway involvement includes upper airway angioedema, necrotic tracheitis and early post-intubation stenosis, bronchial stenosis; small airway obstruction with bronchiolitis is found in the 13% to 21% of patients with the use of high-resolution computed tomography (HRCT) [17] and bronchiectasis as a consequence of direct SLE involvement or as sequelae of bronchopulmonary infections [17–21].

Using pulmonary function tests (PFTs), Andonopoulos et al. found a prevalence of obstructive disorders in 6% of SLE patients and 0% of control group (smokers were excluded) and initial damage of small airways (defined as maximum expiratory flow-volume (MEFV) 25–75 below 60% of predicted value) was present in 24% of SLE patients but the difference was not statistically significant with the control group [22], moreover, surveillance of pulmonary function tests revealed a progressive decline in values indicating small airways damage with time [17].

3. Parenchymal Lung Disease

3.1. Acute Diseases

Acute lupus pneumonitis (ALP) and diffuse alveolar hemorrhage (DAH) are acute and uncommon manifestations of SLE [10].

3.1.1. Acute Lupus Pneumonitis

ALP is a rare, probably under-recognized, manifestation of SLE that occurs in 1–8% of SLE patients, in particular younger patients and patients with a recent diagnosis. Moreover, it can be the first manifestation of a previously unrecognized SLE in 50% of cases [10,17,23–25]. Clinical presentation is non-specific and can simulate infectious pneumonia with sudden onset of fever, cough, dyspnea, pleuritic chest pain and occasionally hemoptysis. Physical examination can reveal tachycardia, tachypnoea hypoxemia, hypocapnia and lung crackles. Occasionally, it can present with acute respiratory failure requiring mechanical ventilation. ALP has been described complicating SLE during pregnancy [10,17,23–26]. Chest X-ray can show multiple, bilateral patchy infiltrations, predominantly in the lower lobes, with or without pleural effusion. However, chest X-ray can be normal, especially in the initial phases or shows only lung nodules. Although these findings are non-specific, CT scan can show ground glass opacities and areas of consolidation, predominantly in the lower lobes [10,23]. Histologically, ALP presents diffuse alveolar damage (DAD) with inflammatory cell infiltration, damage and necrosis of alveolar-capillary unit, edema, hyaline membrane formation and alveolar hemorrhage. Capillaritis and thrombosis have also been described. Alveolar damage may be mediated by the deposition of ICs and complement fractions. However, there are not diagnostic and/or pathognomonic findings specific for ALP. Some data highlight a pathogenetic role of anti-Ro/SSA antibodies, due to an association between ALP and these autoantibodies [10,17,23–26]. Since there are no specific clinical or imaging findings in ALP, the diagnosis is of exclusion and a comprehensive differential diagnosis must be considered with infections, organizing pneumonia, malignancy, DAH, pulmonary edema, lung drug toxicity [23,24]. Infections must always be ruled out, since they may have a similar clinical picture and immunosuppressive treatments needed to treat ALP, could have a deleterious effect on the infection course. In this setting, bronchoscopy with bronchoalveolar lavage fluid (BALF) analysis should be performed and followed by microbiological tests for common and opportunistic pathogens [23]. It seems that the presence of eosinophilia or neutrophilia on BALF carries worse prognosis than lymphocytosis. A marked elevation in C-reactive protein (CRP) and procalcitonin levels in the serum may suggest an infection. Lung biopsy is rarely necessary [23,24,27]. Prognosis is severe, with a high mortality risk; in particular, Matthay et al. reported a mortality rate of 50% among 12 patients treated for ALP [28] while more recently Wan et al. found a mortality of 40% [29]. High doses of CS are the mainstay of treatment. In severe cases daily pulses of methylprednisolone (up to 1000 mg/day for 3 days) can be used, followed by 1–2 mg/kg per day of prednisone and a subsequent tapering according to clinical response. Immunosuppressants such as cyclophosphamide (CYC) and azathioprine, biologics drugs such as rituximab (RTX), intravenous immunoglobulins (IVIg) or plasma exchange can be added in severe refractory cases, but the evidence on their efficacy is scarce. A broad-spectrum antibiotic coverage should be started until an infection is ruled out, and then prophylaxis against opportunistic pathogens (e.g., Pneumocystis jirovecii) can be considered during immunosuppressive treatment [10,17,23–25,28,29]. Factors that seem to contribute to poor outcome include intercurrent infections, aspiration, diaphragmatic dysfunction, cardiac and renal failure, drug and oxygen toxicity [7,29–31]. Of those who recover from the acute episode, 50–100% may eventually develop chronic interstitial pneumonia so a thorough follow-up is advisable [10,31].

3.1.2. Diffuse Alveolar Hemorrhage

DAH, first described by Dr. William Osler in 1904, is a rare, but very severe and potentially fatal complication of SLE [8,32]. It is not exclusive to SLE, occurring in several other conditions such as anti-neutrophil cytoplasmic autoantibody (ANCA)-associated vasculitis, antiphospholipid syndrome (APS), other connective tissue diseases, infections, bone marrow transplantation, and drug toxicity [33,34].

DAH prevalence among SLE patients ranges from 0.5–0.6% to 5.4–5.7% with a femal-to-male ratio of approximately 6:1. DAH was described as initial manifestation of SLE in 11–20% of cases; some autoptic studies in SLE patients have found the presence of red blood cells in the lungs of 30–66% of cases maybe due to the presence of either unidentified or subclinical, paucisymptomatic forms of DAH [10,33]. Mean age of presentation is 27 years, but it can occur at an early stage of the disease [17]. Some patients may have recurrent episodes [33,35].

The clinical picture of DAH is characterized by the sudden onset, within hours or a few days, of dyspnea, hypoxemia with possible acute respiratory failure and need for mechanical ventilation in more than 50% of cases, fever, cough, hemoptysis with a rapid fall in hemoglobin levels, and appearance of new alveolar or interstitial infiltrates. Some patients can present chest pain. Hemoptysis can be of variable severity, dramatic in some cases, or initially absent in up to 33% of cases [8,10,33,36].

Chest X-ray can be normal or show bilateral, rarely unilateral, airspace opacities (patchy, focal or diffuse). CT scan may show diffuse, bilateral and patchy alveolar infiltrates, also asymmetrical, ground glass opacities or diffuse nodular opacities and it is more accurate than chest X-ray to evaluate the extent of the disease. BALF is usually hemorrhagic, and the presence of 20% or more hemosiderin-laden macrophages in BALF is a criterion for DAH diagnosis [8]. However, this pattern can appear only after 48–72 h from symptom onset. BALF culture is mandatory to exclude an infection as a cause of DAH; many pathogens such as Legionella pneumophila, Strongyloides stercoralis and Cytomegalovirus can be associated with DAH [8]. Secondary infections, mainly nosocomial, can complicate the course of DAH thereby worsening the disease prognosis. Zamora et al. found a mortality rate of 100% in 3 patients with secondary infections (1 infected with Aspergillus, 1 with Escherichia coli and 1 with both methicillin-resistant Staphilococcus aureus and Candida) [37]; in a study by Rojas-Serrano et al., bronchoscopic assessment performed during the first 48 h of admission in 13 SLE patients demonstrated infections in 57% of cases including Pseudomonas aeruginosa, Serratia marcescens, Citrobacter freundii, and Aspergillus fumigates [38].

Lung biopsy is rarely necessary, and critically ill patients might not tolerate this invasive procedure. Histologic findings are non-specific with the presence of mild blood extravasation. More severe cases present capillaritis with neutrophil infiltration of alveolar septa [8,10,33,35,36]. Laboratory findings can show a rapid drop in hemoglobin levels, along with other characteristics of an active SLE, such as low complement levels, thrombocytopenia and autoantibodies. A rapid fall in hematocrit levels must alert clinicians to DAH [8]. An increase of carbon monoxide diffusing capacity (DLCO) of 30% or more over baseline values or an absolute elevation over 130% of predictive value is supportive to the diagnosis of DAH, due to the enhanced uptake of carbon monoxide by hemoglobin present in the alveoli [8,10,39].

DAH pathogenesis is not completely known, but it is characterized by an immune mediated damage of small vessels and alveolar septa, with deposition of ICs and complement fractions in the alveolar capillaries. A neutrophil interstitial infiltration with alveolar and capillary walls necrosis (capillaritis) has also been demonstrated. Neutrophils may play a pathogenetic role by the release of neutrophils extracellular traps (NETs) and cytotoxic proteins that contribute to the local damage. The loss of integrity of the alveolar-capillary wall results in the leakage of red blood cells into the alveolar space [3,10,36]. Other proposed mechanisms include: increased apoptosis of the alveolar wall cells with monocyte-macrophage infiltration, diffuse alveolar damage with edema of alveolar septa and formation of hyaline membranes, and fibrinoid necrosis. B-lymphocytes may play a pivotal role in autoantibodies formation [8,36].

Risk factors for the development of DAH include: history of thrombocytopenia, low C3 fraction, high titers of anti-double-stranded (ds)DNA, leucopenia, coexisting neuropsychiatric lupus, high disease activity (e.g., SLE Disease Activity Index (SLEDAI) score >10) and the presence of active renal disease (in particular class III and IV lupus nephritis) [8,10,36].

DAH treatment is based on case reports, expert opinion or derived from other conditions [36]. The treatment's mainstay is the early administration of high dose iv methylprednisolone (usually 1 g/day iv for 3 or more days up to 4–8 g total dose) with subsequent tapering according to clinical evolution. CYC can be added in severe forms but data on its efficacy are contrasting with an increased mortality in the study of Zamora et al. [37], when compared to the beneficial effect in the study of Sun et al. [40]. However, a recent meta-analysis did not confirm an association with CYC and survival [41]. Other immunosuppressants have been used, such as cyclosporine, azathioprine, tacrolimus, mycophenolate mofetil (MMF), without any conclusive evidence. Among biologic drugs, RTX has shown some good results and different schemes and dosages has been used, mainly 375 mg/m^2 weekly × 4 or fortnightly × 2 or 1 g 2 weeks apart, generally in association with CS. In the majority of reports, one course of therapy was sufficient; however, in refractory cases, maintenance therapy with RTX can be needed [8,36,42–46]. The potential role of belimumab remains unknown [8,36].

Plasmapheresis is generally used in patients with refractory and more severe disease, with contrasting results in literature [41]. Adverse events can occur in up to 10% of cases, are more frequent in the first procedure and are generally mild or moderate, including access site or device problems, hypotension and syncope, tingling, urticaria, nausea/vomiting, chills, fever, arrhythmia [47].

Other therapeutic options include IVIg, intrapulmonary administration of recombinant factor VIIa, and umbilical cord mesenchymal stem cell transplantation [36]. Supportive and resuscitative treatments must be guaranteed, in particular in the context of respiratory failure in which patients may require mechanical ventilation up to extracorporeal membrane oxygenation support in more severe cases. Broad spectrum antimicrobic therapy is mandatory, since infections can both initiate or complicate the course of DAH [8,36].

Prognosis is poor, with a mortality rate of up to 70–92%, (average 50%); however, a trend in the reduction of mortality was observed in the recent years, likely due to a better knowledge of the disorder, a more rapid diagnosis and a precocious introduction of novel, targeted therapies [8]. Older age, longer lupus disease duration, acute massive hemoptysis, requirement of mechanical ventilation and plasmapheresis treatment, thrombocytopenia (not universally accepted) and infections are associated with an increased risk of mortality [8,10,41]. However, severe diseases rendered the requirement of plasmapheresis treatment and mechanical ventilation are themselves associated with poor outcome. The presence of other comorbidities must also be considered. Among survivors, 70–90% can eventually develop pulmonary fibrosis therefore a strict follow-up is mandatory [10,41]. Randomized trials of therapeutics are needed to determine the most efficacious strategies for SLE-associated DAH for better management of this life-threatening complication.

3.2. Chronic Diseases

Chronic interstitial lung disease (ILD) in SLE seems to be less frequent in comparison to other connective tissue diseases (CTDs), and it is rarely severe [10,48–50]. The exact prevalence is probably underestimated, because older studies performing chest X-ray have shown the presence of ILD in 6–24% of SLE patients, while in those using a more sensitive method such as HRCT, ILD was found in up to 70% of cases, suggesting that the condition is frequently subclinical [10,49,51]. Risk factors for ILD include older age, late-onset SLE, illness duration ($\geq$1 year), tachypnea, low levels of anti-dsDNA, high level of C3 and male gender [48–52]. The presence of Raynaud's phenomenon, swollen fingers, sclerodactyly, telangiectasia, nailfold capillary abnormalities among SLE patients was associated with a higher prevalence of restrictive deficit and reduced DLCO, probably in the context of overlap syndromes that seem to carry a worse lung prognosis. Some associations were found with anti-U1 RNP, anti-SSB, anti-Scl70 and anti-SSA antibodies and sicca syndrome [10,49–53].

The most common pattern, histologically and radiologically, is non-specific interstitial pneumonia (NSIP); however, usual interstitial pneumonia (UIP) is not uncommon [52]. Lian et al. reported that the most frequent findings were ground glass opacities (84.4%), followed by consolidation (21.1%), honeycombing (15.6%), and traction bronchiectasis (12.8%) [53].

Clinically, ILD can evolve as a consequence a disease with acute onset (ALP or DAH) or follow a more insidious onset with chronic non-productive cough, exertional dyspnea and non-pleuritic chest pain. The mean age of onset is earlier when following an acute condition (mean 38 years) compared to the chronic form (46 years). Patients with a radiologically documented ILD can also be asymptomatic [10,51]. Inspiratory fine crackles may be heard upon physical examination, while the presence of digital clubbing is rare. Pulmonary function tests can show a restrictive pattern with reduced DLCO [10]. The severity of ILD does not correlate with SLE serologic markers [49].

Prognosis for SLE-associated ILD seems more favorable when compared to idiopathic pulmonary fibrosis or RA-associated ILD [50,52,54,55]. Toyoda et al. found a five-year survival rates of 92.9% calculated from the time ILD was diagnosed and the survival rate did not significantly differ between the patients with and without ILD [52].

Lymphocytic interstitial pneumonia (LIP) can complicate many autoimmune conditions and has been described in SLE patients in particular when associated with Sjögren's Syndrome. LIP is characterized by the formation of lung cysts, an infiltration of the interstitium with polyclonal lymphocytes and lymphocytic alveolitis [10,49,56,57]. Prognosis is variable. Approximately 50–60% of patients respond to corticosteroids with stabilization or improvement of the disease, but in others there is progressive decline in pulmonary function and development of honeycomb lung. In general, death occurs in approximately 33 to 50% of patients within 5 years of diagnosis [56,57].

Organizing pneumonia (OP) has also been described as initial manifestation of SLE and regardless of SLE activity [10,49,58–60]. On HRCT, OP shows ground glass opacities, consolidations and peribronchovascular opacities. OP has also been described in rhupus syndrome [61]. CS are the treatment of choice. In the majority of cases patients recover within days of weeks after treatment introduction and radiographic findings show improvement in 50–86% of patients. Spontaneous resolution may occur. However, in a minority of cases, the disease may persist, and up to 30% may have a relapse after treatment withdrawal [62]. Several immunosuppressant agents, such as azathioprine, MMF, cyclosporin, CYC and plasmapheresis, have been used in various case reports. [58–62]. Finally, an association between SLE and pulmonary sarcoidosis has been described [10,63–66]. According to Rajoriya N et al., patients with sarcoidosis have an OR of 8.33 (2.71 to 19.4) for the development of SLE [64].

Placebo-controlled trials to guide the treatment of SLE-associated ILD are lacking. CS are, generally, the mainstay of treatment and patients usually show a good response. Immunosuppressants such as CYC, azathioprine, or MMF can be added in refractory more severe cases [10,23]. Among biologics, RTX can be used in some cases [67].

Treatments are generally well tolerated; with CYC, immuno- and myelosuppression, as well as IgG levels decreased can occur with subsequent infections that are generally non-life-threatening and do not necessitate stopping treatment [68,69]. In particular, in the study of Okada et al., only two sessions of CYC infusions among a total of 141 were postponed because of upper respiratory infections [69]. Interestingly, cumulative data show a higher frequency of adverse events, including hemorrhagic cystitis, premature ovarian failure, herpes zoster and cancer, with the oral administration, in comparison with pulse intravenous infusion of CYC, as found in the lupus nephritis [68–70]. Concerning the use of MMF in SLE-ILD, only one of ten patients with CTD-ILD had a diagnosis of SLE in the case series by Saketkoo et al. [71], while Fisher et al. included four patients with SLE-ILD in their retrospective study [72]. The most common side effects reported in these studies were diarrhea and leucopenia.

4. Vascular Diseases

4.1. Acute Reversible Hypoxemia Syndrome

First described in 1991 by Abramson [73], acute reversible hypoxemia syndrome is characterized by the acute onset of dyspnea, chest pain and hypoxemia. Pleural involvement may be present. It is frequently associated with a flare of SLE. Pulmonary imaging is generally normal, while PFTs may show reduction in vital capacity and DLCO [17,51]. Pathophysiology is not completely understood. An association between endothelium activation, with a high expression of vascular adhesion cell molecule-1 (VACM-1) and intercellular adhesion molecule-1(ICAM-1), and activated neutrophil and platelet sludging mediated by complement activation has been postulated as a pathogenic mechanism. These alterations can ultimately lead to endothelial dysfunction, vascular lumen occlusion by leukocyte aggregates and subsequent hypoxemia [17,51,73,74].

This condition rapidly responds to low doses of CS, usually insufficient to control SLE flares, when present together, so higher doses may be needed. Combination of high doses of aspirin can be useful [17,51], and most cases respond to therapy with rapid improvement of gas exchanges [9].

4.2. Pulmonary Embolism

SLE patients are at increased risk of developing deep vein thrombosis (DVT), occurring in up to 10% of patients [75], and pulmonary embolism (PE) with a 3-fold increased risk in comparison to general population [76]. Vein thromboembolism (VTE) represents the third most common cardiovascular (CV) event after myocardial infarction and stroke [77,78]. PE has a high mortality rate of up to 15%. Many risk factors have been investigated besides "classical" risk factors such as obesity, hyperglycemia and hyperlipidemia [77]. Moreover, You et al. found the following risk factors associated with PE: high body max index, hypoalbuminemia, positivity for anti-phospolipid antibodies (aPL), high levels of high sensitivity CRP and high doses of CS (>0.5 mg/kg/day) [78]. Finally, SLE patients with APS are at increased risk of DVT and PE. The prevalence of APS among SLE patients is about 30% [79].

APS can cause a hypercoagulable state by interacting and activating platelets, neutrophils and endothelial cells [78]. In particular, a metanalysis found that SLE patients with APS have a six times greater risk of developing PE than SLE patients without APS [79]. Moreover, patients with the positivity for lupus anticoagulant (LA) and high titers of IgG anti-cardiolipin (aCL) are at increased risk [80,81].

Clinical manifestations depend on the severity of vasculature occlusion, ranging from asymptomatic small vessels occlusion to massive PE with sudden right ventricular failure and acute circulatory collapse. Other symptoms of PE include pleuritic chest pain, dyspnea, hemoptysis, crepitations, tachypnea and tachycardia. Chronic PE can progress to secondary pulmonary arterial hypertension (PAH) due to the reduction of pulmonary vascular tree [49]. In addition to PAH, other non-thrombotic intrathoracic manifestations of APS associated with SLE are: DAH, adult respiratory distress syndrome (ARDS) and valvular heart disease (e.g., Libman-Sacks endocarditis) [49,82]. A rare, potentially fatal, manifestation of APS is the catastrophic APS (CAPS). CAPS is characterized by the diffuse occlusion of small vessels in three or more organs [81–85]. It generally develops in APS patients in association with a trigger such as infections, neoplasm or surgery. Respiratory failure is often present and can rapidly progress to acute respiratory distress syndrome (ARDS) [81–85].

Treatment of APS includes anticoagulation with the vitamin K antagonists (VKA), to maintain an international normalized ratio (INR) range of 2.0 to 3.0, for a definite period in a first provoked episode, indefinitely in recurrent episodes or in patients with a high-risk profile [81,85]. In patients with recurrent arterial or venous thrombosis, a higher INR range 3.0–4.0 or the addition on low dose aspirin should be considered. Common CV risk factors should be corrected, concurrently. In high-risk anti-phospholipid antibodies (aPL) carriers without history of thrombosis, prophylactic treatment with low dose aspirin can be adopted [81,85]. Hydroxychloroquine may reduce thrombotic risk both in APS and non-APS SLE patients due to its pleiotropic effects but evidence in this regard is still scarce [78,85]. Treatment of CAPS includes: elimination of triggers (e.g., infections), combination therapy with heparin, glucocorticoids and plasma exchange or intravenous immunoglobulins. B-cell depletion (e.g., RTX) or complement inhibition (e.g., eculizumab) can be considered in refractory cases. Supportive treatments in the intensive care unit may be necessary [81,85]. Recent systematic literature reviews and meta-analyses investigating direct oral anticoagulants have recommended against their use in these patients [86,87].

4.3. Pulmonary Arterial Hypertension

Pulmonary hypertension (PH) is classified into five major categories, according to its clinical characteristics and etiology and pulmonary arterial hypertension (PAH) associated with connective tissue diseases (CTDs) belongs to the first group and it is the second most frequent form after idiopathic PAH [88,89]. PAH is defined by the presence of an increase in mean pulmonary arterial pressure (mPAP) $\geq$ 25mmHg at rest (assessed by right heart catheterization (RHC)) with a normal pulmonary capillary wedge pressure ($\leq$15 mmHg) and increased pulmonary vascular resistance (PVR) > 3 wood units (WU) [73]. Less frequently, SLE patients can present PH secondary to chronic pulmonary thromboembolism (group 4), mitral stenosis due to Libman-Sacks endocarditis (group 2), pulmonary veno-occlusive disease (group 1), ILD-associated PH (group 3) [88–92].

According to the REVEAL registry (Registry to Evaluate Early and Long-term Pulmonary Arterial Hypertension disease management), SLE patients display the second highest prevalence of PAH after systemic sclerosis (SSc) [93,94]. The real prevalence of PAH among SLE patients is unknown. Past studies have reported different results due to the method used for diagnosis (right heart catheterization (RHC) versus transthoracic echocardiography (TTE)) and the cut-off value used for the diagnosis [94]. The majority of patients are women with a mean age at PAH diagnosis of about 45 years, and with its prevalence and severity increasing with time from SLE onset. PAH can occasionally be the first manifestation of SLE. Usually, PAH tends to be moderate with systolic PAP of 40–60 mmHg and PVR between 5 and 15 WU [93–95]. Some possible risk factors for PAH are Raynaud's phenomenon, active renal disease, vasculitic manifestations, pleuritis, pericardial effusion, ILD, SLEDAI $\leq$9, lack of rash, low erythrocyte sedimentation rate (ESR) $\leq$ 20 mm/h. Among immunological parameters associated with PAH: aPL, Anti-U1-RNP and anti-SSA/Ro have been described [94]. The pathogenesis of SLE-PAH is probably multifactorial and is not completely understood. Multiple factors such as genetic predisposition, environmental stimuli and immune system dysfunction could lead to an imbalance between vasoconstrictor and vasodilator mediators resulting in an increase in PVR [94,96]. aPL, anti-endothelial cells and anti-endothelin receptor antibodies, vasculitis, vasospasm, inflammation, decreased oxygen saturation, apoptosis and smooth muscle cell proliferation contribute to the development of the typical lesions of idiopathic PAH, such as plexiform lesions, smooth muscle cell hypertrophy, intimal proliferation, and collagen deposition [94,96]. Moreover, in SLE-associated PAH, there is an involvement of pulmonary veins and perivascular inflammatory infiltration [94,96,97].

Clinical presentation is non-specific, progressive and related to right ventricle dysfunction and includes dyspnea, dry cough, fatigue, weakness, exercise intolerance, angina, syncope, and hemoptysis; hoarseness due to recurrent laryngeal nerve compression, wheeze caused by large airway compression, and exercise-induced vomiting can be present in advanced cases. Symptoms are initially exercise-related, but in advanced cases occur at rest. With progression of right ventricle failure, lower limb edema, liver enlargement, abdominal distention and ascites may develop. Exceptionally, severe dilatation of pulmonary artery may complicate with its rupture or dissection leading to a cardiac tamponade. Physical findings may include: accentuated pulmonary component of the second heart sound, left parasternal lift, right ventricle third sound, murmurs indicative of tricuspid and/or pulmonary regurgitation, wheeze, and crackles; elevated jugular pressure may be present in advanced cases [88,94]. The gold standard for the diagnosis is RHC that can show some rough etiologic characterization. TTE is a non-invasive and low-cost method for the screening and follow-up of PAH patients. Other ancillary investigations may be used, such as HRCT of the lungs for the diagnosis of ILD, ventilation/perfusion scintigraphy for the assessment of chronic thromboembolism, pulmonary function tests that may show an isolated reduction of DLCO [88,94].

Early aggressive treatment aimed at normalizing PAP can improve survival. Vasodilators (e.g prostacyclin analogues), endothelin receptor antagonists (ERAs) (e.g., bosentan), phosphodiesterase 5 inhibitors (PDE-5Is) (e.g., sildenafil), guanylate cyclase stimulants (e.g., riociguat), prostacyclin IP receptor agonist (e.g., selexipag) and calcium channel blockers (CCB) (in those with a positive response to acute vasodilator testing) have shown good results. In more severe and/or refractory forms a combination with two or more different classes of drugs can be considered [49,88,94,98–105].

Side effects are in part shared by vasodilators agents. Limiting factors for CCB dose increasing are generally lower limb peripheral oedema and systemic hypotension. In the group of ERAs, ambrisentan and bosentan are associated with abnormal liver function tests (in the 0.8–3% for the former and in the 10% for the latter) with ambrisentan also associated with peripheral oedema [88,100,103]. Macitentan is not associated with liver toxicity, but a reduction in hemoglobin levels ≤8 g/dL was observed in 4.3% of patients in the study of Pulido et al. [88,106]. PDE-5Is side effects are mainly related to vasodilation such as headache, flushing and epistaxis and are mild to moderate [88]. The most frequent adverse events with riociguat were hypotension, dizziness, peripheral oedema, vomiting and anemia [105]. With beraprost the most adverse events (common with other prostanoids) are headache, flushing, jaw pain and diarrhea [88], while epoprostenol also carries the risk of a long-term intravenous catheter [88,102,104]. According to the GRIPHON study, most frequent adverse events with the use of selexipag are similar with therapies that target the prostacycline pathway (e.g., headache, diarrhea, nausea, dizziness) and are more frequent during the titration period [98].

Some studies have reported a beneficial effect of immunosuppressive therapy in SLE-associated PAH. Among immunosuppressants, CYC +/− glucocorticoids showed good response; other small studies evaluated RTX, MMF and cyclosporine. Immunosuppressants can be combined with vasoactive agents in more severe forms. Supportive treatments such as diuretics, anticoagulants and oxygen may be beneficial [88,94,107–110].

PAH affects quality of life and survival of SLE patients. Data from REVEAL registry reveal that CTD-associated PAH has a worse prognosis compared to idiopathic PAH; however, among CTDs-associated PAH, SLE patients seem to have a better prognosis, with a 1-year survival rate of 94% vs. 82% of SSc [93,94,111]. Cardiac failure and arrhythmias are the most frequent causes of death in patients with SLE-PAH [9,94].

5. Pleural Disease

Pleuritis is the most frequent lung manifestation in patients with SLE, occurring, often in association with pericarditis, in about 40–60% of patients during the course of the disease, although in autoptic studies up to 83% of patients can show signs of pleural involvement [10,112]. Of note, it is the only SLE manifestation of the respiratory system included in the diagnostic criteria [5]. Pleuritis, with or without pleural effusion, can be the first manifestation of SLE in the 3% and 1% of SLE patients, respectively [113,114]. Pleural involvement can be present also in overlap syndromes like rhupus syndrome [115]. The clinical picture can vary from asymptomatic, incidental findings on imaging, to pleuritic chest pain that is increased with deep inspiration, dyspnea, dry cough, fever and other systemic manifestations. Pleural effusion can be uni- or bilateral, usually mild to moderate, rarely massive. Occasionally pleuritis can be dry [10,49]. Pathogenesis of pleural effusion is thought to be due to ICs deposition on pleural surfaces. Histopathologic studies have shown the presence of a non-specific lymphoplasmacytic infiltration with rare evidence of IC-mediated vasculitis [115]. Pleuritic fluid is sterile, exudative, and yellow-tinged, but occasionally it can be turbidous or seroematic. It contains inflammatory cells such as neutrophils, but it can show a predominance of mononuclear lymphocytic cells, especially in longstanding cases. It also contains glucose levels similar to those of plasma (60–95 mg/dL), increased levels of adenosine deaminase, decreased levels of complement and ANA, in particular with titer $\geq$ 1:160. It has a greater pH (>7.35) and lower lactate dehydrogenase (LDH) levels (<500 IU/L or <2 times upper limit of normal for serum) than in patients with RA or tuberculosis. LE cells can be seen showing a low sensibility (about 40%) and a specificity of 80%. However, none of these characteristics are specific to SLE pleuritis [10,49,113,115–117]. Differential diagnosis may be difficult, since SLE patients can have pleural effusions for many reasons including infections, renal and cardiac failure, pulmonary embolism, and rarely malignancies. It is interesting to note that in SLE pleuritis CRP can be elevated also in the absence of infections [116]. Pleural biopsy can occasionally be necessary, only to rule out tuberculosis or malignancy [116]. Prognosis is usually favorable, with a good and rapid response to CS at medium dosage, although development of progressive pleural fibrosis leading to fibrothorax has been described. Non-steroidal anti-inflammatory drugs (NSAIDs) can be used for milder cases and spontaneous resolution can also occur. In more severe cases CS can be used (in patients already on steroid therapy an increase of dosages may be needed). In chronic forms, hydroxychloroquine can be used as a glucocorticoid-sparing agent. Major immunosuppressants (e.g., CYC and azathioprine) are not used, unless in the case of a concomitant systemic involvement. An association of IVIg and cyclosporine has been used in chronic, refractory pleural effusion. Chest drainage, pleurodesis and/or pleurectomy are rarely necessary in severe refractory cases [51,113,117–119].

6. Infections

SLE patients are at high risk of severe infections, by either common or opportunistic pathogens, the majority of which are lung infections, but also urinary tract, soft tissue and skin. Bacteria are the most commonly implicated agents, followed by viruses and fungi [120]. In the EuroLupus cohort, 36% of patients developed an infection and about 30% of deaths were related to infections in the five-year follow-up [121]. In addition, SLE patients have a higher incidence of respiratory failure and a high mortality rate for the ones admitted to the intensive care unit (ICU) with pneumonia as the most common cause of death. It is estimated that up to half of SLE patients develop major infections during the course of the disease [121–123].

Different causes accounting for this increased risk have been postulated. A genetic, non-Mendelian predisposition has been hypothesized, since the risk for severe infections seems to be increased prior to the development of SLE and a great number of genetic polymorphisms have been studied. Immunologic dysfunctions can involve both adaptive and innate immunity, in particular: complement deficiency, Ig deficiency, functional asplenia, altered cytokine production, impaired chemotaxis and phagocytosis are the major alterations thought to be involved [97,120–124]. SLE patients can present underlying structural alterations in the respiratory tract, such as respiratory muscle weakness, parenchymal disease, bronchiectasis, atelectasis with impaired local mucociliary clearance and defense against infections [97,120–124].

Immunosuppressants are well known risk factors for infections, both traditional (e.g., CYC, azathioprine) and new biologic agents (e.g., RTX and belimumab). CS are an often-underestimated cause of immunosuppression, especially when used in long term courses (>3 weeks), at relatively high dosage and in association with other immunosuppressants. On the contrary, antimalarials seem to have a protective role against infections both by allowing the reduction of CS dosage and by exerting a direct antimicrobial activity. It is also interesting to note that the risk of infections parallels disease activity [120].

Many pathogens can cause infections in SLE patients: Streptococcus pneumoniae is the most frequent cause of respiratory tract infections. Along with Salmonella, it is also associated with bacteriemia in the context of functional asplenia. Among fungal pathogens, Pneumocystis jiroveci, Criptococcus neoformans, Candida albicans, Aspergillus have been identified in SLE patients. Viral infections have been reported in particular with cytomegalovirus and varicella zoster virus, often in the context of a disseminated infection. SLE patients are also at increased risk for tuberculosis and infections with non-tuberculous mycobacteria [120–126]. Protozoa infections, also with rare pathogens such as Lophomonas blattarum, have been reported [127].

Diagnostic workup for infections in SLE patients may be challenging; infections can have an atypical course due to immunosuppression, moreover lung infections can simulate a lupus flare. In this context, infections must be always ruled out in a SLE patient with lung complaints and/or the appearance of a new infiltrate prior to increase the immunosuppressive therapy. Bronchoscopy with BALF analysis may be very useful for the isolation of pathogens and start of a targeted therapy [120,122]. A reduction of the immunosuppressive therapy for a short period may be necessary in severe cases during antimicrobial therapy in order to improve the immune response.

Prevention of infections can be adopted with seasonal influenza and pneumococcal vaccination and with Pneumocystis jirovecii prophylaxis in at risk patients [128–130].

7. Miscellanea

Shrinking Lung Syndrome

Shrinking lung syndrome (SLS) is a rare manifestation of SLE affecting less than 1% of SLE patients [131], with about 100 cases described to date [132]. Older papers reported a higher prevalence of 18–27%, while a prevalence of up to 7% has been described among patients with refractory SLE [132–134]. It was described for the first time in 1965 by Hoffbrand and Beck [135], and subsequently it has occasionally been described in other autoimmune diseases (e.g., systemic sclerosis, primary Sjögren's syndrome, RA and undifferentiated arthritis) [136,137]. It is characterized by progressive exertional dyspnea, pleuritic chest pain and, less frequently, cough. It can be observed in every phase of the disease but usually it occurs in long standing disease, often as the only main organ involvement of SLE, with women more often affected than men. There is no correlation with SLE activity. Physical findings are often normal, sometimes bibasilar rales can be heard. Chest X-rays show reduced lung volumes, elevated hemidiaphragms (also monolateral) and less commonly basilar atelectasis due to poor chest expansion, pleural effusions and pleural thickening. CT scan is usually negative for parenchymal disease. Ultrasound and fluoroscopy have been proposed to study diaphragm mobility. PFTs show a restrictive pattern (reduced forced expiratory volume in the 1st second, forced vital capacity and total lung capacity) with a deterioration compared to previous tests, while carbon monoxide transfer corrected for lung volume (KCO) is normal. Echocardiography does not show any signs of PAH. No specific association was found between serologic markers and the disease, it was suggested an association with Anti-Ro/SSA. Since there are no specific diagnostic criteria, the diagnosis is one of exclusion [131,132,138–141]. The pathogenesis of this condition is not known, and several mechanisms have been proposed in recent years: micro-atelectasis with surfactant deficiency, phrenic nerve neuropathy, primary respiratory muscle myopathy, diaphragmatic fibrosis, steroid induced myopathy, pleural adhesions, and pleuritic chest pain with reduced chest expansion by an inhibitory reflex [135,140,142–145].

The majority of patients received high dose of CS, even with iv pulses, with improvement occurring in several weeks, but in some cases even in 48 h [140,141]; anecdotal data support the use of immunosuppressive agents such CYC, azathioprine, methotrexate, MMF after CS failure or as CS-sparing agents [132,139,141]. RTX has been shown to improve lung function and pain in some cases [146]. Choudhury et al. reported improvement of one patient treated with belimumab [132]. Theophylline has shown to improve diaphragmatic strength and improve PFT [147], beta-agonists could reduce diaphragmatic fatigue thanks to their positive inotropic effect [148], theophylline and beta agonists may be more efficacious if combined with CS [141]. An improvement in PFT after hematopoietic stem cells transplantation has also been described [149]. Physiotherapy could be useful to improve lung volumes and prevent impaired chest wall expansion, but it could be limited by pain [141]. Antalgic agents may be considered in the initial phase [140], while in severe respiratory weakness ICU admission and mechanical ventilation may be required [141]. Prognosis seems favorable, with a rapid improvement of symptoms, and progressive improvement, stabilization or only minor deterioration of PFTs, although full recovery is rare. Pain can persist for a long time, despite improvement in PFT. Death, due to respiratory failure is unusual [133,140,141]. In this regard, an early diagnosis and an appropriate treatment is mandatory.

8. Conclusions

SLE can affect any part of the respiratory tract, with various degrees of severity and at any phase of the disease course. Respiratory manifestations may display acute and/or chronic course and since most respiratory signs and symptoms are non-specific, differential diagnosis is often challenging. However, the early recognition and management of SLE-related respiratory manifestations is essential to prevent complications and the worsening of disease prognosis.

Author Contributions: Writing—Original Draft Preparation, S.D.B.; Writing—Review & Editing A.A.; Writing—Review & Editing F.C. All authors have read and agreed to the published version of the manuscript.

Funding: This research received no external funding.

Data Availability Statement: No new data were created or analyzed in this study. Data sharing is not applicable to this article.

Conflicts of Interest: The authors declare no conflict of interest.

References

1. Stojan, G.; Petri, M. Epidemiology of Systemic Lupus Erythematosus: An update. *Curr. Opin. Rheumatol.* **2018**, *30*, 144–150. [CrossRef] [PubMed]
2. Zucchi, D.; Elefante, E.; Calabresi, E.; Signorini, V.; Bortoluzzi, A.; Tani, C. One year in review 2019: Systemic lupus erythematosus. *Clin. Exp. Rheumatol.* **2019**, *37*, 715–722.

3. Cervera, R.; Doria, A.; Amoura, Z.; Khamashta, M.; Schneider, M.; Guillemin, F.; Maurel, F.; Garofano, A.; Roset, M.; Perna, A.; et al. Patterns of systemic lupus erythematosus expression in Europe. *Autoimmun. Rev.* **2014**, *13*, 621–629. [CrossRef] [PubMed]
4. Lisnevskaia, L.; Murphy, G.; Isenberg, D. Systemic lupus erythematosus. *Lancet* **2014**, *384*, 1878–1888. [CrossRef]
5. Aringer, M.; Costenbader, K.; Daikh, D.; Brinks, R.; Mosca, M.; Ramsey-Goldman, R.; Smolen, J.S.; Wofsy, D.; Boumpas, D.T.; Kamen, D.L.; et al. 2019 European League Against Rheumatism/American College of Rheumatology classification criteria for systemic lupus erythematosus. *Ann. Rheum. Dis.* **2019**, *78*, 1151–1159. [CrossRef]
6. Fanouriakis, A.; Kostopoulou, M.; Alunno, A.; Aringer, M.; Bajema, I.; Boletis, J.N.; Cervera, R.; Doria, A.; Gordon, C.; Govoniet, M.; et al. 2019 update of the EULAR recommendations for the management of systemic lupus erythematosus. *Ann. Rheum Dis.* **2019**, *78*, 736–745. [CrossRef] [PubMed]
7. Kostopoulou, M.; Fanouriakis, A.; Cheema, K.; Boletis, J.; Bertsias, G.; Jayne, D.; Boumpas, D.T. Management of lupus nephritis: A systematic literature review informing the 2019 update of the joint EULAR and European Renal Association-European Dialysis and Transplant Association (EULAR/ERA-EDTA) recommendations. *RMD Open.* **2020**, *6*, e001263. [CrossRef]
8. Al-Adhoubi, N.K.; Bystrom, J. Systemic lupus erythematosus and diffuse alveolar hemorrhage, etiology and novel treatment strategies. *Lupus* **2020**, *29*, 355–363. [CrossRef]
9. Pego-Reigosa, J.M.; Medeiros, D.A.; Isenberg, D.A. Respiratory manifestations of systemic lupus erythematosus: Old and new concepts. *Best Pract. Res. Clin. Rheumatol.* **2009**, *23*, 469–480. [CrossRef]
10. Torre, O.; Harari, S. Pleural and pulmonary involvement in systemic lupus erythematosus. *Presse Med.* **2011**, *40 Pt 2*, e19–e29. [CrossRef]
11. Fidler, L.; Keen, K.J.; Touma, Z.; Mittoo, S. Impact of pulmonary disease on patient-reported outcomes and patient-performed functional testing in systemic lupus erythematosus. *Lupus* **2016**, *25*, 1004–1011. [CrossRef]
12. Gasparyan, A.Y.; Ayvazyan, L.; Blackmore, H.; Kitas, G.D. Writing a narrative biomedical review: Considerations for authors, peer reviewers, and editors. *Rheumatol. Int.* **2011**, *31*, 1409–1417. [CrossRef]
13. Karim, A.; Ahmed, S.; Siddiqui, R.; Marder, G.S.; Mattana, J. Severe Upper Airway Obstruction from Cricoarytenoiditis as the Sole Presenting Manifestation of a Systemic Lupus Erythematosus Flare. *Chest* **2002**, *121*, 990–993. [CrossRef] [PubMed]
14. Schwartz, I.S.; Grishman, E. Rheumatoid Nodules of the Vocal Cords as the Initial Manifestation of Systemic Lupus Erythematosus. *JAMA* **1980**, *244*, 2751–2752. [CrossRef] [PubMed]
15. Teitel, A.D.; MacKenzie, C.R.; Stern, R.; Paget, S.A. Laryngeal involvement in systemic lupus erythematosus. *Semin. Arthritis Rheum.* **1992**, *22*, 203–214. [CrossRef]
16. Malinvaud, D.; Mukundan, S.; Crevier-Buchman, L.; Bonfils, P.; Laccourreye, O. Glottic Bamboo Nodules from Systemic Lupus Erythematosus. *Ann. Otol. Rhinol. Laryngol.* **2013**, *122*, 496–499. [CrossRef] [PubMed]
17. Carmiera, D.; Marchand-Adam, S.; Diot, P.; Diot, E. Respiratory involvement in systemic lupus erythematosus. *Rev. Mal. Respir.* **2010**, *27*, e66–e78. [CrossRef]
18. Luo, Y.; Fan, X.; Jiang, C.; Ramos-Rodriguez, A.; Wen, Y.; Zhang, J.; Huang, F.; Guan, X.; Xu, J. Systemic Lupus Erythematosus and Angioedema: A Cross-Sectional Study From the National Inpatient Sample. *Arch. Rheumatol.* **2019**, *34*, 301–307. [CrossRef] [PubMed]
19. Kumar, N.; Surendran, D.; Bammigatti, C. Angioedema as the presenting feature of systemic lupus erythematosus. *BMJ Case Rep.* **2018**, *2018*, bcr2018224222. [CrossRef] [PubMed]
20. Todic, J.; Leuchter, I. Lupus of the larynx: When bamboo nodes lead to diagnosis. *BMJ Case Rep.* **2018**. [CrossRef] [PubMed]
21. Lee, J.H.; Sung, I.Y.; Park, J.H.; Roh, J.L. Recurrent laryngeal neuropathy in a systemic lupus erythematosus (SLE) patient. *Am. J. Phys. Med. Rehabil.* **2008**, *87*, 68–70. [CrossRef]
22. Andonopoulos, A.P.; Constantopoulos, S.H.; Galanopoulou, V.; Drosos, A.A.; Acritidis, N.C.; Moutsopoulos, H.M. Pulmonary function of nonsmoking patients with systemic lupus rythematosus. *Chest* **1988**, *94*, 312–315. [CrossRef]
23. Gari, A.G.; Telmesani, A.; Alwithenani, R. Pulmonary Manifestations of Systemic Lupus Erythematosus. In *Systemic Lupus Erythematosus*; InTech: London, UK, 2012.
24. Cantero, C.; Vongthilath, R.; Plojoux, J. Acute lupus pneumonitis as the initial presentation of systemic lupus erythematosus. *BMJ Case Rep.* **2020**, *13*, e234638. [CrossRef]
25. Chattopadhyay, B.; Chatterjee, A.; Maiti, A.; Debnath, N.B. Systemic lupus erythematosus presenting as acute lupus pneumonitis in a young female. *J. Postgrad. Med.* **2015**, *61*, 129–130. [CrossRef] [PubMed]
26. Comer, M.; D'Cruz, D.; Thompson, I.; Erskine, K.; Dacre, J. Pneumonitis in a lupus twin pregnancy: A case report. *Lupus* **1996**, *5*, 146–148. [CrossRef] [PubMed]
27. Witt, C.; Dorner, T.; Hiepe, F.; Borges, A.C.; Fietze, I.; Baumann, G. Diagnosis of alveolitis in interstitial lung manifestation in connective tissue diseases: Importance of late inspiratory crackles, 67 gallium scan and bronchoalveolar lavage. *Lupus* **1996**, *5*, 606–612. [CrossRef] [PubMed]
28. Matthay, R.A.; Schwarz, M.I.; Petty, T.L.; Stanford, R.E.; Gupta, R.C.; Sahn, S.A.; Steigerwald, J.C. Pulmonary manifestations of systemic lupus erythematosus: Review of twelve cases of acute lupus pneumonitis. *Medicine* **1975**, *54*, 397–409. [CrossRef] [PubMed]
29. Wan, S.A.; The, C.L.; Jobli, A.T. Lupus pneumonitis as the initial presentation of systemic lupus erythematosus: Case series from a single institution. *Lupus* **2016**, *25*, 1485–1490. [CrossRef]

30. Cheema, G.S.; Quismorio, F.P., Jr. Interstitial lung disease in systemic lupus Erythematosus. *Curr. Opin. Pulm. Med.* **2000**, *6*, 424–429. [CrossRef] [PubMed]
31. Boulware, D.W.; Hedgpeth, M.T. Lupus pneumonitis and anti-SSA(Ro) antibodies. *J. Rheumatol.* **1989**, *16*, 479–481.
32. Osler, W. On the visceral manifestations of the erythema group of skin diseases [Third Paper] 1904. *Am. J. Med. Sci.* **2009**, *338*, 396–408. [CrossRef] [PubMed]
33. Lara, A.R.; Schwarz, M.I. Diffuse Alveolar Hemorrhage. *Chest* **2010**, *137*, 1164–1171. [CrossRef] [PubMed]
34. Quartuccio, L.; Bond, M.; Isola, M.; Monti, S.; Felicetti, M.; Furini, F.; Murgia, S.; Berti, A.; Silvestri, E.; Pazzola, G.; et al. Alveolar haemorrhage in ANCA-associated vasculitis: Long-term outcome and mortality predictors. *J. Autoimmun.* **2020**, *108*, 102397. [CrossRef] [PubMed]
35. Andrade, C.; Mendonca, T.; Farinha, F.; Correia, J.; Marinho, A.; Almeida, I.; Vasconcelos, C. Alveolar hemorrhage in systemic lupus erythematosus: A cohort review. *Lupus* **2016**, *25*, 75–80. [CrossRef]
36. Morales-Nebreda, L.; Alakija, O.; Ferguson, K.T.; Singer, B.D. Systemic lupus erythematosus-associated diffuse alveolar hemorrhage: A case report and review of the literature. *Clin. Pulm. Med.* **2018**, *25*, 166–169. [CrossRef]
37. Zamora, M.R.; Warner, M.L.; Tuder, R.; Schwarz, M.I. Diffuse alveolar hemorrhage and systemic lupus erythematosus. Clinical presentation, histology, survival, and outcome. *Medicine* **1997**, *76*, 192–202. [CrossRef] [PubMed]
38. Rojas-Serrano, J.; Pedroza, J.; Regalado, J.; Robledo, J.; Reyes, E.; Sifuentes-Osornio, J.; Flores-Suárez, L.F. High prevalence of infections in patients with systemic lupus erythematosus and pulmonary haemorrhage. *Lupus* **2008**, *17*, 295–299. [CrossRef]
39. Ewan, P.W.; Jones, H.A.; Rhodes, C.G.; Hughes, J.M. Detection of intrapulmonary hemorrhage with carbon monoxide uptake. Application in Goodpasture's syndrome. *N. Engl. J. Med.* **1976**, *295*, 1391–1396. [CrossRef]
40. Sun, Y.; Zhou, C.; Zhao, J.; Wang, Q.; Xu, D.; Zhang, S.; Shen, M.; Hou, Y.; Tian, X.; Li, M.; et al. Systemic lupus erythematosus-associated diffuse alveolar hemorrhage: A single-center, matched case-control study in China. *Lupus* **2020**, *29*, 795–803. [CrossRef]
41. Jiang, M.; Chen, R.; Zhao, L.; Zhang, X. Risk factors for mortality of diffuse alveolar hemorrhage in systemic lupus erythematosus: A systematic review and meta-analysis. *Arthritis Res. Ther.* **2021**, *23*, 57. [CrossRef]
42. Tse, J.R.; Schwab, K.E.; McMahon, M.; Simon, W. Rituximab: An emerging treatment for recurrent diffuse alveolar hemorrhage in systemic lupus erythematosus. *Lupus* **2015**, *24*, 756–759. [CrossRef]
43. Wang, C.R.; Liu, M.F.; Weng, C.T.; Lin, W.C.; Li, W.T.; Tsa, H.W. Systemic lupus erythematosus-associated diffuse alveolar haemorrhage: A single-centre experience in Han Chinese patients. *Scand. J. Rheumatol.* **2018**, *47*, 392–399. [CrossRef]
44. Aakjæra, S.; Bendstrupa, E.; Ivarsenb, P.; Madsenc, L.B. Continous Rituximab treatment for recurrent diffuse alveolar hemorrhage in a patient with systemic lupus erythematosus and antiphosholipid syndrome. *Respir. Med. Case Rep.* **2017**, *22*, 263–265. [CrossRef]
45. Na, J.O.; Chang, S.H.; Seo, K.H.; Choi, J.S.; Lee, H.S.; Lyu, J.W.; Nah, S.S. Successful Early Rituximab Treatment in a Case of Systemic Lupus Erythematosus with Potentially Fatal Diffuse Alveolar Hemorrhage. *Respiration* **2015**, *89*, 62–65. [CrossRef]
46. Narshi, C.B.; Haider, S.; Ford, C.M.; Isenberg, D.A.; Giles, I.P. Rituximab as early therapy for pulmonary haemorrhage in systemic lupus erythematosus. *Rheumatology* **2010**, *49*, 392–394. [CrossRef] [PubMed]
47. Henriksson, M.M.; Newman, E.; Witt, V.; Derfler, K.; Leitner, G.; Eloot, S.; Dhondt, A.; Deeren, D.; Rock, G.; Ptak, J.; et al. Review Adverse events in apheresis: An update of the WAA registry data. *Transfus. Apher. Sci.* **2016**, *54*, 2–15. [CrossRef] [PubMed]
48. Chen, Y.; Wang, Y.; Chen, X.; Liang, H.; Yang, X. Association of Interstitial Lung Disease with Clinical Characteristics of Chinese Patients with Systemic Lupus Erythematosus. *Arch. Rheumatol.* **2020**, *35*, 239–246. [CrossRef] [PubMed]
49. Tselios, K.; Urowitz, M.B. Cardiovascular and Pulmonary Manifestations of Systemic Lupus Erythematosus. *Cur. Rheumatol. Rev.* **2017**, *13*, 206–218. [CrossRef]
50. Alunno, A.; Gerli, R.; Giacomelli, R.; Carubbi, F. Clinical, Epidemiological, and Histopathological Features of Respiratory Involvement in Rheumatoid Arthritis. *Biomed. Res. Int.* **2017**, *2017*, 7915340. [CrossRef] [PubMed]
51. Keane, M.P.; Lynch, J.P., III. Pleuropulmonary manifestations of systemic lupus erythematosus. *Thorax* **2000**, *55*, 159–166. [CrossRef] [PubMed]
52. Toyoda, Y.; Koyama, K.; Kawano, H.; Nishimura, H.; Kagawa, K.; Morizumi, S.; Naito, N.; Sato, S.; Yamashita, Y.; Takahashi, N.; et al. Clinical features of interstitial pneumonia associated with systemic lupus erythematosus. *Respir. Investig.* **2019**, *57*, 435–443. [CrossRef]
53. Lian, F.; Zhou, J.; Wang, Y.; Cui, W.; Chen, D.; Li, H.; Qiu, Q.; Zhan, Z.; Ye, Y.; Liang, L.; et al. Clinical features and independent predictors of interstitial lung disease in systemic lupus erythematosus. *Int. J. Clin. Exp. Med.* **2016**, *9*, 4233–4242.
54. Hyldgaard, C.; Hilberg, O.; Pedersen, A.B.; Ulrichsen, S.P.; Løkke, A.; Bendstrup, E.; Ellingsen, T. A population-based cohort study of rheumatoid arthritis-associated interstitial lung disease: Comorbidity and mortality. *Ann. Rheum. Dis.* **2017**, *76*, 1700–1706. [CrossRef]
55. Pérez, E.R.F.; Daniels, C.E.; Sauver, J.S.; Hartman, T.E.; Bartholmai, B.J.; Eunhee, S.Y.; Ryu, J.H.; Schroeder, D.R. Incidence, prevalence, and clinical course of idiopathic pulmonary fibrosis: A population-based study. *Chest* **2010**, *137*, 129–137. [CrossRef] [PubMed]
56. Swigris, J.J.; Berry, G.J.; Raffin, T.A.; Kuschner, W.G. Lymphoid Interstitial Pneumonia. A Narrative Review. *Chest* **2002**, *122*, 2150–2164. [CrossRef]
57. Garcia, D.; Young, L. Lymphocytic interstitial pneumonia as a manifestation of SLE and secondary Sjogren's syndrome. *BMJ Case Rep.* **2013**, *2013*, bcr2013009598. [CrossRef]

58. Min, J.K.; Hong, Y.S.; Park, S.H.; Park, J.H.; Lee, S.H.; Lee, Y.S.; Kim, H.H.; Cho, C.S.; Kim, H.Y. Bronchiolitis obliterans organizing pneumonia as an initial manifestation in patients with systemic lupus erythematosus. *J. Rheumatol.* **1997**, *24*, 2254–2257.
59. Otsuka, F.; Amano, T.; Hashimoto, N.; Takahashi, M.; Hayakawa, N.; Makino, H.; Ota, Z.; Ogura, T. Bronchiolitis obliterans organizing pneumonia associated with systemic lupus erythematosus with antiphospholipid antibody. *Intern. Med.* **1996**, *35*, 341–344. [CrossRef]
60. Gammon, R.B.; Bridges, T.A.; al-Nezir, H.; Alexander, C.B.; Kennedy, J.I., Jr. Bronchiolitis obliterans organizing pneumonia associated with systemic lupus erythematosus. *Chest* **1992**, *102*, 1171–1174. [CrossRef] [PubMed]
61. Gutta, S.; Das, S.; Kodiatte, T.A.; Vimala, L.V. Organising pneumonia in Rhupus syndrome. *BMJ Case Rep.* **2019**, *12*, e232326. [CrossRef] [PubMed]
62. Al-Ghanem, S.; Al-Jahdali, H.; Bamefleh, H.; Khan, A.N. Bronchiolitis obliterans organizing pneumonia: Pathogenesis, clinical features, imaging and therapy review. *Ann. Thorac. Med.* **2008**, *3*, 67–75.
63. Terwiela, M.; Gruttersa, J.C.; Moorsela, C.H.M. Clustering of immune-mediated diseases in sarcoidosis. *Curr. Opin. Pulm. Med.* **2019**, *25*, 539–553. [CrossRef] [PubMed]
64. Rajoriya, N.; Wotton, C.J.; Yeates, D.G.R.; Travis, S.P.L.; Goldacre, M.J. Immune-mediated and chronic inflammatory disease in people with sarcoidosis: Disease associations in a large UK database. *Postgrad Med. J.* **2009**, *85*, 233–237. [CrossRef]
65. Papaioannides, D.; Korantzopoulos, P.; Latsi, P.; Orphanidou, D. Systemic lupus erythematosus developing in a patient with pulmonary sarcoidosis. *Joint Bone Spine* **2004**, *71*, 442–444. [CrossRef] [PubMed]
66. Schnabel, A.; Barth, J.; Schubert, F.; Gross, W.L. Pulmonary Sarcoidosis Coexisting with Systemic Lupus Erythematosus. *Scand. J. Rheumatol.* **1996**, *25*, 109–111. [CrossRef]
67. Robles-Perez, A.; Dorca, J.; Castellvi, I.; Nolla, J.M.; Molina-Molina, M.; Narvaez, J. Rituximab effect in severe progressive connective tissue disease-related lung disease: Preliminary data. *Rheumatol. Int.* **2020**, *40*, 719–726. [CrossRef]
68. Schnabel, A.; Reuter, M.; Gross, W.L. Intravenous pulse cyclophosphamide in the treatment of interstitial lung disease due to collagen vascular diseases. *Arthritis Rheum.* **1998**, *41*, 1215–1220. [CrossRef]
69. Okada, M.; Suzuki, K.; Matsumoto, M.; Nakashima, M.; Nakanishi, T.; Takada, K.; Horikoshi, H.; Matsubara, O.; Ohsuzu, F. Intermittent intravenous cyclophosphamide pulse therapy for the treatment of active interstitial lung disease associated with collagen vascular diseases. *Mod. Rheumatol.* **2007**, *17*, 131–136. [CrossRef]
70. Austin, H.A., III; Klippel, J.H.; Balow, J.E.; le Riche, N.G.; Steinberg, A.D.; Plotz, P.H.; Decker, J.L. Therapy of lupus nephritis. Controlled trial of prednisone and cytotoxic drugs. *N. Engl. J. Med.* **1986**, *314*, 614–619. [CrossRef] [PubMed]
71. Saketkoo, L.A.; Espinoza, L.R. Experience of mycophenolate mofetil in 10 patients with autoimmune-related interstitial lung disease demonstrates promising effects. *Am. J. Med. Sci.* **2009**, *337*, 329–335. [CrossRef]
72. Fischer, A.; Brown, K.K.; Du Bois, R.M.; Frankel, S.K.; Cosgrove, G.P.; Fernandez-Perez, E.R.; Huie, T.J.; Krishnamoorthy, M.; Meehan, R.T.; Olson, A.L.; et al. Mycophenolate mofetil improves lung function in connective tissue disease-associated interstitial lung disease. *J. Rheumatol.* **2013**, *40*, 640–646. [CrossRef] [PubMed]
73. Abramson, S.B.; Dobro, J.; Eberle, M.A.; Benton, M.; Reibman, J.; Epstein, H.; Rapoport, D.M.; Belmont. H.M.; Goldring, R.M. Acute reversible hypoxemia in systemic lupus erythematosus. *Ann. Intern. Med.* **1991**, *114*, 941–947. [CrossRef] [PubMed]
74. Belmont, H.M.; Buyon, J.; Giorno, R.; Abramson, S. Up-regulation of endothelial cell adhesion molecules characterizes disease activity in systemic lupus erythematosus. The Shwartzman phenomenon revisited. *Arthritis Rheum.* **1994**, *37*, 376–383. [CrossRef] [PubMed]
75. Calvo-Alen, J.; Toloza, S.M.A.; Fernandez, M.; Bastian, H.M.; Fessler, B.J.; Roseman, J.M.; McGwin, G., Jr.; Vila, L.M.; Reveille, J.D.; Alarcon, G.S.; et al. Systemic Lupus Erythematosus in a Multiethnic US Cohort (LUMINA) XXV. Smoking, Older Age, Disease Activity, Lupus Anticoagulant, and Glucocorticoid Dose as Risk Factors for the Occurrence of Venous Thrombosis in Lupus Patients. *Arthritis Rheum.* **2005**, *52*, 2060–2068. [CrossRef] [PubMed]
76. Avina-Zubieta, J.A.; Vostretsova, K.; De Vera, M.A.; Sayre, E.C.; Choi, H.K. The risk of pulmonary embolism and deep venous thrombosis in systemic lupus erythematosus: A general population-based study. *Semin. Arthritis Rheum.* **2015**, *45*, 195–201. [CrossRef] [PubMed]
77. Ramirez, G.A.; Efthymiou, M.; Isenberg, D.A.; Cohen, H. Under crossfire: Thromboembolic risk in systemic lupus erythematosus. *Rheumatology* **2019**, *58*, 940–952. [CrossRef]
78. You, H.; Zhao, J.; Wang, Q.; Tian, X.; Li, M.; Zeng, X. Characteristics and risk factors of pulmonary embolism in patients with systemic lupus erythematosus: A case control study. *Clin. Exp. Rheumatol.* **2020**, *38*, 940–948.
79. Wahl, D.G.; Guillemin, F.; de Maistre, E.; Perret, C.; Lecompte, T.; Thibaut, G. Risk for venous thrombosis related to antiphospholipid antibodies in systemic lupus erythematosus: A meta-analysis. *Lupus* **1997**, *6*, 467–473. [CrossRef]
80. Swigris, J.J.; Fischer, A.; Gilles, J.; Meehan, R.T.; Brown, K.K. Pulmonary and Thrombotic Manifestations of Systemic Lupus Erythematosus. *Chest* **2008**, *133*, 271–280. [CrossRef] [PubMed]
81. Tektonidou, M.G.; Andreoli, L.; Limper, M.; Amoura, Z.; Cervera, R.; Costedoat-Chalumeau, N.; Cuadrado, M.J.; Dörner, T.; Ferrer-Oliveras, R.; Hambly, K.; et al. EULAR recommendations for the management of antiphospholipid syndrome in adults. *Ann. Rheum. Dis.* **2019**, *78*, 1296–1304. [CrossRef]
82. Asherson, R.A.; Cervera, R.; Shepshelovich, D.; Shoenfels, Y. Nonthrombotic manifestations of the antiphospholipid syndrome: Away from thrombosis? *J. Rheumatol.* **2006**, *33*, 1038–1044. [PubMed]

83. Asherson, R.A.; Cervera, R.; Piette, J.C.; Shoenfeld, Y.; Espinosa, G.; Petri, M.A.; Lim, E.; Lau, T.C.; Gurjal, A.; Jedryka-Góral, A.; et al. Catastrophic antiphospholipid syndrome: Clues to the pathogenesis from a series of 80 patients. *Medicine* **2001**, *80*, 355–377. [CrossRef] [PubMed]
84. Bucciarelli, S.; Espinosa, G.; Asherson, R.A.; Cervera, R.; Claver, G.; Gómez-Puerta, J.A.; Ramos-Casals, M.; Ingelmo, M. Catastrophic Antiphospholipid Syndrome Registry Project Group, The acute respiratory distress syndrome in catastrophic antiphospholipid syndrome: Analysis of a series of 47 patients. *Ann. Rheum. Dis.* **2006**, *65*, 81–86. [CrossRef] [PubMed]
85. Chaturvedi, S.; McCrae, K.R. Diagnosis and management of the antiphospholipid syndrome. *Blood Rev.* **2017**, *31*, 406–417. [CrossRef]
86. Dufrost, V.; Risse, J.; Zuily, S.; Wahl, D. Direct Oral Anticoagulants Use in Antiphospholipid Syndrome: Are These Drugs an Effective and Safe Alternative to Warfarin? A Systematic Review of the Literature. *Curr. Rheumatol. Rep.* **2016**, *18*, 74. [CrossRef] [PubMed]
87. Sanchez-Redondo, J.; Espinosa, G.; Varillas Delgado, D.; Cervera, R. Recurrent Thrombosis with Direct Oral Anticoagulants in Antiphospholipid Syndrome: A Systematic Literature Review and Meta-analysis. *Clin. Ther.* **2019**, *41*, 1839–1862. [CrossRef]
88. Galiè, N.; Humbert, M.; Vachiery, J.L.; Gibbs, S.; Lang, I.; Torbicki, A.; Simonneau, G.; Peacock, A.; Noordegraaf, A.V.; Beghetti, M.; et al. 2015 ESC/ERS Guidelines for the diagnosis and treatment of pulmonary hypertension. *Eur. Heart J.* **2016**, *37*, 67–119. [CrossRef]
89. Shahane, A. Pulmonary hypertension in rheumatic diseases: Epidemiology and pathogenesis. *Rheumatol. Int.* **2013**, *33*, 1655–1667. [CrossRef]
90. Soler, J.F.; Borg, A.; Mercieca, C. Dyspnoea in lupus. *BMJ Case Rep.* **2017**, *2017*, bcr2017220162. [CrossRef]
91. Kishida, Y.; Kanai, Y.; Kuramochi, S.; Hosoda, Y. Pulmonary venoocclusive disease in a patient with systemic lupus erythematosus. *J. Rheumatol.* **1993**, *20*, 2161–2162.
92. Aparicio, I.J.; Lee, J.S. Connective tissue disease associated interstitial lung diseases: Unresolved issues. *Semin. Respir. Crit. Care Med.* **2016**, *37*, 468–476. [CrossRef]
93. McGoon, M.D.; Miller, D.P. REVEAL: A contemporary US pulmonary arterial hypertension registry. *Eur. Respir. Rev.* **2012**, *21*, 8–18. [CrossRef] [PubMed]
94. Tselios, K.; Gladman, D.D.; Urowitz, M.B. Systemic lupus erythematosus and pulmonary arterial hypertension: Links, risks, and management Strategies. *Open Access Rheumatol.* **2016**, *9*, 1–9. [CrossRef] [PubMed]
95. Winslow, T.M.; Ossipov, M.A.; Fazio, G.P.; Simonson, J.S.; Redberg, R.F.; Schiller, N.B. Five-year follow-up study of the prevalence and progression of pulmonary hypertension in systemic lupus erythematosus. *Am. Heart J.* **1995**, *129*, 510–515. [CrossRef]
96. Dhala, A. Pulmonary Arterial Hypertension in Systemic Lupus Erythematosus: Current Status and Future Direction. *Clin. Dev. Immunol.* **2012**, *2012*, 854941. [CrossRef]
97. Dorfmüller, P.; Humbert, M.; Perros, F.; Sanchez, O.; Simonneau, G.; Müller, K.M.; Capron, F. Fibrous remodeling of the pulmonary venous system in pulmonary arterial hypertension associated with connective tissue diseases. *Hum. Pathol.* **2007**, *38*, 893–902. [CrossRef]
98. Gaine, S.; Chin, K.; Coghlan, G.; Channick, R.; Di Scala, L.; Galiè, N.; Ghofrani, H.A.; Lang, I.M.; McLaughlin, V.; Preiss, R.; et al. Selexipag for the treatment of connective tissue disease-associated pulmonary arterial hypertension. *Eur. Respir. J.* **2017**, *50*, 1602493. [CrossRef]
99. Badesch, D.B.; Hill, N.S.; Burgess, G.; Rubin, L.J.; Barst, R.J.; Galiè, N.; Simonneau, G.; SUPER Study Group. Sildenafil for pulmonary arterial hypertension associated with connective tissue disease. *J. Rheumatol.* **2007**, *34*, 2417–2422.
100. Mok, M.Y.; Tsang, P.L.; Lam, Y.M.; Lo, Y.; Wong, W.S.; Lau, C.S. Bosentan use in systemic lupus erythematosus patients with pulmonary arterial hypertension. *Lupus* **2007**, *16*, 279–285. [CrossRef]
101. Oudiz, R.J.; Schilz, R.J.; Barst, R.J.; Galié, N.; Rich, S.; Rubin, L.J.; Simonneau, G.; Treprostinil Study Group. Treprostinil, a prostacyclin analogue, in pulmonary arterial hypertension associated with connective tissue disease. *Chest* **2004**, *126*, 420–427. [CrossRef]
102. Robbins, I.M.; Gaine, S.P.; Schilz, R.; Tapson, V.F.; Rubin, L.J.; Loyd, J.E. Epoprostenol for treatment of pulmonary hypertension in patients with systemic lupus erythematosus. *Chest* **2000**, *117*, 14–18. [CrossRef]
103. Rubin, L.J.; Badesch, D.B.; Barst, R.J.; Galie, N.; Black, C.M.; Keogh, A.; Pulido, T.; Frost, A.; Roux, S.; Leconte, I.; et al. Bosentan therapy for pulmonary arterial hypertension. *N. Engl. J. Med.* **2002**, *346*, 896–903. [CrossRef]
104. Shirai, Y.; Yasuoka, H.; Takeuchi, T.; Satoh, T.; Kuwana, M. Intravenous epoprostenol treatment of patients with connective tissue disease and pulmonary arterial hypertension at a single center. *Mod. Rheumatol.* **2013**, *23*, 1211–1220. [CrossRef]
105. Humbert, M.; Coghlan, J.G.; Ghofrani, H.A.; Grimminger, F.; He, J.G.; Riemekasten, G.; Vizza, C.D.; Boeckenhoff, A.; Meier, C.; de Oliveira Pena, J.; et al. Riociguat for the treatment of pulmonary arterial hypertension associated with connective tissue disease: Results from PATENT-1 and PATENT-2. *Ann. Rheum. Dis.* **2017**, *76*, 422–426. [CrossRef]
106. Pulido, T.; Adzerikho, I.; Channick, R.N.; Delcroix, M.; Galiè, N.; Ghofrani, H.A.; Jansa, P.; Jing, Z.C.; Le Brun, F.O.; Mehta, S.; et al. SERAPHIN Investigators Macitentan and morbidity and mortality in pulmonary arterial hypertension. *N. Engl. J. Med* **2013**, *369*, 809–818. [CrossRef]
107. Kuzuya, K.; Tsuji, S.; Matsushita, M.; Ohshima, S.; Saeki, Y. Systemic sclerosis and systemic lupus erythematosus overlap syndrome with pulmonary arterial hypertension successfully treated with immunosuppressive therapy and riociguat. *Cureus* **2019**, *11*, e4327. [CrossRef] [PubMed]

108. Gonzalez-Lopez, L.; Cardona-Munoz, E.G.; Celis, A.; García-De la Torre, I.; Orozco-Barocio, G.; Salazar-Paramo, M.; Garcia-Gonzalez, C.; Garcia-Gonzalez, A.; Sanchez-Ortiz, A.; Trujillo-Hernandez, B.; et al. Therapy with intermittent pulse cyclophosphamide for pulmonary hypertension associated with systemic lupus erythematosus. *Lupus* **2004**, *13*, 105–112. [CrossRef] [PubMed]
109. Kommireddy, S.; Bhyravavajhala, S.; Kurimeti, K.; Chennareddy, S.; Kanchinadham, S.; Prasad, I.R.V.; Rajasekhar, L. Pulmonary arterial hypertension in systemic lupus erythematosus may benefit by addition of immunosuppression to vasodilator therapy: An observational study. *Rheumatology* **2015**, *54*, 1673–1679. [CrossRef] [PubMed]
110. Hennigan, S.; Channick, R.N.; Silverman, G.J. Rituximab treatment of pulmonary arterial hypertension associated with systemic lupus erythematosus: A case report. *Lupus* **2008**, *17*, 754–756. [CrossRef] [PubMed]
111. Chung, S.M.; Lee, C.K.; Lee, E.Y.; Yoo, B.; Lee, S.D.; Moon, H.B. Clinical aspects of pulmonary hypertension in patients with systemic lupus erythematosus and in patients with idiopathic pulmonary arterial hypertension. *Clin. Rheumatol.* **2006**, *25*, 866–872. [CrossRef] [PubMed]
112. Crestani, B. The respiratory system in connective tissue disorders. *Allergy* **2005**, *60*, 715–734. [CrossRef] [PubMed]
113. So, C.; Imai, R.; Tomishima, Y.; Nishimura, N. Bilateral Pleuritis as the Initial Symptom of Systemic Lupus Erythematosus: A Case Series and Literature Review. *Intern. Med.* **2019**, *58*, 1617–1620. [CrossRef] [PubMed]
114. Dubois, E.L.; Tuffanelli, D.L. Clinical manifestations of systemic lupus erythematosus: Computer analysis of 520 cases. *JAMA* **1964**, *190*, 104–111. [CrossRef]
115. Saha, K.; Saha, A.; Mitra, M.; Panchadhyayee, P. Bilateral pleural effusion with APLA positivity in a case of rhupus syndrome. *Lung India* **2014**, *31*, 390–393. [CrossRef]
116. Choi, B.Y.; Yoon, M.J.; Shin, K.; Lee, Y.J.; Song, Y.W. Characteristics of pleural effusions in systemic lupus erythematosus: Differential diagnosis of lupus pleuritis. *Lupus* **2015**, *24*, 321–326. [CrossRef] [PubMed]
117. Sharma, S.; Smith, R.; Al-Hameed, F. Fibrothorax and severe lung restriction secondary to lupus pleuritis and its successful treatment by pleurectomy. *Can. Respir. J.* **2002**, *9*, 335–337. [CrossRef]
118. Kao, A.H.; Manzi, S. How to manage patients with cardiopulmonary disease? *Best Pract. Res. Clin. Rheumatol.* **2002**, *16*, 211–227. [CrossRef]
119. Sherer, Y.; Langevitz, P.; Levy, Y.; Fabrizzi, F.; Shoenfeld, Y. Treatment of chronic bilateral pleural effusions with intravenous immunoglobulin and cyclosporine. *Lupus* **1999**, *8*, 324–327. [CrossRef]
120. Esposito, S.; Bosis, S.; Semino, M.; Rigante, D. Infections and systemic lupus erythematosus. *Eur. J. Clin. Microbiol. Infect. Dis.* **2014**, *33*, 1467–1475. [CrossRef]
121. Cervera, R.; Khamashta, M.A.; Font, J.; Sebastiani, G.D.; Gil, A.; Lavilla, P.; Mejía, J.C.; Aydintug, A.O.; Chwalinska-Sadowska, H.; de Ramón, E.; et al. Morbidity and mortality in systemic lupus erythematosus during a 10-year period A comparison of early and late manifestations in a cohort of 1,000 patients. *Medicine* **2003**, *82*, 299–308. [CrossRef]
122. Lai, C.C.; Sun, Y.S.; Lin, F.C.; Yang, C.Y.; Tsai, C.Y. Bronchoalveolar lavage fluid analysis and mortality risk in systemic lupus erythematosus patients with pneumonia and respiratory failure. *J. Microbiol Immunol Infect.* **2020**. [CrossRef] [PubMed]
123. Rúa-Figueroa, I.; Nóvoa, J.; García-Laorden, M.I.; Erausquin, C.; García-Bello, M.; de Castro, F.R.; Herrera-Ramos, E.; Ojeda, S.; Quevedo, J.C.; Francisco, F.; et al. Clinical and Immunogenetic Factors Associated with Pneumonia in Patients with Systemic Lupus Erythematosus: A Case-Control Study. *J. Rheumatol.* **2014**, *41*, 1801–1807. [CrossRef]
124. Scerpella, E.G. Functional Asplenia and Pneumococcal Sepsis in Patients with Systemic Lupus Erythematosus. *Clin. Infect. Dis.* **1995**, *20*, 194–195. [CrossRef]
125. Gaiba, R.; O'Neill, E.; Lakshmi, S. Pulmonary cryptococcosis complicating interstitial lung disease in a patient with systemic lupus erythematosus. *BMJ Case Rep.* **2019**, *12*, e229403. [CrossRef]
126. Hardie, R.; James-Goulbourne, T.; Rashid, M.; Sullivan, J.; Homsi, Y. Fatal Disseminated Aspergillosis in a Patient with Systemic Lupus Erythematosus. *Case Rep. Infect. Dis.* **2020**, *2020*, 9623198. [CrossRef]
127. Wahid, W.; Fahmi, N.A.A.; Salleh, A.F.M.; Yasin, A.M. Case report Bronchopulmonary lophomoniasis: A rare cause of pneumonia in an immunosuppressed host. *Respir Med. Case Rep.* **2019**, *28*, 100939. [PubMed]
128. Elkayam, O.; Paran, D.; Caspi, D.; Litinsky, I.; Yaron, M.; Charboneau, D.; Rubins, J.B. Immunogenicity and safety of pneumococcal vaccination in patients with rheumatoid arthritis or systemic lupus erythematosus. *Clin. Infect. Dis.* **2002**, *34*, 147–153. [CrossRef]
129. Furer, V.; Rondaan, C.; Heijstek, M.W.; Agmon-Levin, N.; van Assen, S.; Bijl, M.; Breedveld, F.C.; D'Amelio, R.; Dougados, M.; Kapetanovic, M.C.; et al. 2019 update of EULAR recommendations for vaccination in adult patients with autoimmune inflammatory rheumatic diseases. *Ann. Rheum Dis.* **2020**, *79*, 39–52. [CrossRef] [PubMed]
130. Park, J.W.; Curtis, J.R.; Kim, M.J.; Lee, H.; Song, Y.W.; Lee, E.B. Pneumocystis pneumonia in patients with rheumatic diseases receiving prolonged, non-high-dose steroids-clinical implication of primary prophylaxis using trimethoprim-sulfamethoxazole. *Arthritis Res. Ther.* **2019**, *21*, 207. [CrossRef]
131. Hannah, J.R.; D'Cruz, D.P. Pulmonary Complications of Systemic Lupus Erythematosus. *Semin. Respir. Crit. Care Med.* **2019**, *40*, 227–234. [CrossRef]
132. Choudhury, S.; Ramos, M.; Anjum, H.; Ali, M.; Surani, S. Shrinking Lung Syndrome: A Rare Manifestation of Systemic Lupus Erythematosus. *Cureus* **2020**, *12*, e8216. [CrossRef] [PubMed]
133. Warrington, K.J.; Moder, K.G.; Brutinel, W.M. The Shrinking Lungs Syndrome in Systemic Lupus Erythematosus. *Mayo Clin. Proc.* **2000**, *75*, 467–472. [CrossRef]

134. Muñoz-Rodríguez, F.J.; Font, J.; Badia, J.R.; Miret, C.; Barberà, J.A.; Cervera, R.; Ingelmo, M. Shrinking lungs syndrome in systemic lupus erythematosus: Improvement with inhaled beta-agonist therapy. *Lupus* **1997**, *6*, 412–414. [CrossRef] [PubMed]
135. Hoffbrand, B.I.; Beck, E.R. "Unexplained" Dyspnoea and Shrinking Lungs in Systemic Lupus Erythematosus. *Br. Med. J.* **1965**, *1*, 1273–1277. [CrossRef]
136. Scire, C.A.; Caporali, R.; Zanierato, M.; Mojoli, F.; Braschi, A.; Montecucco, C. Shrinking lung syndrome in systemic sclerosis. *Arthritis Rheum.* **2003**, *48*, 2999–3000. [CrossRef] [PubMed]
137. Tavoni, A.; Vitali, C.; Cirigliano, G.; Frigelli, S.; Stampacchia, G.; Bombardieri, S. Shrinking lung in primary Sjögren's syndrome. *Arthritis Rheum.* **1999**, *42*, 2249–2250. [CrossRef]
138. Ciaffi, J.; Gegenava, M.; Ninaber, M.K.; Huizinga, T.W.J. Shrinking Lung Syndrome Diagnostic and Therapeutic Challenges in 3 Patients With Systemic Lupus Erythematosus. *J. Clin. Rheumatol.* **2019**. [CrossRef]
139. Borrell, H.; Narváez, J.; Alegre, J.J.; Castellví, I.; Mitjavila, F.; Aparicio, M.; Armengol, E.; Molina-Molina, M.; Nolla, J.N. Shrinking lung syndrome in systemic lupus erythematosus A case series and review of the literature. *Medicine* **2016**, *95*, e4626. [CrossRef]
140. Duron, L.; Cohen-Aubart, F.; Diot, E.; Borie, R.; Abad, S.; Richez, C.; Banse, C.; Vittecoq, O.; Saadoun, D.; Haroche, J.; et al. Shrinking lung syndrome associated with systemic lupus erythematosus: A multicenter collaborative study of 15 new cases and a review of the 155 cases in the literature focusing on treatment response and long-term outcomes. *Autoimmun. Rev.* **2016**, *15*, 994–1000. [CrossRef]
141. Carmier, D.; Diot, D.; Diot, P. Shrinking lung syndrome: Recognition, pathophysiology and therapeutic strategy. *Expert Rev. Respir. Med.* **2011**, *5*, 33–39. [CrossRef]
142. Karim, M.Y.; Miranda, L.C.; Tench, C.M.; Gordon, P.A.; D'Cruz, D.P.; Khamashta, M.A.; Hughes, G.R.V. Presentation and Prognosis of the Shrinking Lung Syndrome in Systemic Lupus Erythematosus. *Semin. Arthritis Rheum.* **2002**, *31*, 289–298. [CrossRef] [PubMed]
143. Hardy, K.; Herry, I.; Attali, V.; Cadranel, J.; Similowski, T. Bilateral Phrenic Paralysis in a Patient with Systemic lupus erythematosus. *Chest* **2001**, *119*, 1274–1277. [CrossRef] [PubMed]
144. Wilcox, P.G.; Stein, H.B.; Clarke, S.D.; Pare, P.D.; Pardy, R.L. Phrenic Nerve Function in Patients with Diaphragmatic Weakness and Systemic Lupus Erythematosus. *Chest* **1988**, *93*, 352–358. [CrossRef] [PubMed]
145. Toya, S.P.; Tzelepis, G.E. Association of the shrinking lung syndrome in systemic lupus erythematosus with pleurisy: A systematic review. *Semin. Arthritis Rheum.* **2009**, *39*, 30–37. [CrossRef]
146. Benham, H.; Garske, L.; Vecchio, P.; Eckert, B.W. Successful treatment of shrinking lung syndrome with rituximab in a patient with systemic lupus erytematosus. *J. Clin. Rheumatol.* **2010**, *16*, 68–70. [CrossRef]
147. Van Veen, S.; Peeters, A.J.; Sterk, P.J.; Breedveld, F.C. The "shrinking lung syndrome" in SLE, treatment with theophylline. *Clin. Rheumatol.* **1993**, *12*, 462–465. [CrossRef]
148. Thompson, P.J.; Dhillon, D.P.; Ledingham, J.; Turner-Warwick, M. Shrinking Lungs, Diaphragmatic Dysfunction, and Systemic Lupus Erythematosus. *Am. Rev. Respir. Dis.* **1985**, *132*, 926–928.
149. Traynor, A.E.; Corbridge, T.C.; Eagan, A.E.; Barr, W.G.; Liu, Q.; Oyama, Y.; Burt, R.K. Prevalence and Reversibility of Pulmonary Dysfunction in Refractory Systemic Lupus Improvement Correlates With Disease Remission Following Hematopoietic Stem Cell Transplantation. *Chest* **2005**, *127*, 1680–1689. [CrossRef]

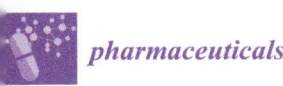

Review

Pharmacological Interventions for Pulmonary Involvement in Rheumatic Diseases

Eun Ha Kang [1] and Yeong Wook Song [2],*

[1] Division of Rheumatology, Department of Internal Medicine, Seoul National University Bundang Hospital, Seongnam 13620, Korea; kangeh@snubh.org
[2] Division of Rheumatology, Department of Internal Medicine, Seoul National University Hospital, Seoul 03080, Korea
* Correspondence: ysong@snu.ac.kr

Abstract: Among the diverse forms of lung involvement, interstitial lung disease (ILD) and pulmonary arterial hypertension (PAH) are two important conditions in patients with rheumatic diseases that are associated with significant morbidity and mortality. The management of ILD and PAH is challenging because the current treatment often provides only limited patient survival benefits. Such challenges derive from their common pathogenic mechanisms, where not only the inflammatory processes of immune cells but also the fibrotic and proliferative processes of nonimmune cells play critical roles in disease progression, making immunosuppressive therapy less effective. Recently, updated treatment strategies adopting targeted agents have been introduced with promising results in clinical trials for ILD ad PAH. This review discusses the epidemiologic features of ILD and PAH among patients with rheumatic diseases (rheumatoid arthritis, myositis, and systemic sclerosis) and the state-of-the-art treatment options, focusing on targeted agents including biologics, antifibrotic agents, and vasodilatory drugs.

Keywords: rheumatic; interstitial lung disease; pulmonary arterial hypertension; targeted therapy

1. Introduction

Lung involvement is common in patients with rheumatic diseases (RDs), causing substantial morbidity and mortality in these patients. Individual RDs tend to be associated with a characteristic lung disease pattern where the key structure of the injury, as well as the critical cells and cytokines involved, are different [1].

Among the diverse forms of lung involvement, interstitial lung disease (ILD) and pulmonary arterial hypertension (PAH) are the two most important manifestations in patients with RD, leading to grave prognoses [2]. Of note, rheumatoid arthritis (RA), myositis, and systemic sclerosis (SSc) are the major systemic RDs, in which a significant proportion of the patients develop and die from ILD and/or PAH. However, recent advances in pharmacologic interventions have been shown to delay the disease progression of these lung conditions and also improve patient survival. In this review, we introduced updated knowledge on the treatment options for ILD and PAH in RDs, focusing on targeted therapies.

2. Interstitial Lung Disease (ILD)

Lung involvement in RDs most commonly takes the form of ILD. In particular, more than two thirds of the patients exhibit ILD in SSc and myositis [3,4]. Clinically symptomatic ILD is less frequent in RA than SSc and myositis, found only in about 10% of the patients [5]. However, the associated morbidity and mortality are never less. RD-associated ILD (RD-ILD) can be classified as usual interstitial pneumonia (UIP), nonspecific interstitial pneumonia (NSIP), organizing pneumonia (OP), diffuse alveolar damage (DAD), lymphoid interstitial pneumonia (LIP) and others, according to the radiologic and/or pathologic–morphologic patterns presented by the revised 2013 American Thoracic Society/European

Respiratory Society classification of idiopathic interstitial pneumonias [6]. In RDs, the two most predominant types of ILDs are NISP and UIP [1]. While the prognosis is similar between RD-NISP and idiopathic NSIP, the prognosis of the RD-UIP other than RA-UIP is better than that of idiopathic UIP or idiopathic pulmonary fibrosis (IPF) [7].

2.1. Rheumatoid Arthritis Associated ILD (RA-ILD)

Potential targets of the lung injury in RA include almost all components of the lung structures. Thus, lung injury associated with RA encompasses a wide spectrum of disorders such as parenchymal (ILD), airway (bronchiectasis or bronchiolitis), pleural (pleurisy), and vascular diseases. Among them, ILD is most common.

2.1.1. Clinical Features of RA-ILD

Approximately 10% of RA patients suffer clinically significant RA-ILD [5], with 8–9 times the lifetime risk of ILD development among RA patients compared to that of the general population (7.7% vs. 0.9%, respectively) [8]. Thirty-four percent of RA-ILD was found to occur within one year of RA diagnosis [9] and the risk of RA-ILD increases with RA duration and autoantibody (rheumatoid factor and/or anticitrullinated protein antibody) titers [10,11].

Unlike other RD-ILDs in which NSIP is the most prevalent histopathologic pattern, up to half of the RA-ILD cases show the UIP pattern, with NSIP as the second most common pattern [1]. With a heterogeneous progression rate across individuals, symptoms of RA-ILD usually progress over time once clinically present. The UIP patterns tend to demonstrate extensive disease at baseline and more rapid pulmonary function decline during follow-up, thus are associated with a worse prognosis [1,12]. The mortality of the patients with RA-ILD was as high as three times that of the patients with RA alone, with more than one third of RA-ILD patients being dead at five-years after ILD diagnosis [8,9].

Although it is considered that the natural progression of RA-ILD is heterogeneous, as in IPF, and a subgroup of those whose lung function progressively declines would show a grave prognosis, the exact natural history of RA-ILD is not fully known, particularly regarding acute exacerbation. In addition to the chronic lung function loss, acute exacerbation is another cause of the mortality associated with RA-ILD. However, a substantial proportion of patients with RA-ILD would suffer mixed patterns.

Acute exacerbation is a fatal condition characterized by a rapidly progressive respiratory failure. It has been well recognized not only in IPF and NSIP [6], but also in RD-ILD, particularly RA-ILD [13]. The radiographic characteristics of the acute exacerbation are defined as ground-glass opacities (GGOs) or consolidations newly overlaid on the background reticular abnormalities. Two thirds of RA-ILD patients with acute exacerbation died during the initial episode, causing a 2.5-fold increased mortality among RA-ILD patients [14]. The risk factors for the acute exacerbation of RA-ILD include UIP histology, old age, and methotrexate (MTX) use [14]. In IPF, more advanced lung fibrosis is also known as a reliable risk factor of the acute exacerbation [15].

2.1.2. Pharmacologic Treatment of RA-ILD

Unfortunately, there have been no randomized controlled trials (RCTs) for RA-ILD and the EULAR and ACR recommendations do not specify how to treat RA-ILD yet [16,17]. In general, physicians either adopt the treatment strategies against the corresponding pattern of idiopathic interstitial pneumonia or practice empirical therapies with immunosuppressives. However, due to the heterogeneous clinical behaviors of RA-ILD, the treatment goal is hard to define: treatment to achieve recovery versus treatment to stabilize or slow progression. In the case of acute exacerbation, most therapies are immunosuppressants with potent anti-inflammatory effects, assuming reversibility of the lesions, while in case of chronic progression, the antifibrotic approach will take the priority [2]. Therefore, physicians need to understand the dominant pathogenic mechanism underlying the clinical behavior of individual cases of RA-ILD, which can vary at different time points even in the same patient.

Treatment with Conventional Agents

The data on the effect of individual immunosuppressive agents on RA-ILD are limited. Mycophenolate mofetil (MMF) was associated with a modest improvement in forced vital capacity (FVC) and the diffusing capacity of carbon monoxide (DLCO), reducing prednisone dosage in an observational study on 125 patients with RD-ILD including 18 RA-ILD cases [18]. In the case of the acute exacerbation of RA-ILD, high dose steroid therapy is delivered in combination with other immunosuppressive agents including MMF, azathioprine, or cyclophosphamide (CYC) [13,14].

Treatment with Targeted Agents

Although hope has been placed on biologics for RA-ILD treatment based on their excellent efficacy against articular inflammation, the evidence suggests that the safety profile of biologics including TNF inhibitors and others is uncertain for ILD treatment. Since biologics could, albeit rarely, exacerbate or cause the de novo development of ILD [19], experts recommend carefully assessing patients before and after treatment. While anti-TNF therapy has been suspected to aggravate ILD or induce its development [19], clear causal evidence is lacking [20,21]. Rituximab and abatacept have been more favorably suggested for patients with RA-ILD over anti-TNF therapy [22,23]. However, even these drugs have also been associated with lung toxicity and their data are scarce due to the less common use compared to TNF inhibitors [19].

Besides biologics, there are targeted agents with antifibrotic effects, recently introduced to treat IPF and RD-ILD (Table 1). These agents include nintedanib and pirfenidone.

Nintedanib is a competitive inhibitor of the nonreceptor and receptor tyrosine kinases that shows an antifibrotic effect [24]. The nonreceptor targets of nintedanib include Lck, Lyn, and Src and the receptor targets include platelet-derived growth factor receptors (PDGFR) α/β, fibroblast growth factor receptors (FGFR) 1/2/3, vascular endothelial growth factor receptors (VEGFR) 1/2/3, and fms-related tyrosine kinase 3 (FLT3). The targets of both categories play important roles in fibrosis [24]. In the phase II proof-of-concept TOMORROW study on patients with IPF diagnosed based on biopsy and/or high resolution computed tomography (HRCT) whose % predicted FVC of $\geq 50\%$ and DLCO of 30–79% [25], 52-week nintedanib treatment (150 mg twice/day) was associated with less FVC decline, fewer acute exacerbations, and the preservation of health-related quality of life compared to placebo in patients with IPF. The antifibrotic effect of nintedanib on IPF was also replicated in phase 3 INPULSIS 1 and 2 trials, which showed significant reductions in the annual FVC decline in the treated group compared to the placebo (between-group difference of 125.3 and 93.7 mL/year in INPULSIS 1 and 2 trials, respectively, $p < 0.001$ in both results) [26]. Unlike treatment consistency on lung function preservation, however, the benefits on acute exacerbation were only observed in the INPULSIS 2. Nintedanib reduced the FVC decline among diverse subgroups defined by sex, age (<65 or ≥ 65 years), race (White or Asian), the baseline FVC% predicted ($\leq 70\%$ or >70%) and DLCO% ($\leq 40\%$ or >40%), composite physiologic index at baseline (≤ 45 or >45), the total baseline score on St George's Respiratory Questionnaire (≤ 40 or >40), smoking status (never-smoker or current/ex-smoker), corticosteroids for systemic use at baseline (yes or no), and bronchodilator use at baseline (yes or no) [27,28].

The recent INBUILD study, an RCT that assessed the efficacy and safety of nintedanib in patients with non-IPF ILD (entry criteria: % predicted FVC of $\geq 45\%$ and DLCO of 30–79%), included a subgroup of patients with RD-ILDs, mostly RA-ILD [29]. In the RD subgroup, nintedanib reduced the rate of FVC decline compared to placebo at 52 weeks with a between-group difference of 104 mL/year ($p < 0.001$) [29]. Based on the INBUILD trial, nintedanib was approved by the U.S. Food and Drug Administration (FDA) for progressive-ILD, including RA-ILD in March 2020.

Table 1. Recent clinical trials on targeted drugs for idiopathic pulmonary fibrosis and rheumatic disease-associated interstitial lung disease.

Targeted Therapy	Mechanism of Therapy	Target Disease	Key RCT Name	Primary Outcome	Treatment Duration	Proven Efficacy
Nintedanib	Tyrosine kinase inhibition	IPF	TOMORROW	Annual FVC decline	52 weeks	Reduced FVC decline
		IPF	INPULSIS 1 and 2	Annual FVC decline	52 weeks	Reduced FVC decline
		Non-IPF ILD (e.g., RA-ILD)	INBUILD	Annual FVC decline	52 weeks	Reduced FVC decline
		SSc-ILD	SENSIS	Annual FVC decline	52 weeks	Reduced FVC decline
Pirfenidone	Unknown	IPF	Japanese RCT Capacity 004	Annual VC decline FVC change at 72 weeks	52 weeks 72 weeks	Reduced FVC decline
		IPF	ASCEND	Annual FVC change or death	52 weeks	Reduced FVC decline
		Non-IPF ILD (e.g., RA-ILD)	Multinational RCT	FVC change at 24 weeks	24 weeks	Reduced FVC decline
		RA-ILD	TRAIL1	Annual FVC decline >10% or death	52 weeks	Awaited
Rituximab	B cell depletion	RD-ILD	RECITAL	FVC change at 24 weeks	48 weeks	Awaited
Tocilizumab	IL-6 blockade	SSc-ILD	faSScinate	Modified Rodnan skin score; FVC decline as a secondary outcome	24 weeks	Numerically greater reduction of skin fibrosis; seemed to reduce FVC decline
		SSc-ILD	FocuSSced	Modified Rodnan skin score; FVC decline as a secondary outcome	48 weeks	No primary endpoint was met; seemed to reduce FVC decline

FVC = forced vital capacity, ILD = interstitial lung disease, IPF = idiopathic pulmonary fibrosis, RD = rheumatic disease, RA = rheumatoid arthritis, RCT = randomized controlled trial, SSc = systemic sclerosis.

Pirfenidone, another antifibrotic drug approved for IPF, might show similar benefits for patients with the RA-UIP as the drug did for patients with IPF. Unlike nintedanib, the mechanism of the action of pirfenidone is not well known. Among the three phase 3 clinical trials in patients with IPF [30,31], the Japanese trial showed that pirfenidone reduced the decline in vital capacity at week 52 (between-group difference, 0.07 L/year) and improved progression-free survival compared to placebo [30]. In the remaining two CAPACITY trials (004 and 006) on patients with multinational backgrounds (entry criteria: % predicted FVC of 50–90% and DLCO of 35–90%), the primary endpoint (% predicted FVC change from baseline to week 72) was met in trial 004 (-8.0% vs. -12.4%, $p < 0.05$) but not in 006 (-9.0% vs. -9.6%, $p = 0.501$) [31]. In the ASCEND trial [32], there was a relative reduction of 47.9% in the proportion of IPF patients who had an absolute decline of $\geq 10\%$ in the FVC or who died (16.5% vs. 31.8%, $p < 0.001$). There was also a relative increase of 132.5% in the proportion of patients with no decline in FVC (22.7% vs. 9.7%, $p < 0.001$). In another multinational clinical trial on non-IPF ILD, the use of pirfenidone was associated with a lower risk of FVC decline greater than 10% (odds ratio = 0.44, 95% CI: 0.23–0.84) with a between-group difference in FVC of 95.3 mL/year at 24 weeks [33]. TRAIL1 is a 52-week multicenter randomized, double-blind, placebo-controlled, phase 2 study (ClinicalTrials.gov number, NCT02808871) of the safety, tolerability, and efficacy of pirfenidone in patients with RA-ILD, aiming to enroll as many as 270 subjects with RA-ILD and the results are awaited [34].

There is an overlap of adverse event profiles between nintedanib and pirfenidone [35]. In patients treated with nintedanib, gastrointestinal adverse events (e.g., diarrhea) were most common with mild-to-moderate intensity, accounting for the majority of the drug discontinuation [25,26,29]. Similarly, the most common adverse event of pirfenidone was gastrointestinal including nausea and vomiting, experienced by 40% and 18% of treated patients, respectively, out of 2059 person-years of exposure [36]. However, the two drugs have different pharmacokinetic profiles. Nintedanib is metabolized predominantly by ester cleavage and then glucuronidated to be excreted via the biliary system [35]. The use of nintedanib is associated with liver function test abnormalities in less than 5% of patients, and is not recommended for those with moderate-to-severe hepatic dysfunction. Regular liver function monitoring is required. Nintedanib has a low potential for drug–drug interactions, especially with drugs metabolized by cytochrome P450 enzymes. Pirfenidone is metabolized by various cytochrome P450 enzymes in the liver and predominantly excreted via the urine [35]. Similar rates of liver function test abnormalities were observed with pirfenidone as with nintedanib [25,26,31,32]. Pharmacokinetically, no drug–drug interaction was observed between nintedanib and pirfenidone. There are RCTs that examined the effect of nintedanib added on pirfenidone treatment [37,38]. More reports of nausea and vomiting were observed with nintedanib added on pirfenidone than used alone. However, most of them were mild-to-moderate as with the single drug treatment and the combination did not provide a new safety signal.

General Treatment Strategy for RA-ILD

Due to the heterogeneous progression patterns across individuals, it is hard to define an optimal treatment strategy in RA-ILD. Although the baseline extent of lung injury has been acknowledged as the most reliable risk factor of both progression and acute exacerbation, the cut-off extent to initiate treatment is not well defined. The international guidelines on RA management have yet to specify when to initiate treatment and what to be the first line agent [16,17]. Moreover, the treatment of acute exacerbation should be different from that of chronic progression [2]. However, it seems reasonable to use nintedanib when FVC loss is progressive enough to deteriorate symptoms (e.g., dyspnea or exercise capacity) or of when the current status is severe enough to qualify for the previous RCTs including the INBUILD trial (FVC of $\geq 45\%$, DLCO of 30–79%) [29].

2.2. Systemic Sclerosis Associated Interstitial Lung Disease (SSc-ILD)

The pulmonary manifestations of SSc can be both direct and indirect. The former category includes parenchymal (ILD) and vascular diseases (PAH) and the latter includes aspiration due to gastroesophageal reflux associated with esophageal sphincter fibrosis.

2.2.1. Clinical Features of SSc-ILD

The key pathophysiology of SSc encompasses a triad of immune activation, vasculopathy, and fibrosis. Due to fibrosis and vasculopathy, the lung involvement of SSc most often manifests as ILD and/or PAH. ILD develops more frequently in the diffuse than limited cutaneous subset, particularly in the presence of antitopoisomerase I antibodies. SSc-specific anti-U3 RNP and anti-Th/To are also associated with SSc-ILD [39].

As many as 90% of SSc patients show ILD [3]. Among 3656 SSc patients from the European Scleroderma Trials and Research group, ILD was observed by plain chest radiography in approximately half of the patients with the diffuse cutaneous SSc and in one third of the patients with the limited cutaneous SSc [40]. Regarding severity, moderate (FVC of 50–75%) to severe (FVC < 50%) restrictive lung disease was found in 40% of SSc patients [41]. The pulmonary function of SSc-ILD patients mostly declines during the first several years after the onset of non-Raynaud's symptoms, but the progression rate of decline is best predicted by the baseline severity of the lung function or fibrosis [1]. A greater impairment at baseline predicts more progression in the future. Further, there are a significant proportion of patients not treated without progression [42], suggesting that the clinical course of SSc-ILD is variable [43].

The predominant histologic pattern of SSc-ILD is NSIP based on biopsy and/or HRCT [1,3,44]. However, the histologic pattern does not affect the clinical outcome of SSc-ILD [1,7,44]. Because fibrosis is the main histologic finding other than inflammation, even GGO represents fine reticulation and is rarely reversed but replaced later by overt fibrotic findings such as reticulation or honeycombing [45,46].

The mortality of SSc patients showed an overall three-fold increased standardized mortality ratio compared to the general population [47]: the survival of SSc patients was 74.9% at 5 years and 62.5% at 10 years from the diagnosis, with the mortality risk in the presence of ILD being 2.9-fold compared to in the absence of ILD [47].

2.2.2. Pharmacologic Treatment of SSc-ILD

The lung function of SSc patients with FVC of $\geq$80% at baseline rarely declines [43]. Thus, symptomatic patients are the primary target of treatments, particularly those whose ILD is moderate-to-severe or shows progression. The recent European consensus statements presented an agreement on screening of ILD for all SSc patients at baseline particularly in the presence of risk factors (diffuse cutaneous subset, antitopoisomerase antibody, low DLCO) preferably by HRCT but also with pulmonary function test (PFT) and clinical assessment as supporting tools [48]. The statements recommend treatment for all severe cases defined by PFT or HRCT, and for those who progress based on clinical assessment, HRCT, and/or PFT. However, the statements did not specify the threshold to define severe ILD or when to initiate or escalate treatment. Those who have symptoms that are progressively deteriorating (newly developed functional class II and more), whose FVC and/or DLCO decline is large enough ($\geq$10% and $\geq$15%, respectively) [49,50], or whose FVC or DLCO is severe enough to justify treatment-related adverse events (refer to the inclusion criteria for Scleroderma Lung Study or SENSCIS trial below) [51–53] would be reasonable candidates to initiate or escalate treatment.

Treatment with Conventional Agents

Until recently, the treatment SSc-ILD has relied on immunosuppressants such as CYC and MMF based on the RCT data [51,52,54]. Since GGO of SSc-ILD often indicates fine fibrosis rather than inflammation [45,46], these immunosuppressive treatments stabilize rather than improve such lesions.

In the Scleroderma Lung Study (SLS) I on 158 SSc patients with symptomatic ILD (active alveolitis on imaging and FVC ranging between 45–85%) [51], the mean absolute difference of FVC% predicted at 12 months (2.53%, $p < 0.03$) was significantly in favor of oral CYC over placebo. When the patients were followed for another one year after stopping the medication, the effect was maintained or even greater at six months after treatment termination but disappeared by one year [52]. According to the subgroup analysis, a greater response to CYC was linked to more severe lung disease at baseline [52]. In SLS II, the efficacy of the two-year treatment with MMF was comparable to that of the one-year treatment with oral CYC at 24 months (mean FVC improvement from baseline of 2.17% in the MMF group versus 2.86% in the CYC group) [54]. The adverse events were less with the former drug. The 2017 updated EULAR recommendations still suggest CYC preferentially over MMF [55], but MMF is a viable first line treatment for patients who are susceptible to the toxicity of CYC.

Treatment with Targeted Agents

Antifibrotics

The SENSCIS trial was performed on 576 patients with SSc-ILD (mean age 54.6 years, 74–76% female) of at least 10% extent of the lung [53]. The entry criteria of ILD required % predicted FVC $\geq$ 40% and % predicted DLCO ranging in 30–90%. The % predicted FVC of included patients was 72% and DLCO 53% at baseline. Of the patients included in the study, 48.4% were taking background MMF. After 52 weeks of treatment, nintedanib (150mg twice daily) was associated with a lower annual rate of FVC decline compared to the placebo treatment (-52.4 mL/year versus -93.3 mL/year). The curves for the FVC change from the baseline separated by 12 weeks and continued to diverge until the end of study. The effect of nintedanib was additive when combined with MMF: the annual rates of change in FVC among the patients receiving mycophenolate were -40.2 mL/year in the nintedanib group and -66.5 mL/year in the placebo group, and the corresponding rates among the patients who were not receiving mycophenolate were -63.9 mL/year and -119.3 mL/year. Of note, the SENSCIS trial did not show any treatment effect on the skin fibrosis. According to the subgroup analysis, the effect of nintedanib was consistent regardless of the use of MMF, suggesting that there is no synergy but additive effect between nintedanib and MMF [56]. The gastrointestinal adverse (e.g., diarrhea) events were more common in the SENSCIS trial compared to the INPULSIS trials probably due to the gastrointestinal involvement by SSc itself [26,53]. The post hoc analysis on the SENSCIS trial showed that the effect of nintedanib was significant to prevent % predicted FVC decline of >10% but not of >5% [57]. An open label extension study is ongoing to provide long term data on nintedanib use in patients with SSc-ILD (ClinicalTrials.gov number, NCT03313180). Based on the SENSCIS trial [53], nintedanib was approved to treat SSc-ILD by the FDA in 2019 and by the European Medicines Agency (EMA) in 2020.

The acceptable safety and tolerability of the antifibrotic agent pirfenidone were reported among patients with SSc-ILD [58], but its efficacy needs to be assessed in further clinical trials. There are two ongoing RCTs on SSc-ILD. The efficacy and safety of pirfenidone is now being assessed in a phase 3 study on 144 SSc-ILD patients (ClinicalTrials.gov number, NCT03856853). In addition, the SLS III study (phase 2) will randomize 150 patients with SSc-ILD to pirfenidone versus placebo, with background MMF, over 18 months of follow-up (ClinicalTrials.gov number, NCT03221257), to assess the effect of combination treatment of pirfenidone and MMF versus MMF alone.

Biologics

Promising benefits in SSc-ILD from biologics have recently been suggested. In the phase II faSScinate trial that assessed the skin fibrosis as the primary outcome and lung function as the secondary outcome, 48-week treatment with tocilizumab (TCZ) provided an encouraging numerical improvement in the modified Rodnan skin scores and evidence of less decline in lung function [59]. During another 48-week open-label extension period of TCZ treatment, skin score improvement and FVC stabilization were observed in the placebo-treated patients who transitioned to tocilizumab [60]. In the faSScinate study, the patient population showing benefits from TCZ had a shorter duration of disease (mean disease duration, 1.6 years), increased serum acute phase reactants, progressive skin disease, and low normal mean FVC levels (mean predicted FVC%, 81%) at the study baseline. These findings may suggest that more inflammatory process is involved during the early phase of the disease, where immunosuppressive or anti-inflammatory treatment can provide more benefits. In the subsequent focuSSced study of the multinational background on 210 patients with early diffuse cutaneous SSc (duration $\leq$ 5 years) [61], TCZ and placebo were compared regarding skin fibrosis (primary outcome) and lung function (secondary outcome). After 48 weeks, the skin fibrosis endpoint was not met but the FVC loss was more in favor of the TCZ group than the placebo (between-group difference, 241 mL, p = 0.002). The results of the focuSSced study on FVC should be interpreted with caution because the SSc-ILD was not the primary outcome and only 65% of enrolled patients had SSc-ILD at baseline. Controlled studies are awaited to assess whether TCZ has an effect in patients with severe established SSc lung disease. In addition, the paradoxical response of aggravating ILD has been also reported from TCZ treatment [19], indicating that meticulous monitoring of ILD is mandatory before and after treatment despite the overall benefits of TCZ in patients with ILD.

Rituximab has also been used to treat SSc-ILD. In an open-label RCT on 60 patients with SSc-ILD, the RTX treatment showed a significantly better patient response than the CYC treatment in terms of improvement in FVC and skin fibrosis [62]. However, a propensity score matched observational study showed that the proportion of patients with FVC decline of ≥10% was similar regardless of RTX treatment. Nevertheless, patients treated with RTX were more likely to stop or decrease steroid use [63]. According to the experts, rituximab was considered as one of the first induction agents for SSc-ILD in addition to MMF or CYC [64]. An ongoing trial (RECITAL) is comparing rituximab and CYC for RD-ILD including SSc-ILD [65].

General Treatment Strategy for SSc-ILD

For those who are asymptomatic with minimal extent of ILD (e.g., FVC > 80%), watchful monitoring without treatment is justified [42,43]. For those who need treatment, the EULAR guidelines endorse CYC over MMF as the first line treatment for SSc-ILD [55] while the European consensus statements consider CYC and MMF, and nintedanib as equivalent options for treatment initiation or escalation [48]. The subgroup analysis of SENSCIS showed a comparable FVC change between placebo with baseline MMF group (−66.5 mL/year) versus nintedanib without baseline MMF group (−63.5 mL/year) [53]. Thus, whether to use antifibrotics as a first line treatment needs further data (e.g., head-to-head comparison between immunosuppressants versus antifibrotics) and discussion. A reasonable approach would be to switch to or add nintedanib when refractory to CYC or MMF. Although some evidence emerged suggestive of the benefits with TCZ and RTX on lung function, such evidence is only exploratory and needs to be confirmed in an RCT that examines lung function as the primary end point.

2.3. Myositis Associated Interstitial Lung Disease (Myositis-ILD)

As in SSc, the pulmonary manifestations of myositis can be categorized as direct and indirect. The direct involvements are mostly ILD. The indirect involvements consist of aspiration pneumonia due to pharyngeal muscle weakness and hypoventilation due to respiratory muscle weakness [66].

2.3.1. Clinical Course of Myositis-ILD

A majority of myositis-associated lung involvement manifests as ILD. Unlike in SSc, isolated PAH is rare in myositis [67]. ILD manifests early in the course of myositis, often found at the time of diagnosis [4,68,69]. Being prevalent in up to two thirds of myositis patients [4,69], more than 90% of myositis patients develop ILD in the presence of antiaminoacyl tRNA synthetase (ARS) antibody [70]. The clinical course of myositis-ILD is diverse but distinguished from SSc-ILD in that as many as 20% of myositis-ILD cases manifest as a rapidly progressive form that challenges successful treatment [69]. This contrasts with SSc-ILD, where fibrosis is the hallmark of the disease, causing more chronic progression. Such difference indicates that inflammatory process is a dominant process in myositis-ILD, generally in proportion to symptom deterioration rate, and culminates in the rapidly progressive form in which respiratory failure can occur even within days [71,72].

While NSIP is most common for myositis-ILD in general [1], DAD is more common in case of the rapidly progressive type [70]. The rapidly progressive ILD tends to cluster in patients with either classic DM or amyopathic dermatomyositis than polymyositis, particularly in the presence of antimelanoma differentiation-associated gene 5 (anti-MDA5) [73]. Myositis-ILD of the rapidly progressive type is refractory to treatment leading to a high mortality [72].

The treatment response of myositis-ILD follows the underlying histological pattern [69,74,75]. OP is well treated by steroids alone, whereas DAD and UIP respond poorly even to combination therapy [69,74]. The treatment response of NSIP depends upon the degree of inflammation compared to fibrosis [75]. Biomarker studies showed that high serum levels of ferritin, IL-18, or soluble CD206 (macrophage mannose receptor) were associated with a poor treatment response among patients with anti-MDA5-positive ILD [76,77].

2.3.2. Pharmacologic Treatment of Myositis-ILD

Due to the rarity of the disease and the heterogeneous clinical subsets within the disease, the treatment of myositis-ILD most often relies upon empirical therapy consisting of steroids combined with conventional immunosuppressives such as CYC, cyclosporine, or MMF without sufficient data supported by RCTs [1]. Even more limited are the data for targeted treatments. A recent Japanese study showed that the initial combination treatment with high dose steroid, tacrolimus, and CYC with or without plasmapheresis was associated with a better response in anti-MDA5-positive ILD patients compared to step-up therapy from initial high-dose steroids [78]. This finding also put emphasis on the early aggressive treatment for anti-MDA5-positive, rapidly progressive ILD. Moreover, a Spanish expert group agreed that anti-MDA5-positive ILD should be similarly treated [79]. Of note, despite the disease-specific anti-MDA5 autoantibody, successful treatment with rituximab has only been anecdotally reported [80].

2.4. Future Treatment Strategies for Rheumatic Disease Associated Interstitial Lung Disease

Nintedanib and pirfenidone slow but do not halt the progression of IPF. Thus, interest in the combination of the two drugs is growing, but more data are needed on the safety and efficacy of combination therapy. There are a few studies that showed relatively acceptable tolerability and safety of the two drugs combined for a short-term period (12~24 weeks) [37,38]: the combination was completed in two thirds of patients despite a higher adverse event rate compared to the single drug treatment. However, there have yet to be large randomized controlled trials assessing whether combination therapy has increased efficacy compared to treatment with a single antifibrotic drug.

Several clinical trials evaluating the efficacy of the new drugs on pulmonary outcomes are underway. The ISABELA 1 and 2 trials are now ongoing to examine the effect of autotaxin inhibitor GB-0998 among patients with IPF (ClinicalTrials.gov number, NCT03711162; NCT03733444) [81]. A phase 2 RCT of bortezomib plus MMF versus MMF alone on patients with SSc-ILD is currently ongoing (ClinicalTrials.gov number, NCT02370693). Romilkimab, a monoclonal antibody targeting IL-4 and IL-13, showed efficacy after 24 weeks on skin fibrosis associated with diffuse SSc under background immunosuppressive agents in a phase 2 pilot study [82]. However, it failed to show benefits in the of IPF after 52 weeks [83]. Guselkumab (monoclonal antibody that blocks IL-23) is under investigation in SSc patients with skin fibrosis as the primary outcome of and lung function as one of the secondary outcomes (ClinicalTrials.gov number, NCT04683029).

3. Pulmonary Arterial Hypertension (PAH)

Abnormal proliferation, vasoconstriction, and thrombosis of the pulmonary vasculature are the main pathogenic mechanisms of PAH. Right heart catheterization (RHC) is the gold standard to diagnose PAH using the criteria of a mean pulmonary arterial pressure of ≥ 25 mmHg and a pulmonary capillary wedge pressure of ≤ 15 mmHg [84].

3.1. Systemic Sclerosis Associated Pulmonary Arterial Hypertension (SSc-PAH)

Not only isolated PAH but also PH secondary to either left heart dysfunction or ILD progression can occur in SSc, either separately or in combination. The SSc-PAH shows a unique phenotype of PAH with a worst prognosis compared to idiopathic or non-SSc RD-PAH [85,86].

3.1.1. Clinical Features of SSc-PAH

The mortality risk of SSc patients increases by 3-fold in the presence of PAH, showing PAH is a deadly complication of SSc patients [87]. Therefore, patients should be screened for PAH based on symptoms, echocardiography, and DLCO patterns and undergo RHC if identified as high-risk [88,89]. With RHC, SSc-PAH was found in approximately 10% of these high-risk candidates. The limited rather than the diffuse cutaneous subset shows a higher prevalence of SSc-PAH, which was observed in up to half of the patients with CREST syndrome [90]. It was reported that 50% of SSc-PAH occurs within five years from the first non-Raynaud phenomenon symptom with the mean interval from SSc diagnosis to PAH occurrence of 6.3 years [91].

Like those with idiopathic PAH, patients with SSc-PAH are either clinically silent or show only nonspecific symptoms until their disease is advanced. Therefore, active surveillance is the key to early intervention, which indeed led to better survival compared to passive identification [92]. In SSc patients, male sex, old age, overt vasculopathy such as telangiectasia and digital ulcers, anticentromere or anti-U3 RNP antibodies, and the limited cutaneous subset (e.g., CREST syndrome) were identified as risk factors for PAH [93]. However, both the sensitivity and the specificity of these risk factors are limited. Other findings suggestive of PAH include elevated levels of the N-terminal probrain natriuretic peptide (NT-proBNP) or disproportionately low DLCO [94,95]. In particular, echocardiographic measures are one of the important screening tools to identify candidates for RHC. For example, a tricuspid regurgitation (TR) velocity of ≥ 2.5 m/s is considered one of the findings highly suggestive of PAH [96]. However, the sensitivity at this TR velocity threshold is limited, missing 20% of the mild PAH patients [96,97]. DETECT is a multidimensional algorithm to identify SSc patients at a high risk of PAH, used as the active surveillance strategy to avoid the delayed diagnosis of PAH [1,96]. Among 57 DETECT enrollees with SSc-PAH, 44% progressed during a median follow-up of 12.6 months [98]. The factors associated with progression were male gender, disproportionately low DLCO, and poor functional capacity. A more simplified and practical algorithm proposed in 2013 to initially screen SSc patients uses PFT, echocardiography, and NT-proBNP for referral for RHC [99] (Table 2).

In a recent prospective observational study, 93 SSc-ILD patients were screened and underwent RHC following the above 2013 algorithm. Of these, 31.2% were found to have RHC-proven PAH, and the survival rate was 91% at three years [100]. This improved survival is striking compared to the exceptionally grave prognosis (survival of 39% at three years) previously reported for SSc patients with coexisting ILD and PAH [101]. Based on this finding, the poor prognosis of SSc-PAH patients compared to patients with idiopathic or PAH of other rheumatic diseases could be due to delayed diagnosis and treatment [85,86], and early treatment is paramount for better survival.

3.1.2. Pharmacological Treatment of SSc-PAH

Treatment with Conventional Agents

Immunosuppression against the hyperimmune state of SSc is never sufficient to stop SSc-PAH progression due to fibrotic and proliferative pathways driven by nonimmune cells. An acute vasoreactive response is observed in 10% of the patients with RD-PAH, but the response to calcium channel blockers beyond 3–4 months is preserved in less than 1% of these patients [102].

Table 2. Screening algorithm for SSc-PAH proposed in 2013 [a].

			Quality of Evidence
All patients with SSc should be screened for PAH			Moderate
Initial screening evaluation in patients with SSc or SSc-spectrum disorders			
▶ Pulmonary function test (PFT) with diffusion capacity of carbon monoxide (DLCO)			High
▶ Transthoracic echocardiography (TTE)			High
▶ N-terminal probrain natriuretic peptide (NT-proBNP)			Moderate
▶ DETECT algorithm if DLCO% < 60% and >3 years disease duration from non-RP			Moderate
Recommendations for right heart catheterization for SSc or SSc-spectrum disorders			
Screening method	Parameter cut-off	Signs/symptoms requirement [b]	
PFT [c]	FVC/DLCO ratio > 1.6 and/or DLCO < 60%	Yes	High
	FVC/DLCO ratio > 1.6 and/or DLCO < 60% plus NT-proBNP > 2 x upper limit of normal	No	High
TTE	TR velocity	Yes	High
	2.5–2.8 m/s	No	High
	>2.8 m/s	No	High
	Cavity enlargements irrespective of TR velocity RA major dimension > 53 mm or RV mid-cavity dimension > 35 mm		
Composite	Meets DETECT algorithm with DLCO% < 60% and >3 years of disease duration	No	Moderate

[a] Cited and modified from "Recommendations for screening and detection of connective tissue disease-associated pulmonary arterial hypertension" by Khanna D, et al. Arthritis Rheum 2013; 65: 3194–3201 [99]. [b] Symptoms: dyspnea upon rest or exercise, fatigue, presyncope/syncope, chest pain, palpitations, dizziness, lightheadedness. Signs: loud pulmonic sound, peripheral edema. [c] Without overt systolic dysfunction, greater than grade I diastolic dysfunction, greater than mild mitral or aortic valve disease, or evidence of PAH in echocardiography. DLCO = diffusion capacity of carbon monoxide; FVC = forced vital capacity; NT-proBNP = N-terminal probrain natriuretic peptide; PAH = pulmonary arterial hypertension; PFT = pulmonary function test; RA = right atrium; RV = right ventricle; SSc = systemic sclerosis; TTE = transthoracic echocardiography.

Treatment with Targeted Agents and Risk Stratification

Although the autoimmune process may be the fundamental mechanism orchestrating the initiation and progression of RD-PAH, its downstream effects involve nonimmune components as well, leading to pulmonary vascular remodeling. In particular, the treatment effect of anti-inflammatory agents is limited in lung diseases associated with SSc, indicating that noninflammatory pathways play a dominant role. In PAH, endothelial dysfunction due to abnormally regulated vasoactive and/or proliferative mediators induces vascular constriction and remodeling. Currently, three pathways important in endothelial function are targeted by PAH treatments, endothelin-1, nitric oxide (NO), and prostacyclin pathways [103]. Endothelin receptor antagonist (ERA), phosphodiesterase 5 inhibitor (PDE5i), and soluble guanylate cyclase (sGC) stimulator, which potentiate the effect of nitric oxide (NO), as well as prostacyclin analogs (PCA), are commercially available (Table 3).

Table 3. Efficacy of drug monotherapy for group 1 PAH according to WHO functional class [a].

			Class [b]-Level [c]					
			WHO-FC II		**WHO-FC III**		**WHO-FC IV**	
ERA		Ambrisentan	I	A	I	A	IIb	C
		Bosentan	I	A	I	A	IIb	C
		Macitentan	I	B	I	B	IIb	C
PDE5i		Sildenafil	I	A	I	A	IIb	C
		Tadalafil	I	B	I	B	IIb	C
		Vardenafil	IIb	B	IIb	B	IIb	C
sGC stimulator		Riociguat	I	B	I	B	IIb	C
PCA	Epoprostenol	Intravenous	-	-	I	A	I	A
	Iloprost	Inhaled	-	-	I	B	IIb	C
		Intravenous	-	-	IIa	C	IIb	C
	Treprostinil	Subcutaneous	-	-	I	B	IIb	C
		Inhaled	-	-	I	B	IIb	C
		Intravenous	-	-	IIa	C	IIb	C
		Oral	-	-	IIb	B	-	-
	Beraprost		-	-	IIb	IIb	-	-
	Selexipag [oral]		I	B	I	B	-	-

[a] Cited and modified from "2015 European Society of Cardiology (ESC)/European Respiratory Society (ERS) guidelines for the diagnosis and treatment of pulmonary hypertension" by Galiè N et al. Eur Heart J. 2016; 37:67–119 [97], [b] Class of recommendation, [c] level of evidence, ERA = endothelin receptor antagonist; PDE5i = phosphodiesterase 5 inhibitor; sGC = soluble guanylate cyclase; PAH = pulmonary arterial hypertension; PCA = prostacyclin analog or receptor antagonist; WHO = World Health Organization; FC = functional class.

According to the 2017 EULAR recommendations [55], ERA (ambrisentan, bosentan, and macitentan), PDE5i (sildenafil and tadalafil), and an sGC stimulator (riociguats) are considered the first-line options for treating SSc-PAH based on high-quality RCTs that showed improvement in exercise capacity, the time to clinical worsening (defined as a composite of death, hospitalization, and disease progression), and/or PAH-related hemodynamics in heterogeneous patients with PAH including RD-PAH. These studies were not powered to show the independent efficacy of the SSc-PAH subgroup, but the EULAR recommendations are based on the extrapolation of the high-quality RCT results. In the subgroup analyses, the direction of the results was not different between patients with idiopathic PAH and RD-PAH. In the idiopathic PAH, significant improvements in exercise capacity and reductions in mortality (pooled effect, 44% reduction; $p < 0.041$) by these treatments were demonstrated [104].

A high-quality RCT showed that continuous intravenous epoprostenol (a prostacyclin analog) administration improved exercise capacity, functional class, and hemodynamics in patients with SSc-PAH [105]. The administration of continuous intravenous epoprostenol requires an indwelling central venous catheter and abrupt cessation of the drug may cause PAH rebound that can be fatal. Thus, the EULAR recommendations suggest that this treatment should be considered for severe SSc-PAH of class III and IV [55]. In addition to epoprostenol, other PCAs (iloprost and treprostinil) showed similar results in high-quality RCTs on heterogeneous patients with PAH including RD-PAH and are also approved for the treatment of PAH including RD-PAH [55]. Although not commented in EULAR recommendations, selexipag, an oral selective prostacyclin IP receptor agonist, has shown efficacy in the phase 3 GRIPHON trial of reducing the risk of a primary composite endpoint of morbidity and mortality by 40% and 41% in PAH and RD-PAH (majority, SSc-PAH), respectively [106,107]. Selexipag is the only oral prostacyclin receptor agonist that showed a reduction of morbidity and mortality in a RCT.

In addition to the application of individual drugs that target each corresponding pathway, the advancements in recent treatment strategies include the risk assessment of PAH patients and linking the baseline severity of PAH to the subsequent treatment intensity or escalation [97,103]. According to the 2015 European Society of Cardiology (ESC)/European Respiratory Society (ERS) pulmonary hypertension guidelines [97], a multiparametric approach should be considered to stratify patients into low-, intermediate- or high-risk groups for 1-year mortality using clinical (clinical signs of right heart failure, the progression of symptoms, and syncope), functional class (WHO or NYHA class), exercise (6-min walking distance and cardiopulmonary exercise testing), biochemical (NT-proBNP), and echocardiographic/hemodynamic parameters (Table 4).

Table 4. 2015 European Society of Cardiology (ESC)/European Respiratory Society (ERS) guidelines for the risk assessment of patients with PAH [a].

Parameters of Prognosis	Estimated 1-Year Mortality		
	Low Risk < 5%	Low Risk < 5%	Low Risk < 5%
Clinical signs of right heart failure	Absent	Absent	Present
Progression of symptoms	No	Slow	Rapid
Syncope	No	Occasional syncope [b]	Repeated syncope [c]
WHO functional class	I, II	III	IV
6MWD	>440 m	165–440 m	<165 m
Cardiopulmonary exercise testing	Peak VO$_2$ > 15 mL/min/kg (>65% predicted) VE/VCO$_2$ slope < 36	Peak VO$_2$ >15 mL/min/kg (35–65% predicted) VE/VCO$_2$ slope < 36	Peak VO$_2$ <11 mL/min/kg (<35% predicted) VE/VCO$_2$ slope $\geq$ 45
NT-proBNP levels	BNP < 50 ng/L NT-proBNP < 300 ng/L	BNP 50–300 ng/L NT-proBNP 300–1400 ng/L	BNP >300 ng/L NT-proBNP > 1400 ng/L
Imaging (echocardiography, CMR imaging)	RA area <18 cm^2 No pericardial effusion	VE/VCO$_2$ slope < 36	RA area > 26 cm^2 pericardial effusion
Hemodynamics	RAP < 8 mmHg CI $\geq$ 2.5 L/min/m^2 S$_v$O$_2$ > 65%	RAP 8–14 mmHg CI 2.0–2.4 L/min/m^2 S$_v$O$_2$ 60–65%	RAP > 14 mmHg CI < 2.0 L/min/m^2 S$_v$O$_2$ < 60%

[a] Cited and modified from "2015 European Society of Cardiology (ESC)/European Respiratory Society (ERS) guidelines for the diagnosis and treatment of pulmonary hypertension" Galiè N, et al. Eur Heart J. 2016;37:67–119 [97]. [b] Occasional syncope during brisk or heavy exercise, or occasional orthostatic syncope in an otherwise stable patient. [c] Repeated episodes of syncope even with little or regular physical activity. 6MWD = 6-min walking distance; BNP = brain natriuretic peptide; CI = cardiac index; CMR = cardiac magnetic resonance; NT-proBNP = N-terminal probrain natriuretic peptide; PAH = pulmonary arterial hypertension; RA = right atrium; RAP = right atrial pressure; S$_v$O$_2$ = mixed venous oxygen saturation; VE/VCO$_2$ = ventilatory equivalents for carbon dioxide; VO$_2$ = oxygen consumption; WHO = World Health Organization.

Another important feature of the 2015 ESC/ERS guidelines for PAH is the endorsement of pre-emptive combination therapy targeting different endothelial pathways, particularly for high-risk patients [97]. The most compelling evidence for such strategy came from the recent AMBITION trial where a 50% reduction in the composite endpoint of clinical failure events at 24 weeks was seen from treatment with the upfront combination of ambrisentan and tadalafil compared to either drug alone in patients with PAH and RD-PAH [108]. Similarly, the add-on effect of a study drug (either macitentan, selexipag, or riociguat) was observed in other RCTs when combined with a background PAH treatment using a different class [106,109,110], also endorsing sequential combination therapy. Similar evidence for upfront or initial combination or sequential combination therapy was also observed in patients with RD-PAH including SSc-PAH [107,111,112]. The 2015 ESC/ERS guidelines also depict a treatment algorithm that recommends treatment escalation (double to triple, maximal medical therapy including intravenous PCA) when the reassessment in 3–6 months shows an insufficient response such as residual intermediate- or high-risk status [97]. However, the evidence for the benefits of combination therapy remains to be replicated, specifically for SSc-PAH in future studies.

4. Pulmonary Manifestations of Other Rheumatic Diseases

Other than RA, SSc, and myositis, Sjogren's syndrome (SjS) and mixed connective tissue disease (MCTD) also show a substantial prevalence of pulmonary manifestations including ILD and PAH. Although the data on the epidemiology are growing in SjS and MCTD, RCT data regarding the treatments are very limited. However, we may be able to apply similar treatment strategies in SjS and MCTD as in other RDs described in this review, based on the dominant underlying mechanism of fibrosis versus inflammation or chronic progression versus acute exacerbation.

4.1. Sjogren's Syndrome Associated Pulmonary Involvements

SjS is a systemic autoimmune disease primarily affecting exocrine glands, which ultimately leads to the destruction of the given tissue [113]. The autoimmunity of SjS activates both immune cells and glandular epithelial cells showing a histological lesion of focal lymphocytic infiltrates, enriched in CD4+ T-cells, around the salivary and lachrymal ducts and even in lung tissues [114]. Of note, the focus score of salivary glands has been shown to correlate with the increased prevalence of airway disease and ILD in SjS [115]. These findings may suggest that the glandular and extraglandular lesions of SjS share similar pathogenic pathways involving autoimmunity to epithelial cells.

The prevalence of pulmonary involvement in patients with SjS has been estimated to range from 10% to 20% [116]. Airway disease and ILD are the predominant forms of lung involvement among the pulmonary manifestations of SjS, but lymphoproliferative disorders as well as cystic lesions are also observed [116]. The most common histologic type of ILD associated with SjS was found to be NSIP followed by UIP and LIP [117,118], with NSIP present in up to 45% of biopsied cases [117] and mostly of the fibrotic type [118]. Unlike RA-UIP, SjS-UIP tends to have a better response to immunotherapy as compared to IPF [119]. LIP constitutes 15% of SjS-ILD, of which clinical course is variable from complete resolution without treatment to progression and possible death or transformation to lymphoma [120].

4.2. Mixed Connective Tissue Disease Associated Pulmonary Involvements

MCTD is characterized by mixed features of two or more RDs including but not limited to SSc, myositis or systemic lupus erythematosus, with disease specific high titer anti-U1 RNP antibodies [121]. The common pulmonary manifestations of MCTD are ILD and PAH. A Norwegian nationwide cross-sectional study showed that 35% of MCTD patients had lung fibrosis in HRCT after a mean disease duration 9 years [122]. A higher rate of ILD was found (up to two thirds of the patients) in the hospital-based study [123]. In the Norwegian study, 19% of MCTD associated ILD (MCTD-ILD) was severe in extent involving >50% of lung parenchyma [122]. However, the retrospective cohort study on unselected 53 patients with a mean disease duration of 9 years in Brazil showed that 51% of the patients had ILD at baseline with a mean FVC that remained stable at around 77% over 10 years of follow-up and a mean DLCO that declined from 84% to 71% [124]. Such discrepant findings leave a debate on the natural course of MCTD-ILD, and further cohort studies at a larger scale are needed. Together with ILD, PAH is a major prognostic factor of MCTD [125,126]. The Norwegian population-based prevalence of pulmonary hypertension was reported to be less than 5% over 5.6 years [125], but PAH has been recognized as the leading cause of death in patients with MCTD, explaining 41% of all deaths [126].

5. Conclusions

ILD and PAH are the two most important prognostic factors in patients with RD and are associated with significant morbidity and mortality. Early diagnosis and early treatment are the key steps to the successful management of these two conditions, improving survival. In addition to conventional immunosuppressants, new targeted treatments are under investigation and some have already been incorporated into the international recommendations for treating RD-related ILD or PAH. However, more data are needed to ensure that the efficacy and safety of drugs used to treat RD as a whole are demonstrated for a specific RD.

Funding: This research received no external funding.

Institutional Review Board Statement: Not applicable.

Informed Consent Statement: Not applicable.

Data Availability Statement: Not applicable.

Conflicts of Interest: The authors declare no conflict of interest.

Abbreviations

CYC = cyclophosphamide, DAD = diffuse alveolar damage, DLCO = diffusion capacity of carbon monoxide, FVC = forced vital capacity, GGO = ground glass opacity, HRCT = high resolution computed tomography, ILD = interstitial lung disease, IPF = idiopathic pulmonary fibrosis, LIP = lymphoid interstitial pneumonia, MCTD = mixed connective tissue disease, MMF = mycophenolate, NSIP = nonspecific interstitial pneumonia, OP = organizing pneumonia, PAH = pulmonary arterial hypertension, RA = rheumatoid arthritis, RCT = randomized controlled trial, RD = rheumatic disease, SjS = Sjogren's syndrome, SSc = systemic sclerosis, UIP = usual interstitial pneumonia

References

1. Ha, Y.-J.; Lee, Y.J.; Kang, E.H. Lung involvements in rheumatic diseases: Update on the epidemiology, pathogenesis, clinical features, and treatment. *BioMed Res. Int.* **2018**, *2018*, 6930297. [CrossRef]
2. Mathai, S.C.; Danoff, S.K. Management of interstitial lung disease associated with connective tissue disease. *BMJ* **2016**, *352*, h6819. [CrossRef]
3. Schurawitzki, H.; Stiglbauer, R.; Graninger, W.; Herold, C.; Pölzleitner, D.; Burghuber, O.C.; Tscholakoff, D. Interstitial lung disease in progressive systemic sclerosis: High-resolution CT versus radiography. *Radiology* **1990**, *176*, 755–759. [CrossRef]
4. Fathi, M.; Dastmalchi, M.; Rasmussen, E.; Lundberg, I.; Tornling, G. Interstitial lung disease, a common manifestation of newly diagnosed polymyositis and dermatomyositis. *Ann. Rheum. Dis.* **2004**, *63*, 297–301. [CrossRef] [PubMed]
5. Olson, A.L.; Swigris, J.J.; Sprunger, D.B.; Fischer, A.; Fernandez-Perez, E.R.; Solomon, J.; Murphy, J.; Cohen, M.; Raghu, G.; Brown, K.K. Rheumatoid arthritis—Interstitial lung disease—Associated mortality. *Am. J. Respir. Crit. Care Med.* **2011**, *183*, 372–378. [CrossRef]
6. Travis, W.D.; Costabel, U.; Hansell, D.M.; King, T.E., Jr.; Lynch, D.A.; Nicholson, A.G.; Ryerson, C.J.; Ryu, J.H.; Selman, M.; Wells, A.U. An official American Thoracic Society/European Respiratory Society statement: Update of the international multidisciplinary classification of the idiopathic interstitial pneumonias. *Am. J. Respir. Crit. Care Med.* **2013**, *188*, 733–748. [CrossRef]
7. Park, J.H.; Kim, D.S.; Park, I.-N.; Jang, S.J.; Kitaichi, M.; Nicholson, A.G.; Colby, T.V. Prognosis of fibrotic interstitial pneumonia: Idiopathic versus collagen vascular disease-related subtypes. *Am. J. Respir. Crit. Care Med.* **2007**, *175*, 705–711. [CrossRef] [PubMed]
8. Bongartz, T.; Nannini, C.; Medina-Velasquez, Y.F.; Achenbach, S.J.; Crowson, C.S.; Ryu, J.H.; Vassallo, R.; Gabriel, S.E.; Matteson, E.L. Incidence and mortality of interstitial lung disease in rheumatoid arthritis: A population-based study. *Arthritis Rheumatol.* **2010**, *62*, 1583–1591. [CrossRef] [PubMed]
9. Hyldgaard, C.; Hilberg, O.; Pedersen, A.B.; Ulrichsen, S.P.; Løkke, A.; Bendstrup, E.; Ellingsen, T. A population-based cohort study of rheumatoid arthritis-associated interstitial lung disease: Comorbidity and mortality. *Ann. Rheum. Dis.* **2017**, *76*, 1700–1706. [CrossRef] [PubMed]
10. Restrepo, J.F.; Del Rincón, I.; Battafarano, D.F.; Haas, R.W.; Doria, M.; Escalante, A. Clinical and laboratory factors associated with interstitial lung disease in rheumatoid arthritis. *Clin. Rheumatol.* **2015**, *34*, 1529–1536. [CrossRef] [PubMed]
11. Rocha-Muñoz, A.D.; Ponce-Guarneros, M.; Gamez-Nava, J.I.; Olivas-Flores, E.M.; Mejía, M.; Juárez-Contreras, P.; Martínez-García, E.A.; Corona-Sánchez, E.G.; Rodríguez-Hernández, T.M.; Vázquez-del Mercado, M. Anti-cyclic citrullinated peptide antibodies and severity of interstitial lung disease in women with rheumatoid arthritis. *J. Immunol. Res.* **2015**, *2015*, 151626. [CrossRef]

12. Solomon, J.J.; Chung, J.H.; Cosgrove, G.P.; Demoruelle, M.K.; Fernandez-Perez, E.R.; Fischer, A.; Frankel, S.K.; Hobbs, S.B.; Huie, T.J.; Ketzer, J. Predictors of mortality in rheumatoid arthritis-associated interstitial lung disease. *Eur. Respir. J.* **2016**, *47*, 588–596. [CrossRef] [PubMed]
13. Suda, T.; Kaida, Y.; Nakamura, Y.; Enomoto, N.; Fujisawa, T.; Imokawa, S.; Hashizume, H.; Naito, T.; Hashimoto, D.; Takehara, Y. Acute exacerbation of interstitial pneumonia associated with collagen vascular diseases. *Respir. Med.* **2009**, *103*, 846–853. [CrossRef] [PubMed]
14. Hozumi, H.; Nakamura, Y.; Johkoh, T.; Sumikawa, H.; Colby, T.V.; Kono, M.; Hashimoto, D.; Enomoto, N.; Fujisawa, T.; Inui, N. Acute exacerbation in rheumatoid arthritis-associated interstitial lung disease: A retrospective case control study. *BMJ Open* **2013**, *3*, e003132. [CrossRef] [PubMed]
15. Kolb, M.; Bondue, B.; Pesci, A.; Miyazaki, Y.; Song, J.W.; Bhatt, N.Y.; Huggins, J.T.; Oldham, J.M.; Padilla, M.L.; Roman, J.; et al. Acute exacerbations of progressive-fibrosing interstitial lung diseases. *Eur. Respir. Rev.* **2018**, *27*, 180071. [CrossRef] [PubMed]
16. Singh, J.A.; Saag, K.G.; Bridges Jr, S.L.; Akl, E.A.; Bannuru, R.R.; Sullivan, M.C.; Vaysbrot, E.; McNaughton, C.; Osani, M.; Shmerling, R.H.; et al. 2015 American College of Rheumatology guideline for the treatment of rheumatoid arthritis. *Arthritis Rheumatol.* **2016**, *68*, 1–26. [CrossRef]
17. Smolen, J.S.; Landewé, R.; Bijlsma, J.; Burmester, G.; Chatzidionysiou, K.; Dougados, M.; Nam, J.; Ramiro, S.; Voshaar, M.; Van Vollenhoven, R.; et al. EULAR recommendations for the management of rheumatoid arthritis with synthetic and biological disease-modifying antirheumatic drugs: 2016 update. *Ann. Rheum. Dis.* **2017**, *76*, 960–977. [CrossRef]
18. Fischer, A.; Brown, K.K.; Du Bois, R.M.; Frankel, S.K.; Cosgrove, G.P.; Fernandez-Perez, E.R.; Huie, T.J.; Krishnamoorthy, M.; Meehan, R.T.; Olson, A.L. Mycophenolate mofetil improves lung function in connective tissue disease-associated interstitial lung disease. *J. Rheumatol.* **2013**, *40*, 640–646. [CrossRef]
19. Roubille, C.; Haraoui, B. Interstitial lung diseases induced or exacerbated by DMARDS and biologic agents in rheumatoid arthritis: A systematic literature review. *Semin. Arthritis Rheum.* **2014**, *43*, 613–626. [CrossRef]
20. Herrinton, L.J.; Harrold, L.R.; Liu, L.; Raebel, M.A.; Taharka, A.; Winthrop, K.L.; Solomon, D.H.; Curtis, J.R.; Lewis, J.D.; Saag, K.G. Association between anti-TNF-α therapy and interstitial lung disease. *Pharmacoepidemiol. Drug Saf.* **2013**, *22*, 394–402. [CrossRef]
21. Dixon, W.; Hyrich, K.; Watson, K.; Lunt, M.; Consortium, B.C.C.; Symmons, D. Influence of anti-TNF therapy on mortality in patients with rheumatoid arthritis-associated interstitial lung disease: Results from the British Society for Rheumatology Biologics Register. *Ann. Rheum. Dis.* **2010**, *69*, 1086–1091. [CrossRef] [PubMed]
22. Keir, G.J.; Maher, T.M.; Ming, D.; Abdullah, R.; de Lauretis, A.; Wickremasinghe, M.; Nicholson, A.G.; Hansell, D.M.; Wells, A.U.; Renzoni, E.A. Rituximab in severe, treatment-refractory interstitial lung disease. *Respirology* **2014**, *19*, 353–359. [CrossRef] [PubMed]
23. Fernández-Díaz, C.; Castañeda, S.; Melero-González, R.B.; Ortiz-Sanjuán, F.; Juan-Mas, A.; Carrasco-Cubero, C.; Casafont-Solé, I.; Olivé, A.; Rodríguez-Muguruza, S.; Almodóvar-González, R. Abatacept in interstitial lung disease associated with rheumatoid arthritis: National multicenter study of 263 patients. *Rheumatology* **2020**, *59*, 3906–3916. [CrossRef] [PubMed]
24. Wollin, L.; Wex, E.; Pautsch, A.; Schnapp, G.; Hostettler, K.E.; Stowasser, S.; Kolb, M. Mode of action of nintedanib in the treatment of idiopathic pulmonary fibrosis. *Eur. Respir. J.* **2015**, *45*, 1434–1445. [CrossRef]
25. Richeldi, L.; Costabel, U.; Selman, M.; Kim, D.S.; Hansell, D.M.; Nicholson, A.G.; Brown, K.K.; Flaherty, K.R.; Noble, P.W.; Raghu, G. Efficacy of a tyrosine kinase inhibitor in idiopathic pulmonary fibrosis. *N. Engl. J. Med.* **2011**, *365*, 1079–1087. [CrossRef]
26. Richeldi, L.; Du Bois, R.M.; Raghu, G.; Azuma, A.; Brown, K.K.; Costabel, U.; Cottin, V.; Flaherty, K.R.; Hansell, D.M.; Inoue, Y. Efficacy and safety of nintedanib in idiopathic pulmonary fibrosis. *N. Engl. J. Med.* **2014**, *370*, 2071–2082. [CrossRef] [PubMed]
27. Costabel, U.; Inoue, Y.; Richeldi, L.; Collard, H.R.; Tschoepe, I.; Stowasser, S.; Azuma, A. Efficacy of nintedanib in idiopathic pulmonary fibrosis across prespecified subgroups in INPULSIS. *Am. J. Respir. Crit. Care Med.* **2016**, *193*, 178–185. [CrossRef] [PubMed]
28. Brown, K.K.; Flaherty, K.R.; Cottin, V.; Raghu, G.; Inoue, Y.; Azuma, A.; Huggins, J.T.; Richeldi, L.; Stowasser, S.; Stansen, W. Lung function outcomes in the INPULSIS® trials of nintedanib in idiopathic pulmonary fibrosis. *Respir. Med.* **2019**, *146*, 42–48. [CrossRef]
29. Wells, A.U.; Flaherty, K.R.; Brown, K.K.; Inoue, Y.; Devaraj, A.; Richeldi, L.; Moua, T.; Crestani, B.; Wuyts, W.A.; Stowasser, S. Nintedanib in patients with progressive fibrosing interstitial lung diseases—Subgroup analyses by interstitial lung disease diagnosis in the INBUILD trial: A randomised, double-blind, placebo-controlled, parallel-group trial. *Lancet Respir. Med.* **2020**, *8*, 453–460. [CrossRef]
30. Taniguchi, H.; Ebina, M.; Kondoh, Y.; Ogura, T.; Azuma, A.; Suga, M.; Taguchi, Y.; Takahashi, H.; Nakata, K.; Sato, A. Pirfenidone in idiopathic pulmonary fibrosis. *Eur. Respir. J.* **2010**, *35*, 821–829. [CrossRef]
31. Noble, P.W.; Albera, C.; Bradford, W.Z.; Costabel, U.; Glassberg, M.K.; Kardatzke, D.; King, T.E., Jr.; Lancaster, L.; Sahn, S.A.; Szwarcberg, J. Pirfenidone in patients with idiopathic pulmonary fibrosis (CAPACITY): Two randomised trials. *Lancet* **2011**, *377*, 1760–1769. [CrossRef]
32. King, T.E., Jr.; Bradford, W.Z.; Castro-Bernardini, S.; Fagan, E.A.; Glaspole, I.; Glassberg, M.K.; Gorina, E.; Hopkins, P.M.; Kardatzke, D.; Lancaster, L. A phase 3 trial of pirfenidone in patients with idiopathic pulmonary fibrosis. *N. Engl. J. Med.* **2014**, *370*, 2083–2092. [CrossRef]

33. Maher, T.M.; Corte, T.J.; Fischer, A.; Kreuter, M.; Lederer, D.J.; Molina-Molina, M.; Axmann, J.; Kirchgaessler, K.-U.; Samara, K.; Gilberg, F. Pirfenidone in patients with unclassifiable progressive fibrosing interstitial lung disease: A double-blind, randomised, placebo-controlled, phase 2 trial. *Lancet Respir. Med.* **2020**, *8*, 147–157. [CrossRef]
34. Solomon, J.J.; Danoff, S.K.; Goldberg, H.J.; Woodhead, F.; Kolb, M.; Chambers, D.C.; DiFranco, D.; Spino, C.; Haynes-Harp, S.; Hurwitz, S. The design and rationale of the trail1 trial: A randomized double-blind phase 2 clinical trial of pirfenidone in rheumatoid arthritis-associated interstitial lung disease. *Adv. Ther.* **2019**, *36*, 3279–3287. [CrossRef] [PubMed]
35. Ogura, T.; Taniguchi, H.; Azuma, A.; Inoue, Y.; Kondoh, Y.; Hasegawa, Y.; Bando, M.; Abe, S.; Mochizuki, Y.; Chida, K.; et al. Safety and pharmacokinetics of nintedanib and pirfenidone in idiopathic pulmonary fibrosis. *Eur. Respir. J.* **2015**, *45*, 1382–1392. [CrossRef]
36. Valeyre, D.; Albera, C.; Bradford, W.Z.; Costabel, U.; King, T.E., Jr.; Leff, J.A.; Noble, P.W.; Sahn, S.A.; du Bois, R.M. Comprehensive assessment of the long-term safety of pirfenidone in patients with idiopathic pulmonary fibrosis. *Respirology* **2014**, *19*, 740–747. [CrossRef]
37. Flaherty, K.R.; Fell, C.D.; Huggins, J.T.; Nunes, H.; Sussman, R.; Valenzuela, C.; Petzinger, U.; Stauffer, J.L.; Gilberg, F.; Bengus, M.; et al. Safety of nintedanib added to pirfenidone treatment for idiopathic pulmonary fibrosis. *Eur. Respir. J.* **2018**, *52*, 1800230. [CrossRef]
38. Vancheri, C.; Kreuter, M.; Richeldi, L.; Ryerson, C.J.; Valeyre, D.; Grutters, J.C.; Wiebe, S.; Stansen, W.; Quaresma, M.; Stowasser, S.; et al. Nintedanib with add-on pirfenidone in idiopathic pulmonary fibrosis. Results of the INJOURNEY trial. *Am. J. Respir. Crit. Care Med.* **2018**, *197*, 356–363. [CrossRef]
39. Hamaguchi, Y. Autoantibody profiles in systemic sclerosis: Predictive value for clinical evaluation and prognosis. *J. Dermatol.* **2010**, *37*, 42–53. [CrossRef] [PubMed]
40. Walker, U.; Tyndall, A.; Czirjak, L.; Denton, C.; Farge-Bancel, D.; Kowal-Bielecka, O.; Müller-Ladner, U.; Bocelli-Tyndall, C.; Matucci-Cerinic, M. Clinical risk assessment of organ manifestations in systemic sclerosis: A report from the EULAR Scleroderma Trials And Research group database. *Ann. Rheum. Dis.* **2007**, *66*, 754–763. [CrossRef] [PubMed]
41. Steen, V.D.; Conte, C.; Owens, G.R.; Medsger, T.A., Jr. Severe restrictive lung disease in systemic sclerosis. *Arthritis Rheum.* **1994**, *37*, 1283–1289. [CrossRef]
42. Kwon, H.M.; Kang, E.H.; Park, J.K.; Go, D.J.; Lee, E.Y.; Song, Y.W.; Lee, H.-J.; Lee, E.B. A decision model for the watch-and-wait strategy in systemic sclerosis–associated interstitial lung disease. *Rheumatology* **2015**, *54*, 1792–1796. [CrossRef]
43. Man, A.; Davidyock, T.; Ferguson, L.T.; Ieong, M.; Zhang, Y.; Simms, R.W. Changes in forced vital capacity over time in systemic sclerosis: Application of group-based trajectory modelling. *Rheumatology* **2015**, *54*, 1464–1471. [CrossRef] [PubMed]
44. Bouros, D.; Wells, A.U.; Nicholson, A.G.; Colby, T.V.; Polychronopoulos, V.; Pantelidis, P.; Haslam, P.L.; Vassilakis, D.A.; Black, C.M.; Du Bois, R.M. Histopathologic subsets of fibrosing alveolitis in patients with systemic sclerosis and their relationship to outcome. *Am. J. Respir. Crit. Care Med.* **2002**, *165*, 1581–1586. [CrossRef]
45. Shah, R.M.; Jimenez, S.; Wechsler, R. Significance of ground-glass opacity on HRCT in long-term follow-up of patients with systemic sclerosis. *J. Thorac. Imaging* **2007**, *22*, 120–124. [CrossRef] [PubMed]
46. Launay, D.; Remy-Jardin, M.; Michon-Pasturel, U.; Mastora, I.; Hachulla, E.; Lambert, M.; Delannoy, V.; Queyrel, V.; Duhamel, A.; Matran, R. High resolution computed tomography in fibrosing alveolitis associated with systemic sclerosis. *J. Rheumatol.* **2006**, *33*, 1789–1801.
47. Rubio-Rivas, M.; Royo, C.; Simeón, C.P.; Corbella, X.; Fonollosa, V. Mortality and survival in systemic sclerosis: Systematic review and meta-analysis. *Semin. Arthritis Rheum.* **2014**, *44*, 208–219. [CrossRef]
48. Hoffmann-Vold, A.-M.; Maher, T.M.; Philpot, E.E.; Ashrafzadeh, A.; Barake, R.; Barsotti, S.; Bruni, C.; Carducci, P.; Carreira, P.E.; Castellví, I.; et al. The identification and management of interstitial lung disease in systemic sclerosis: Evidence-based European consensus statements. *Lancet Rheumatol.* **2020**, *2*, e71–e83. [CrossRef]
49. Khanna, D.; Mittoo, S.; Aggarwal, R.; Proudman, S.M.; Dalbeth, N.; Matteson, E.L.; Brown, K.; Flaherty, K.; Wells, A.U.; Seibold, J.R.; et al. Connective tissue disease-associated interstitial lung diseases (CTD-ILD)—Report from OMERACT CTD-ILD Working Group. *J. Rheumatol.* **2015**, *42*, 2168–2171. [CrossRef] [PubMed]
50. Goh, N.S.; Hoyles, R.K.; Denton, C.P.; Hansell, D.M.; Renzoni, E.A.; Maher, T.M.; Nicholson, A.G.; Wells, A.U. Short-term pulmonary function trends are predictive of mortality in interstitial lung disease associated with systemic sclerosis. *Arthritis Rheumatol.* **2017**, *69*, 1670–1678. [CrossRef]
51. Tashkin, D.P.; Elashoff, R.; Clements, P.J.; Goldin, J.; Roth, M.D.; Furst, D.E.; Arriola, E.; Silver, R.; Strange, C.; Bolster, M. Cyclophosphamide versus placebo in scleroderma lung disease. *N. Engl. J. Med.* **2006**, *354*, 2655–2666. [CrossRef] [PubMed]
52. Tashkin, D.P.; Elashoff, R.; Clements, P.J.; Roth, M.D.; Furst, D.E.; Silver, R.M.; Goldin, J.; Arriola, E.; Strange, C.; Bolster, M.B. Effects of 1-year treatment with cyclophosphamide on outcomes at 2 years in scleroderma lung disease. *Am. J. Respir. Crit. Care Med.* **2007**, *176*, 1026–1034. [CrossRef]
53. Distler, O.; Highland, K.B.; Gahlemann, M.; Azuma, A.; Fischer, A.; Mayes, M.D.; Raghu, G.; Sauter, W.; Girard, M.; Alves, M. Nintedanib for systemic sclerosis-associated interstitial lung disease. *N. Engl. J. Med.* **2019**, *380*, 2518–2528. [CrossRef]
54. Tashkin, D.P.; Roth, M.D.; Clements, P.J.; Furst, D.E.; Khanna, D.; Kleerup, E.C.; Goldin, J.; Arriola, E.; Volkmann, E.R.; Kafaja, S. Mycophenolate mofetil versus oral cyclophosphamide in scleroderma-related interstitial lung disease (SLS II): A randomized controlled, double-blind, parallel group trial. *Lancet Respir. Med.* **2016**, *4*, 708–719. [CrossRef]

55. Kowal-Bielecka, O.; Fransen, J.; Avouac, J.; Becker, M.; Kulak, A.; Allanore, Y.; Distler, O.; Clements, P.; Cutolo, M.; Czirjak, L. Update of EULAR recommendations for the treatment of systemic sclerosis. *Ann. Rheum. Dis.* **2017**, *76*, 1327–1339. [CrossRef] [PubMed]
56. Highland, K.B.; Distler, O.; Kuwana, M.; Allanore, Y.; Assassi, S.; Azuma, A.; Bourdin, A.; Denton, C.P.; Distler, J.H.; Hoffmann-Vold, A.M.; et al. Efficacy and safety of nintedanib in patients with systemic sclerosis-associated interstitial lung disease treated with mycophenolate: A subgroup analysis of the SENSCIS trial. *Lancet Respir. Med.* **2021**, *9*, 96–106. [CrossRef]
57. Maher, T.M.; Mayes, M.D.; Kreuter, M.; Volkmann, E.R.; Aringer, M.; Castellvi, I.; Cutolo, M.; Stock, C.; Schoof, N.; Alves, M.; et al. Effect of nintedanib on lung function in patients with systemic sclerosis-associated interstitial lung disease: Further analyses of the SENSCIS trial. *Arthritis Rheumatol.* **2020**. [CrossRef]
58. Khanna, D.; Albera, C.; Fischer, A.; Khalidi, N.; Raghu, G.; Chung, L.; Chen, D.; Schiopu, E.; Tagliaferri, M.; Seibold, J.R. An open-label, phase II study of the safety and tolerability of pirfenidone in patients with scleroderma-associated interstitial lung disease: The LOTUSS trial. *J. Rheumatol.* **2016**, *43*, 1672–1679. [CrossRef]
59. Khanna, D.; Denton, C.P.; Jahreis, A.; van Laar, J.M.; Frech, T.M.; Anderson, M.E.; Baron, M.; Chung, L.; Fierlbeck, G.; Lakshminarayanan, S. Safety and efficacy of subcutaneous tocilizumab in adults with systemic sclerosis (faSScinate): A phase 2, randomised, controlled trial. *Lancet* **2016**, *387*, 2630–2640. [CrossRef]
60. Khanna, D.; Denton, C.P.; Lin, C.J.; van Laar, J.M.; Frech, T.M.; Anderson, M.E.; Baron, M.; Chung, L.; Fierlbeck, G.; Lakshminarayanan, S. Safety and efficacy of subcutaneous tocilizumab in systemic sclerosis: Results from the open-label period of a phase II randomised controlled trial (faSScinate). *Ann. Rheum. Dis.* **2018**, *77*, 212–220. [CrossRef]
61. Khanna, D.; Lin, C.J.F.; Furst, D.E.; Goldin, J.; Kim, G.; Kuwana, M.; Allanore, Y.; Matucci-Cerinic, M.; Distler, O.; Shima, Y.; et al. Tocilizumab in systemic sclerosis: A randomised, double-blind, placebo-controlled, phase 3 trial. *Lancet Respir. Med.* **2020**, *8*, 963–974. [CrossRef]
62. Sircar, G.; Goswami, R.P.; Sircar, D.; Ghosh, A.; Ghosh, P. Intravenous cyclophosphamide vs. rituximab for the treatment of early diffuse scleroderma lung disease: Open label, randomized, controlled trial. *Rheumatology* **2018**, *57*, 2106–2113. [CrossRef] [PubMed]
63. Elhai, M.; Boubaya, M.; Distler, O.; Smith, V.; Matucci-Cerinic, M.; Sancho, J.J.A.; Truchetet, M.-E.; Braun-Moscovici, Y.; Iannone, F.; Novikov, P.I. Outcomes of patients with systemic sclerosis treated with rituximab in contemporary practice: A prospective cohort study. *Ann. Rheum. Dis.* **2019**, *78*, 979–987. [CrossRef]
64. Fernández-Codina, A.; Walker, K.M.; Pope, J.E. Treatment algorithms for systemic sclerosis according to experts. *Arthritis Rheumatol.* **2018**, *70*, 1820–1828. [CrossRef] [PubMed]
65. Saunders, P.; Tsipouri, V.; Keir, G.J.; Ashby, D.; Flather, M.D.; Parfrey, H.; Babalis, D.; Renzoni, E.A.; Denton, C.P.; Wells, A.U. Rituximab versus cyclophosphamide for the treatment of connective tissue disease-associated interstitial lung disease (RECITAL): Study protocol for a randomised controlled trial. *Trials* **2017**, *18*, 1–11. [CrossRef] [PubMed]
66. Fathi, M.; Lundberg, I.E.; Tornling, G. Pulmonary complications of polymyositis and dermatomyositis. *Semin. Respir. Crit. Care. Med.* **2007**, *28*, 451–458. [CrossRef]
67. Sanges, S.; Yelnik, C.M.; Sitbon, O.; Benveniste, O.; Mariampillai, K.; Phillips-Houlbracq, M.; Pison, C.; Deligny, C.; Inamo, J.; Cottin, V. Pulmonary arterial hypertension in idiopathic inflammatory myopathies: Data from the French pulmonary hypertension registry and review of the literature. *Medicine* **2016**, *95*, e4911. [CrossRef] [PubMed]
68. Cottin, V.; Thivolet-Béjui, F.; Reynaud-Gaubert, M.; Cadranel, J.; Delaval, P.; Ternamian, P.; Cordier, J.-F. Interstitial lung disease in amyopathic dermatomyositis, dermatomyositis and polymyositis. *Eur. Respir. J.* **2003**, *22*, 245–250. [CrossRef] [PubMed]
69. Marie, I.; Hachulla, E.; Cherin, P.; Dominique, S.; Hatron, P.Y.; Hellot, M.F.; Devulder, B.; Herson, S.; Levesque, H.; Courtois, H. Interstitial lung disease in polymyositis and dermatomyositis. *Arthritis Rheum.* **2002**, *47*, 614–622. [CrossRef] [PubMed]
70. Mimori, T.; Nakashima, R.; Hosono, Y. Interstitial lung disease in myositis: Clinical subsets, biomarkers, and treatment. *Curr. Rheumatol. Rep.* **2012**, *14*, 264–274. [CrossRef]
71. Dickey, B.F.; Myers, A.R. Pulmonary disease in polymyositis/dermatomyositis. *Semin. Arthritis Rheum.* **1984**, *14*, 60–76. [CrossRef]
72. Kang, E.H.; Lee, E.B.; Shin, K.C.; Im, C.; Chung, D.; Han, S.; Song, Y.-W. Interstitial lung disease in patients with polymyositis, dermatomyositis and amyopathic dermatomyositis. *Rheumatology* **2005**, *44*, 1282–1286. [CrossRef]
73. Kang, E.H.; Nakashima, R.; Mimori, T.; Kim, J.; Lee, Y.J.; Lee, E.B.; Song, Y.W. Myositis autoantibodies in Korean patients with inflammatory myositis: Anti-140-kDa polypeptide antibody is primarily associated with rapidly progressive interstitial lung disease independent of clinically amyopathic dermatomyositis. *BMC Musculoskelet. Disord.* **2010**, *11*, 223. [CrossRef]
74. Tazelaar, H.D.; Viggiano, R.W.; Pickersgill, J.; Colby, T.V. Interstitial lung disease in polymyositis and dermatomyositis. *Am. Rev. Respir Dis* **1990**, *141*, 727–731. [CrossRef] [PubMed]
75. Tansey, D.; Wells, A.; Colby, T.; Ip, S.; Nikolakoupolou, A.; Du Bois, R.; Hansell, D.; Nicholson, A. Variations in histological patterns of interstitial pneumonia between connective tissue disorders and their relationship to prognosis. *Histopathology* **2004**, *44*, 585–596. [CrossRef] [PubMed]
76. Gono, T.; Sato, S.; Kawaguchi, Y.; Kuwana, M.; Hanaoka, M.; Katsumata, Y.; Takagi, K.; Baba, S.; Okamoto, Y.; Ota, Y. Anti-MDA5 antibody, ferritin and IL-18 are useful for the evaluation of response to treatment in interstitial lung disease with anti-MDA5 antibody-positive dermatomyositis. *Rheumatology* **2012**, *51*, 1563–1570. [CrossRef] [PubMed]

77. Horiike, Y.; Suzuki, Y.; Fujisawa, T.; Yasui, H.; Karayama, M.; Hozumi, H.; Furuhashi, K.; Enomoto, N.; Nakamura, Y.; Inui, N. Successful classification of macrophage-mannose receptor CD206 in severity of anti-MDA5 antibody positive dermatomyositis associated ILD. *Rheumatology* **2019**, *58*, 2143–2152. [CrossRef]
78. Tsuji, H.; Nakashima, R.; Hosono, Y.; Imura, Y.; Yagita, M.; Yoshifuji, H.; Hirata, S.; Nojima, T.; Sugiyama, E.; Hatta, K. Multicenter prospective study of the efficacy and safety of combined immunosuppressive therapy with high-dose glucocorticoid, tacrolimus, and cyclophosphamide in interstitial lung diseases accompanied by anti-melanoma differentiation-associated gene 5-positive dermatomyositis. *Arthritis Rheumatol.* **2020**, *72*, 488–498.
79. Romero-Bueno, F.; del Campo, P.D.; Trallero-Araguás, E.; Ruiz-Rodríguez, J.; Castellvi, I.; Rodriguez-Nieto, M.; Martínez-Becerra, M.; Sanchez-Pernaute, O.; Pinal-Fernandez, I.; Solanich, X. Recommendations for the treatment of anti-melanoma differentiation-associated gene 5-positive dermatomyositis-associated rapidly progressive interstitial lung disease. *Semin. Arthritis Rheum.* **2020**, *50*, 776–790. [CrossRef]
80. Ogawa, Y.; Kishida, D.; Shimojima, Y.; Hayashi, K.; Sekijima, Y. Effective administration of rituximab in anti-MDA5 antibody-positive dermatomyositis with rapidly progressive interstitial lung disease and refractory cutaneous involvement: A case report and literature review. *Case Rep. Rheumatol.* **2017**, *2017*, 5386797. [CrossRef]
81. Maher, T.M.; Kreuter, M.; Lederer, D.J.; Brown, K.K.; Wuyts, W.; Verbruggen, N.; Stutvoet, S.; Fieuw, A.; Ford, P.; Abi-Saab, W.; et al. Rationale, design and objectives of two phase III, randomised, placebo-controlled studies of GLPG1690, a novel autotaxin inhibitor, in idiopathic pulmonary fibrosis (ISABELA 1 and 2). *BMJ Open Respir. Res.* **2019**, *6*, e000422. [CrossRef] [PubMed]
82. Allanore, Y.; Wung, P.; Soubrane, C.; Esperet, C.; Marrache, F.; Bejuit, R.; Lahmar, A.; Khanna, D.; Denton, C.P. A randomised, double-blind, placebo-controlled, 24-week, phase II, proof-of-concept study of romilkimab (SAR156597) in early diffuse cutaneous systemic sclerosis. *Ann. Rheum. Dis.* **2020**, *79*, 1600–1607. [CrossRef] [PubMed]
83. Raghu, G.; Richeldi, L.; Crestani, B.; Wung, P.; Bejuit, R.; Esperet, C.; Antoni, C.; Soubrane, C. SAR156597 in idiopathic pulmonary fibrosis: A phase 2 placebo-controlled study (DRI11772). *Eur. Respir. J.* **2018**, *52*, 1130. [CrossRef] [PubMed]
84. Hoeper, M.M.; Bogaard, H.J.; Condliffe, R.; Frantz, R.; Khanna, D.; Kurzyna, M.; Langleben, D.; Manes, A.; Satoh, T.; Torres, F. Definitions and diagnosis of pulmonary hypertension. *J. Am. Coll. Cardiol.* **2013**, *62*, D42–D50. [CrossRef] [PubMed]
85. Chung, L.; Liu, J.; Parsons, L.; Hassoun, P.M.; McGoon, M.; Badesch, D.B.; Miller, D.P.; Nicolls, M.R.; Zamanian, R.T. Characterization of connective tissue disease-associated pulmonary arterial hypertension from REVEAL: Identifying systemic sclerosis as a unique phenotype. *Chest* **2010**, *138*, 1383–1394. [CrossRef]
86. McLaughlin, V.; Humbert, M.; Coghlan, G.; Nash, P.; Steen, V. Pulmonary arterial hypertension: The most devastating vascular complication of systemic sclerosis. *Rheumatology* **2006**, *48*, iii25–iii31. [CrossRef]
87. Komócsi, A.; Vorobcsuk, A.; Faludi, R.; Pintér, T.; Lenkey, Z.; Költő, G.; Czirják, L. The impact of cardiopulmonary manifestations on the mortality of SSc: A systematic review and meta-analysis of observational studies. *Rheumatology* **2012**, *51*, 1027–1036. [CrossRef]
88. Hachulla, E.; Gressin, V.; Guillevin, L.; Carpentier, P.; Diot, E.; Sibilia, J.; Kahan, A.; Cabane, J.; Frances, C.; Launay, D. Early detection of pulmonary arterial hypertension in systemic sclerosis: A French nationwide prospective multicenter study. *Arthritis Rheum.* **2005**, *52*, 3792–3800. [CrossRef]
89. Mukerjee, D.; St George, D.; Coleiro, B.; Knight, C.; Denton, C.; Davar, J.; Black, C.; Coghlan, J. Prevalence and outcome in systemic sclerosis associated pulmonary arterial hypertension: Application of a registry approach. *Ann. Rheum. Dis.* **2003**, *62*, 1088–1093. [CrossRef]
90. Ungerer, R.G.; Tashkin, D.P.; Furst, D.; Clements, P.J.; Gong Jr, H.; Bein, M.; Smith, J.W.; Roberts, N.; Cabeen, W. Prevalence and clinical correlates of pulmonary arterial hypertension in progressive systemic sclerosis. *Am. J. Med.* **1983**, *75*, 65–74. [CrossRef]
91. Hachulla, E.; Launay, D.; Mouthon, L.; Sitbon, O.; Berezne, A.; Guillevin, L.; Hatron, P.-Y.; Simonneau, G.; Clerson, P.; Humbert, M. Is pulmonary arterial hypertension really a late complication of systemic sclerosis? *Chest* **2009**, *136*, 1211–1219. [CrossRef]
92. Humbert, M.; Yaici, A.; de Groote, P.; Montani, D.; Sitbon, O.; Launay, D.; Gressin, V.; Guillevin, L.; Clerson, P.; Simonneau, G. Screening for pulmonary arterial hypertension in patients with systemic sclerosis: Clinical characteristics at diagnosis and long-term survival. *Arthritis Rheum.* **2011**, *63*, 3522–3530. [CrossRef] [PubMed]
93. Solomon, J.J.; Olson, A.L.; Fischer, A.; Bull, T.; Brown, K.K.; Raghu, G. Scleroderma lung disease. *Eur. Respir. Rev.* **2013**, *22*, 6–19. [CrossRef] [PubMed]
94. Williams, M.H.; Handler, C.E.; Akram, R.; Smith, C.J.; Das, C.; Smee, J.; Nair, D.; Denton, C.P.; Black, C.M.; Coghlan, J.G. Role of N-terminal brain natriuretic peptide (N-TproBNP) in scleroderma-associated pulmonary arterial hypertension. *Eur. Heart J.* **2006**, *27*, 1485–1494. [CrossRef] [PubMed]
95. Steen, V.; Medsger, T.A., Jr. Predictors of isolated pulmonary hypertension in patients with systemic sclerosis and limited cutaneous involvement. *Arthritis Rheum.* **2003**, *48*, 516–522. [CrossRef] [PubMed]
96. Coghlan, J.G.; Denton, C.P.; Grünig, E.; Bonderman, D.; Distler, O.; Khanna, D.; Müller-Ladner, U.; Pope, J.E.; Vonk, M.C.; Doelberg, M. Evidence-based detection of pulmonary arterial hypertension in systemic sclerosis: The DETECT study. *Ann. Rheum. Dis.* **2014**, *73*, 1340–1349. [CrossRef]
97. Galiè, N.; Humbert, M.; Vachiery, J.-L.; Gibbs, S.; Lang, I.; Torbicki, A.; Simonneau, G.; Peacock, A.; Vonk-Noordegraaf, A.; Beghetti, M. 2015 ESC/ERS guidelines for the diagnosis and treatment of pulmonary hypertension: The Joint Task Force for the Diagnosis and Treatment of Pulmonary Hypertension of the European Society of Cardiology (ESC) and the European Respiratory

Society (ERS): Endorsed by: Association for European Paediatric and Congenital Cardiology (AEPC), International Society for Heart and Lung Transplantation (ISHLT). *Eur. Heart J.* **2016**, *37*, 67–119.
98. Mihai, C.; Antic, M.; Dobrota, R.; Bonderman, D.; Chadha-Boreham, H.; Coghlan, J.G.; Denton, C.P.; Doelberg, M.; Grünig, E.; Khanna, D. Factors associated with disease progression in early-diagnosed pulmonary arterial hypertension associated with systemic sclerosis: Longitudinal data from the DETECT cohort. *Ann. Rheum. Dis.* **2018**, *77*, 128–132. [CrossRef] [PubMed]
99. Khanna, D.; Gladue, H.; Channick, R.; Chung, L.; Distler, O.; Furst, D.E.; Hachulla, E.; Humbert, M.; Langleben, D.; Mathai, S.C. Recommendations for screening and detection of connective tissue disease–associated pulmonary arterial hypertension. *Arthritis Rheum.* **2013**, *65*, 3194–3201. [CrossRef]
100. Young, A.; Vummidi, D.; Visovatti, S.; Homer, K.; Wilhalme, H.; White, E.S.; Flaherty, K.; McLaughlin, V.; Khanna, D. Prevalence, treatment, and outcomes of coexistent pulmonary hypertension and interstitial lung disease in systemic sclerosis. *Arthritis Rheumatol.* **2019**, *71*, 1339–1349. [CrossRef] [PubMed]
101. Mathai, S.C.; Hummers, L.K.; Champion, H.C.; Wigley, F.M.; Zaiman, A.; Hassoun, P.M.; Girgis, R.E. Survival in pulmonary hypertension associated with the scleroderma spectrum of diseases: Impact of interstitial lung disease. *Arthritis Rheum.* **2009**, *60*, 569–577. [CrossRef] [PubMed]
102. Montani, D.; Savale, L.; Natali, D.; Jaïs, X.; Herve, P.; Garcia, G.; Humbert, M.; Simonneau, G.; Sitbon, O. Long-term response to calcium-channel blockers in non-idiopathic pulmonary arterial hypertension. *Eur. Heart J.* **2010**, *31*, 1898–1907. [CrossRef] [PubMed]
103. Galiè, N.; Channick, R.N.; Frantz, R.P.; Grünig, E.; Jing, Z.C.; Moiseeva, O.; Preston, I.R.; Pulido, T.; Safdar, Z.; Tamura, Y. Risk stratification and medical therapy of pulmonary arterial hypertension. *Eur. Respir. J.* **2019**, *53*, 1801889. [CrossRef] [PubMed]
104. Galie, N.; Manes, A.; Negro, L.; Palazzini, M.; Bacchi-Reggiani, M.L.; Branzi, A. A meta-analysis of randomized controlled trials in pulmonary arterial hypertension. *Eur. Heart J.* **2009**, *30*, 394–403. [CrossRef]
105. Badesch, D.B.; Tapson, V.F.; McGoon, M.D.; Brundage, B.H.; Rubin, L.J.; Wigley, F.M.; Rich, S.; Barst, R.J.; Barrett, P.S.; Kral, K.M. Continuous intravenous epoprostenol for pulmonary hypertension due to the scleroderma spectrum of disease: A randomized, controlled trial. *Ann. Intern. Med.* **2000**, *132*, 425–434. [CrossRef] [PubMed]
106. Sitbon, O.; Channick, R.; Chin, K.M.; Frey, A.; Gaine, S.; Galiè, N.; Ghofrani, H.-A.; Hoeper, M.M.; Lang, I.M.; Preiss, R.; et al. Selexipag for the treatment of pulmonary arterial hypertension. *N. Engl. J. Med.* **2015**, *373*, 2522–2533. [CrossRef]
107. Gaine, S.; Chin, K.; Coghlan, G.; Channick, R.; Di Scala, L.; Galiè, N.; Ghofrani, H.-A.; Lang, I.M.; McLaughlin, V.; Preiss, R. Selexipag for the treatment of connective tissue disease-associated pulmonary arterial hypertension. *Eur. Respir. J.* **2017**, *50*, 1602493. [CrossRef]
108. Galiè, N.; Barberà, J.A.; Frost, A.E.; Ghofrani, H.-A.; Hoeper, M.M.; McLaughlin, V.V.; Peacock, A.J.; Simonneau, G.; Vachiery, J.-L.; Grünig, E. Initial use of ambrisentan plus tadalafil in pulmonary arterial hypertension. *N. Engl. J. Med.* **2015**, *373*, 834–844. [CrossRef] [PubMed]
109. Pulido, T.; Adzerikho, I.; Channick, R.N.; Delcroix, M.; Galiè, N.; Ghofrani, H.-A.; Jansa, P.; Jing, Z.-C.; Le Brun, F.-O.; Mehta, S. Macitentan and morbidity and mortality in pulmonary arterial hypertension. *N. Engl. J. Med.* **2013**, *369*, 809–818. [CrossRef]
110. Ghofrani, H.-A.; Galiè, N.; Grimminger, F.; Grünig, E.; Humbert, M.; Jing, Z.-C.; Keogh, A.M.; Langleben, D.; Kilama, M.O.; Fritsch, A. Riociguat for the treatment of pulmonary arterial hypertension. *N. Engl. J. Med.* **2013**, *369*, 330–340. [CrossRef]
111. Coghlan, J.G.; Galiè, N.; Barberà, J.A.; Frost, A.E.; Ghofrani, H.-A.; Hoeper, M.M.; Kuwana, M.; McLaughlin, V.V.; Peacock, A.J.; Simonneau, G. Initial combination therapy with ambrisentan and tadalafil in connective tissue disease-associated pulmonary arterial hypertension (CTD-PAH): Subgroup analysis from the AMBITION trial. *Ann. Rheum. Dis.* **2017**, *76*, 1219–1227. [CrossRef]
112. Humbert, M.; Coghlan, J.G.; Ghofrani, H.-A.; Grimminger, F.; He, J.-G.; Riemekasten, G.; Vizza, C.D.; Boeckenhoff, A.; Meier, C.; de Oliveira Pena, J. Riociguat for the treatment of pulmonary arterial hypertension associated with connective tissue disease: Results from PATENT-1 and PATENT-2. *Ann. Rheum. Dis.* **2017**, *76*, 422–426. [CrossRef]
113. Shiboski, C.H.; Shiboski, S.C.; Seror, R.; Criswell, L.A.; Labetoulle, M.; Lietman, T.M.; Rasmussen, A.; Scofield, H.; Vitali, C.; Bowman, S.J.; et al. 2016 ACR-EULAR classification criteria for primary Sjögren's syndrome: A consensus and data-driven methodology involving three international patient cohorts. *Arthritis Rheumatol.* **2017**, *69*, 35–45. [CrossRef]
114. Papiris, S.A.; Saetta, M.; Turato, G.; La Corte, R.; Trevisani, L.; Mapp, C.E.; Maestrelli, P.; Fabbri, L.M.; Potena, A. CD4-positive T-lymphocytes infiltrate the bronchial mucosa of patients with Sjogren's syndrome. *Am. J. Respir. Crit. Care Med.* **1997**, *156*, 637–641. [CrossRef] [PubMed]
115. Kakugawa, T.; Sakamoto, N.; Ishimoto, H.; Shimizu, T.; Nakamura, H.; Nawata, A.; Ito, C.; Sato, S.; Hanaka, T.; Oda, K.; et al. Lymphocytic focus score is positively related to airway and interstitial lung diseases in primary Sjögren's syndrome. *Respir. Med.* **2018**, *137*, 95–102. [CrossRef] [PubMed]
116. Gupta, S.; Ferrada, M.A.; Hasni, S.A. Pulmonary manifestations of primary Sjögren's syndrome: Underlying immunological mechanisms, clinical presentation, and management. *Front. Immunol.* **2019**, *10*, 1327. [CrossRef]
117. Ramos-Casals, M.; Brito-Zerón, P.; Seror, R.; Bootsma, H.; Bowman, S.J.; Dörner, T.; Gottenberg, J.-E.; Mariette, X.; Theander, E.; Bombardieri, S.; et al. Characterization of systemic disease in primary Sjögren's syndrome: EULAR-SS Task Force recommendations for articular, cutaneous, pulmonary and renal involvements. *Rheumatology* **2015**, *54*, 2230–2238. [CrossRef]
118. Enomoto, Y.; Takemura, T.; Hagiwara, E.; Iwasawa, T.; Fukuda, Y.; Yanagawa, N.; Sakai, F.; Baba, T.; Nagaoka, S.; Ogura, T. Prognostic factors in interstitial lung disease associated with primary Sjögren's syndrome: A retrospective analysis of 33 pathologically-proven cases. *PLoS ONE* **2013**, *8*, e73774. [CrossRef]

119. Enomoto, Y.; Takemura, T.; Hagiwara, E.; Iwasawa, T.; Okudela, K.; Yanagawa, N.; Baba, T.; Sakai, F.; Fukuda, Y.; Nagaoka, S.; et al. Features of usual interstitial pneumonia in patients with primary Sjögren's syndrome compared with idiopathic pulmonary fibrosis. *Respir. Investig.* **2014**, *52*, 227–235. [CrossRef]
120. Swigris, J.J.; Berry, G.J.; Raffin, T.A.; Kuschner, W.G. Lymphoid interstitial pneumonia: A narrative review. *Chest* **2002**, *122*, 2150–2164. [CrossRef]
121. Gunnarsson, R.; Hetlevik, S.O.; Lilleby, V.; Molberg, Ø. Mixed connective tissue disease. *Best Pract. Res. Clin. Rheumatol.* **2016**, *30*, 95–111. [CrossRef] [PubMed]
122. Gunnarsson, R.; Aaløkken, T.M.; Molberg, Ø.; Lund, M.B.; Mynarek, G.K.; Lexberg, Å.S.; Time, K.; Dhainaut, A.S.S.; Bertelsen, L.-T.; Palm, Ø.; et al. Prevalence and severity of interstitial lung disease in mixed connective tissue disease: A nationwide, cross-sectional study. *Ann. Rheum. Dis.* **2012**, *71*, 1966–1972. [CrossRef] [PubMed]
123. Bodolay, E.; Szekanecz, Z.; Devenyi, K.; Galuska, L.; Csípo, I.; Vègh, J.; Garai, I.; Szegedi, G. Evaluation of interstitial lung disease in mixed connective tissue disease (MCTD). *Rheumatology* **2005**, *44*, 656–661. [CrossRef]
124. Kawano-Dourado, L.; Baldi, B.G.; Kay, F.U.; Dias, O.M.; Gripp, T.E.; Gomes, P.S.; Fuller, R.; Caleiro, M.T.; Kairalla, R.A.; Carvalho, C.R. Pulmonary involvement in long-term mixed connective tissue disease: Functional trends and imaging findings after 10 years. *Clin. Exp. Rheumatol.* **2015**, *33*, 234–240. [PubMed]
125. Alves, M.R.; Isenberg, D.A. "Mixed connective tissue disease": A condition in search of an identity. *Clin. Exp. Med.* **2020**, *20*, 159–166. [CrossRef]
126. Hajas, A.; Szodoray, P.; Nakken, B.; Gaal, J.; Zöld, E.; Laczik, R.; Demeter, N.; Nagy, G.; Szekanecz, Z.; Zeher, M.; et al. Clinical course, prognosis, and causes of death in mixed connective tissue disease. *J. Rheumatol.* **2013**, *40*, 1134–1142. [CrossRef]

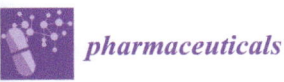

Review

The Relationship between Pulmonary Damage and Peripheral Vascular Manifestations in Systemic Sclerosis Patients

Barbara Ruaro [1,*], Marco Confalonieri [1], Francesco Salton [1], Barbara Wade [2], Elisa Baratella [3], Pietro Geri [1], Paola Confalonieri [1], Metka Kodric [1], Marco Biolo [1] and Cosimo Bruni [4]

1. Department of Pulmonology, University Hospital of Cattinara, 34149 Trieste, Italy; marco.confalonieri@asugi.sanita.fvg.it (M.C.); francesco.salton@gmail.com (F.S.); pietrogeri@gmail.com (P.G.); paola.confalonieri.24@gmail.com (P.C.); metka.kodric@asuits.sanita.fvg.it (M.K.); marcobiolo@gmail.com (M.B.)
2. AOU City of Health and Science of Turin, Department of Science of Public Health and Pediatrics, University of Torino, 10126 Torino, Italy; barbarawade@hotmail.com
3. Department of Radiology, Cattinara Hospital, University of Trieste, 34149 Trieste, Italy; elisa.baratella@gmail.com
4. Department of Experimental and Clinical Medicine, Division of Rheumatology, University of Firenze, 50121 Florence, Italy; cosimobruni85@gmail.com
* Correspondence: barbara.ruaro@yahoo.it; Tel.: +39-(347)-0502-3914

Citation: Ruaro, B.; Confalonieri, M.; Salton, F.; Wade, B.; Baratella, E.; Geri, P.; Confalonieri, P.; Kodric, M.; Biolo, M.; Bruni, C. The Relationship between Pulmonary Damage and Peripheral Vascular Manifestations in Systemic Sclerosis Patients. *Pharmaceuticals* **2021**, *14*, 403. https://doi.org/10.3390/ph14050403

Academic Editor: Antoni Camins Espuny

Received: 21 March 2021
Accepted: 19 April 2021
Published: 23 April 2021

Publisher's Note: MDPI stays neutral with regard to jurisdictional claims in published maps and institutional affiliations.

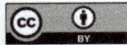

Copyright: © 2021 by the authors. Licensee MDPI, Basel, Switzerland. This article is an open access article distributed under the terms and conditions of the Creative Commons Attribution (CC BY) license (https://creativecommons.org/licenses/by/4.0/).

Abstract: Systemic sclerosis (SSc) is an autoimmune disease, characterized by the presence of generalized vasculopathy and tissue fibrosis. Collagen vascular disorder in SSc is due to fibroblast and endothelial cell dysfunctions. This leads to collagen overproduction, vascular impairment and immune system abnormalities and, in the last stage, multi-organ damage. Thus, to avoid organ damage, which has a poor prognosis, all patients should be carefully evaluated and followed. This is particularly important in the initial disease phase, so as to facilitate early identification of any organ involvement and to allow for appropriate therapy. Pulmonary disease in SSc mainly involves interstitial lung disease (ILD) and pulmonary arterial hypertension (PAH). High-resolution computed tomography (HRCT) and pulmonary function tests (PFT) have been proposed to monitor parenchymal damage. Although transthoracic echocardiography is the most commonly used screening tool for PAH in SSc patients, definitive diagnosis necessitates confirmation by right heart catheterization (RHC). Moreover, some studies have demonstrated that nailfold videocapillaroscopy (NVC) provides an accurate evaluation of the microvascular damage in SSc and is able to predict internal organ involvement, such as lung impairment. This review provides an overview of the correlation between lung damage and microvascular involvement in SSc patients.

Keywords: systemic sclerosis; pulmonary involvement; microvascular involvement; pulmonary arterial hypertension; interstitial lung disease; nailfold capillaroscopy

1. Introduction

Systemic sclerosis (SSc), a heterogeneous disease, is characterized by immune dysfunction, often leading to organ damage due to inflammation, endothelial dysfunction and fibrosis [1–4]. SSc involves microcirculation structural and functional alterations [5–9]. The main cause of death in SSc patients is not only collagen overproduction but also the effects collagen overproduction has on the pulmonary system. This includes fibrosis or pulmonary artery hypertension (PAH) [10–15]. Recent guidelines have recommend screening with high resolution computed tomography (HRCT) to diagnose interstitial lung diseases (ILD) in SSc patients at the baseline visit and once the diagnosis of ILD has been established [16,17], whilst a combination of HRCT and pulmonary function tests is recommended to quantify the extent and severity of ILD [16–19]. Screening for PAH in SSc is transthoracic echocardiography, which has a sensitivity of 90%, even if definitive diagnosis is to be confirmed by right heart catheterization (RHC) [20–25]. Although nailfold videocapillaroscopy (NVC) is the validated method for assessing peripheral vascular damage [26–29], several studies have demonstrated that NVC is capable of predicting internal organ involvement [27–35].

This review aims at providing updated information on the link between pulmonary damage, i.e., ILD and PAH, and peripheral vascular manifestations, evaluated by NVC, in SSc patients.

2. Pulmonary Manifestations

Pulmonary disease in SSc includes interstitial lung disease (ILD) and pulmonary arterial hypertension (PAH) [36–38]. All SSc patients should be screened to detect any ILD and PAH development, at diagnosis and periodically thereafter. Indeed, although there has been no statistically significant change in the SSc mortality rate over the past 40 years, the proportion of deaths due to ILD and PAH has increased [36–41]. ILD and PAH are the two main causes of death in SSc patients and account for 33% and 28% of deaths, respectively [36–41]. Although ILD is reported to be more common in diffuse cutaneous SSc (dcSSc) whilst PAH is reportedly more common in limited cutaneous SSc (lcSSc), both pulmonary manifestations have been described in each of the disease subsets. Patients with rarer phenotypes associated with antiTh/To and anti U3RNP antibodies may have PAH and ILD concomitantly. Pulmonary disease may even occur in SSc with no skin involvement, i.e., scleroderma sine scleroderma [36–41].

Although the clinical course varies from mild and asymptomatic to severely debilitating, most patients have some degree of pulmonary fibrosis [39,40]. The most common early symptoms related to SSc pulmonary manifestations are exertional dyspnea and dry cough and, in most cases, are non-specific findings [42–46]. Should this be the case, then a differential diagnosis should be made to investigate/exclude SSc-ILD, PAH, deconditioning, chronic anemia and/or left heart involvement with a reduced or preserved ejection fraction [42–46]. Considering the frequency of lung involvement in SSc and its impact on prognosis, early recognition of lung involvement and prompt appropriate treatment is a must [36–41]. Although there are inherent challenges in the management of both PAH and ILD, with the early diagnosis, treatment may have a higher chance of efficacy for each of these lung complications [2,10].

The etiologic or enhancing factors of pulmonary involvement in SSc patients are still a question of debate. A previous study implicated genetic factors, i.e., HLA class II (1–3). Others have implicated immunologic factors for which certain autoantibodies such as anti–topoisomerase I (anti–topo I) may be markers [1–3]. The few studies that have addressed the impact of race or ethnicity on lung involvement in early SSc suggest a worse prognosis for nonwhite groups (e.g., African Americans, the Japanese population and Choctaw Indians). However, ethnicity is not only defined by racial or genetic factors but also by sociodemographic and cultural factors [1–4].

3. Interstitial Lung Disease

ILD complicates diffuse cutaneous SSc (dcSSc) in 53% of cases but may also be associated in 35% of cases with limited cutaneous SSc (lcSSc), as reported by the European Scleroderma Trials and Research group (EUSTAR) [39,42]. Furthermore, several autopsy studies reported that parenchymal involvement, in the form of ILD, was present in up to 90% of SSc patients. Risk factors for ILD development include African American ethnicity, skin score, serum creatinine and creatine phosphokinase levels, hypothyroidism and cardiac involvement [1,2,42–44]. Genetic factors, specific serological findings and anti-topoisomerase and anti-endothelial cell antibodies can predict the presence of lung involvement [1,2,42–44]. It is also reported that the patients with dcSSc have a higher incidence of interstitial disease [1–3]. Predictors of severe restrictive lung disease (defined by a forced vital capacity (FVC) of 50% predicted) include African American ethnicity, male gender, the degree of physiological abnormalities at diagnosis (FVC and diffusing lung capacity for carbon monoxide (DLCO)) and a younger age [1,2,46–48].

Unfortunately, there are limited treatment options for this manifestation. This is due to the paucity of high-quality, randomized, controlled trials that specifically target SSc-ILD. Moreover, historically, studies have favored cyclophosphamide (CYC) for SSc-ILD treatment, as also suggested in the most recent European League against Rheumatism (EULAR) recommendations [2,49]. Supportive data have shown that nintedanib, a multi-tyrosine kinase inhibitor, and tocilizumab (TCZ) significantly inhibit the progressive functional decline [2,49]. Current innovative proposals have also recently been made on the basis of clinical and preclinical evidence for rituximab (RTX) and pirfenidone (PIRF), as well as hematopoietic stem cell and lung transplantation [2,49]. However, the safety and efficacy of emerging experimental therapies for SSc-ILD do require further investigation.

Other findings were that high-resolution computed tomography (HRCT) evidenced interstitial abnormalities in as many as 90% of patients, and 40–75% had changes in pulmonary function tests (PFT) [46–52].

4. Imaging

SSc-ILD is diagnosed by HRCT, which is a simple non-invasive, sensitive investigation, able to detect parenchymal lung disease [53–60]. However, despite its high sensitivity, HRCT may be normal in some patients with pulmonary function test abnormalities or abnormal chest auscultation (i.e., crackles) [46–48,58]. The absence of lung involvement in HRCT at the time of disease presentation may lower the long-term risk of developing SSc-ILD, as 85% of patients have a normal HRCT at an average 5 year follow-up [46–55]. These factors stress the importance of making an SSc-ILD diagnosis by combining clinical findings, pulmonary function tests and HRCT abnormalities.

A common HRCT pattern of SSc-ILD is characterized by a greater proportion of ground-glass opacities with a lower degree of reticulation, suggestive of nonspecific interstitial pneumonia (NSIP). The predominant observations in the basal areas of the lungs are low lung volumes and interstitial reticular thickening. In the late lung involvement stages, pulmonary fibrosis manifests as traction bronchiectasis and honeycomb cysts, a marker for usual interstitial pneumonia (UIP) [55–64] (Figure 1). These two alterations have been observed in up to 33% of SSc-ILD patients, suggesting that these patients may have a mixture (or overlap) of UIP and NSIP patterns [55–64].

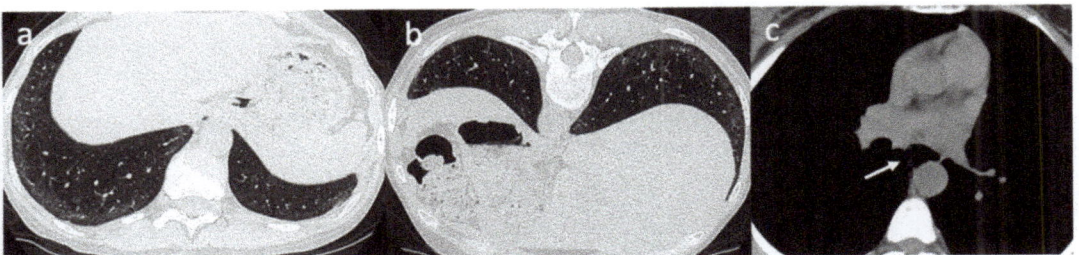

Figure 1. A 43-year-old female with a diagnosis of systemic sclerosis. Axial high-resolution CT scan obtained in the supine position shows subtle ground-glass opacities in the subpleural regions of the lung bases, suspicious for NSIP (non-specific interstitial pneumonia) (**a**). When these findings are not prominent, an additional scan can be acquired in the prone position to differentiate ground-glass opacities due to gravitational phenomena from interstitial lung disease. In this patient the ground-glass opacities persist in the prone position, confirming the interstitial lung involvement (**b**). Additional systemic sclerosis-related findings should be searched for, such as a dilated esophagus on images reconstructed using an appropriate mediastinal window setting (**c**).

Even when treated, ground-glass opacities progress to fibrosis and lead to honeycombing/traction bronchiectasis and/or bronchiectasis formation over time in up to 60% of patients [55–64]. There is a correlation between ground-glass opacities/consolidation and active inflammation, whilst reticular opacities/honeycombing correlate with fibrotic lesions. There is a better treatment response in patients with HRCT features of ground-glass opacities, as they are markers of inflammation and reversible lung injury [50–52,64–67].

Although the HRCT pattern correlates well with histology, nowadays lung biopsies are rarely performed, except for the exclusion of other parenchymal processes [52–55]. However, when performed, histology analysis shows interstitial fibrosis with temporal homogeneity and a modest inflammatory cell infiltrate (i.e., fibrotic NSIP) [42–44,52–55].

It has been observed that HRCT is more sensitive than chest radiography (CR) in diagnosing and characterizing SSc-related lung diseases, as there may be a normal CR in early lung involvement and even in some patients with pulmonary symptoms [58,64,67]. Moreover, ILD HRCT findings correlate more closely with pulmonary function test abnormalities, demonstrating that SSc-related lung injury is a restrictive disorder, associated with low lung volumes, and a diffusion disorder, which impairs carbon monoxide diffusion capacity [55,58].

Chest HRCT findings also have prognostic implications in SSc and SSc-ILD. The absence of lung involvement in HRCT at the time of disease presentation is a good long-term prognostic indicator of SSc-ILD [42,64]. Conversely, the presence of SSc-ILD and its extent, quantified by both visual semi-quantitative and software-based quantitative methods, are able to predict disease-related mortality [64,65]. Along with parenchymal features, lung vessels have also been recently investigated on HRCT. It was observed that the extent of lung volume occupied by vessels has a statistically significant correlation with the extent of SSc-ILD, ILD-related restrictive functional changes and decline in the diffusion capacity of carbon monoxide (DLCO) among SSc patients with or without ILD [51,65–67].

Recently, various radiation-free modalities have been tested, and it seems that lung MRI may be a promising tool for SSc-ILD detection and prognostication [68]. This may be due to the fact that MRI is capable of differentiating inflammation-predominant versus fibrosis-predominant lesions, offering information as to the choice for more anti-inflammatory or more anti-fibrotic targeting medications [68]. Moreover, ultrasound lung investigations are becoming widespread in the SSc-ILD field due to their potential for ILD screening [69–71]. Ultrasound correlates well with ILD extent and lung impairment and has a significant prognostic value in the evaluation of lung involvement, even if further studies are required to support the use of the technique [69–71].

5. Pulmonary Function Tests

Pulmonary function tests (PFT) are essential, readily available non-invasive tests able to detect SSc-related pulmonary changes. PFT in SSc-ILD is characterized by a restrictive ventilatory defect with a decrease in functional vital capacity (FVC) and/or total lung capacity (TLC), a preserved forced expiratory volume in 1 s (FEV1), a normal or increased FEV1/FVC ratio and a DLCO reduction [72–77]. SSc survival has been inversely correlated with the degree of restrictive ventilatory defect on pulmonary function tests. Several studies have reported an 87% 10-year survival rate in patients with minimal to absent restriction and a 75% and 58% 10-year survival rate in patients with moderate or severe restriction [72–77]. Both FVC and DLCO have been identified as adverse prognostic markers in SSc-related lung injury. Indeed, almost all patients have a reduced DLCO, along with other pulmonary function test abnormalities. However, a reduced DLCO is the single most significant marker of poor outcome and correlates with the extent of lung disease on HRCT [72–77]. An important factor, not to be overlooked, is the fact that although patients with early SSc-ILD may have signs of lung disease at HRCT and a DLCO decrease, they may also have preserved lung volumes [72–77].

Recent studies have demonstrated that more than 60% of SSc-ILD patients had normal PFT at HRCT [72–77]. Therefore, although PFT is an important diagnostic tool for SSc-ILD, it is not sensitive enough make an early detection [72–77]. Regular annual PFT after SSc diagnosis may be useful to evidence any changes in lung function that are indicative of ILD [72–77].

The reduced DLCO levels observed in SSc-ILD are due to a variable combination of a reduction in alveolar volume and/or thickening of the alveolar–capillary membrane. Impaired DLCO in SSc-induced lung injury is usually secondary to two main pathological conditions, i.e., ILD and PAH, even if it may be observed without these complications. Indeed, an isolated DLCO impairment, with reduced FVC/TLC and clinical and/or radiological signs of parenchymal lung involvement, has been attributed to lung vasculopathy and could be considered a good prognostic sign, even it may rarely be associated with the future development of PAH or SSc-ILD [72–78].

Up until 2010, the most common outcome test used in clinical lung disease studies was the DLCO evaluation, which was later surpassed by FVC. Indeed, the FVC percentage predicted the primary endpoint in 70.4% of studies, whilst only 11.3% of DLCO evaluations were predictive. To the best of our knowledge, only five studies specifically aimed to validate PFT: two concluded that the extent of SSc-ILD was best measured by DLCO whilst the other three did not favor any PFT parameter. These studies also showed validity measures for total lung capacity (TLC). Despite the current preference for FVC, available evidence suggests that DLCO and TLC should not yet be discounted as potential surrogate markers for SSc-ILD progression [55,72–78].

6. Pulmonary Arterial Hypertension

The highest prevalence of PAH amongst the various connective tissue diseases is observed in SSc patients, and it may occur in all forms [20–25]. The main pathophysiological alteration in SSc-PAH is small vessel vasculopathy [20–25,43,51]. This is usually diagnosed 10 to 15 years after SSc onset and is associated with early mortality [20–25,51]. PAH was previously defined as an average pulmonary artery pressure (mPAP) of $\geq$ 25 mmHg, assessed by right heart catheterization (RHC), with an mPAP between 21 mmHg and 24 mmHg, which was considered "borderline pulmonary hypertension" (Bo-PAH) [19,78]. At the 6th World Symposium of Pulmonary Hypertension, PAH was finally defined as an mPAP of $\geq$ 21 mmHg with a peripheral vascular resistance (PRV) of $\geq$ 3 Woods Units (WU) [19,78].

The presence of PAH in SSc may be the result of vaso-occlusive pulmonary artery hypertension (SSc-PAH), left ventricular heart dysfunction or pulmonary hypoxic disease, classified as group 1, 2 and 3 PAH, respectively [19,78]. Group 1 includes patients with isolated PAH without ILD, whilst PAH patients with ILD are classified into group 3, in the PH classification [19,78].

7. Screening

Our understating of this condition has been changed by the development of systematic algorithms for early diagnosis over the last decade and the data from the follow-up cohorts of incidental SSc-PAH [24]. Indeed, echocardiograph assessment is the most frequently used screening tool to identify candidates for RHC, and a tricuspid regurgitation (TR) velocity of $\geq$ 2.5 m/s is considered to be highly suggestive of PAH [78]. However, the sensitivity at this TR velocity threshold is limited and misses 20% of mild PAH patients [19,78].

Other studies documented that 55–86% of patients with an echocardiography finding suggestive of pulmonary hypertension (e.g., a right ventricular systolic pressure (RVSP) of 30 to 40 mmHg or higher, with or without symptoms) will have pulmonary hypertension on RHC. When the measurement of RVSP is combined with an increase in right atrial or right ventricular size, reduced pulmonary artery acceleration and decreased right ventricular function, the specificity of echocardiography for pulmonary hypertension diagnosis will be higher [78–84].

The multi-dimensional DETECT algorithm, the forced vital capacity (FVC)/diffusion capacity for carbon monoxide (DLCO) ratio or N-terminal-pro-brain natriuretic peptide (NT-pro-BNP) are all proven screening tools that support the early diagnosis of SSc-PAH [24,75,79]. Reduced DLCO levels in PAH are due to vascular remodeling, which leads to vessel wall tightening and arterial stiffness. The presence of a baseline isolated marked reduction in DLCO (<55% of predicted) in SSc patients might characterize a peculiar SSc subset that may precede the development of PAH, and the progression of pulmonary vascular disease can be linked to decreasing DLCO trends [66,72–74].

8. Right Heart Catheterization

Right heart catheterization (RHC) is the gold standard investigation for making a definitive diagnosis of pulmonary arterial hypertension (PAH) [80–84]. The RHC provides useful information on the degree of hemodynamic impairment, determines response to PAH therapy and establishes prognosis, providing information for clinical decision-making in PAH management [80–84] (Figure 2). Despite widespread acceptance, there are no internationally accepted clinical guidelines presenting the best practice for performing RHC. Therefore, to ensure the correct evaluation of directly measured hemodynamic or calculated parameters from RHC, procedures such as the position of the pressure transducer and catheter balloon inflation volume should be standardized with care [80–84]. The assessment of pulmonary arterial wedge pressure is particularly vulnerable to over- or under-wedging, which may lead to false readings. Moreover, errors in RHC measurement and data interpretation can complicate the differentiation of PAH from other disorders and lead to a misdiagnosis. Apart from diagnosis, the role of RHC in conjunction with non-invasive tests is on continuous expansion, encompassing the monitoring of treatment response and establishing the prognosis of patients diagnosed with PAH. However, it has been proposed that further standardization of RHC is warranted if we are to ensure its optimal use in routine clinical practice [80–84].

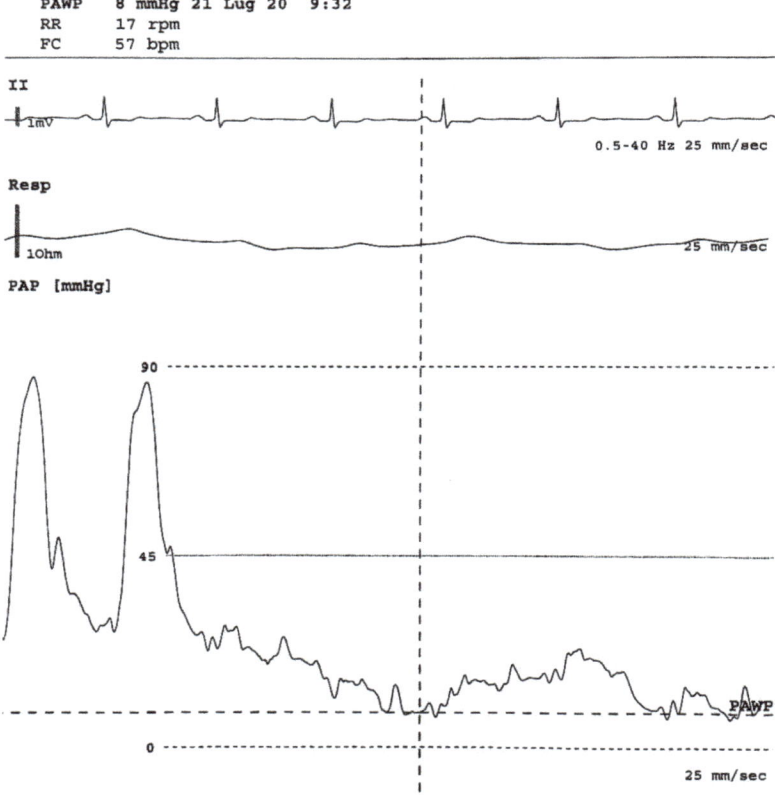

Figure 2. From below: pulmonary arterial pressure, respiratory and EKG waveforms during arterial catheterization. The first part of the pressure trace reflects the pressure in a pulmonary artery (large swings, dicrotic notch), then the balloon is inflated and the tip of the Swan Ganz catheter floats until it wedges in a small artery (small swings synchronous with respiratory rate), allowing a pulmonary arterial wedge pressure (PAWP) to be obtained, which is an indirect measure of left ventricle pressure.

9. Peripheral Vascular Manifestations

Raynaud's phenomenon (RP), secondary to SSc, is the most frequent vascular manifestation in SSc patients. Secondary RP, the most common presenting feature of the disease, is observed in 95% of scleroderma patients and may precede diagnosis by many years [85–88]. During RP, the skin usually turns white (ischemia), blue (deoxygenation) and then red (reperfusion) [85–88].

Secondary Raynaud's phenomenon (SRP) occurs in response to cold temperature or emotional stress, in the setting of underlying vascular disturbance, and is often associated with digital pain and ischemic ulcers [89–92]. However, it may occasionally lead to gangrene with tissue loss or the need for digital amputation [89,90].

As there is an obliterative vasculopathy of the peripheral arteries and microcirculation in SRP, it often leads to critical ischemia in scleroderma. There is often a luminal narrowing of >75% of digital arteries due to underlying intimal fibrosis and luminal occlusion caused by thrombi [85–88]. Endothelial cell injury and activation lead to vascular dysfunction and vasospasm that may quickly obstruct the already limited blood flow of the vasculopathic digital arteries [41].

Conversely, primary RP (PRP) is an isolated finding without underlying pathology (idiopathic). The suggested criteria for PRP include symmetric attacks, the absence of tissue necrosis, ulceration or gangrene, the absence of a secondary cause, negative tests for antinuclear antibodies and a normal erythrocyte sedimentation rate [85,86].

As a diagnosis of PRP is made at a time when no underlying disease has yet been identified, predicting whether or when it may turn into SRP is a difficult task [93–96]. As NVC detects morphological microcirculation abnormalities, it is able to distinguish SRP from both PRP and healthy subjects [97–100]. Therefore, primary RP patients should be carefully followed-up by NVC so as to allow for an early detection of the first signs of any transition to the secondary form of RP in the most reliable manner [101–104].

10. Nailfold Videocapillaroscopy

Morphological signs that represent the microvascular damage can be observed in nailfold videocapillaroscopy (NVC) images in SRP patients; these alterations include giant capillaries, microhemorrhages, capillary loss, the presence of avascular areas and angiogenesis [105–107]. These sequential capillaroscopic changes are typical of the microvascular involvement observed in more than 95% of SSc patients and are described as an "SSc pattern" [93–95,105]. The nailfold capillaries in PRP patients usually have a normal shape without any specific alterations. Whilst the presence of abnormal capillaroscopic findings, i.e., giant capillaries and microhemorrhages, are diagnostic of the early NVC pattern of scleroderma microangiography [105], the NVC technique is able to identify three morphological patterns specific to various SSc stages (early, active and late patterns) [105]. As reported hereafter, the early NVC pattern is characterized by a few enlarged/giant capillaries and capillary microhemorrhages, no evident capillary loss and a relatively well-preserved capillary distribution [105]. The most frequent alterations in the active NVC pattern are giant capillaries and capillary microhemorrhages, with a moderate capillary loss and a mild disorganization of the capillary architecture. There is severe capillary loss with evident avascular areas and disorganization of the normal capillary array in the late NVC pattern [105]. NVC provides a quantitative assessment of the microvascular damage, i.e., a quantification of certain characteristics and a semi-quantitative scoring. The characteristic capillaroscopic diagnostic parameters, i.e., irregularly enlarged capillaries, giant capillaries, microhemorrhages and progression parameters, which include fewer capillaries, capillary ramifications and capillary architectural disorganization, can be scored from 0 to 3 according to increasing severity and have been combined to create a semi-quantitative scale [105].

In healthy and primary RP subjects, NVC evaluation is characterized by morphological/structural homogeneity, evidencing 10–12 capillaries per linear millimeter. morphology of the capillary to "U" or "hairpin shape" and diameters of capillary branches of <20 μm [93–95]. Although it is quite common to observe normal nailfold capillaries in primary RP, capillaries with efferent branch enlargement or tortuosity may also be present [93–95].

The European League Against Rheumatism (EULAR) Study Group on Microcirculation in Rheumatic Diseases (EULAR SG MC/RD) has recently reported a simple consensus definition to name a single capillary as "(ab)normal". The authors tried to standardize and clarify the differences between scleroderma and non-scleroderma patterns, avoiding confusion caused by the various different definitions used to describe non-scleroderma abnormal capillary morphology (e.g., "ramifications", "neoangiogenesis" or "meandering") [28].

In conclusion NVC, which combines a microscope (with system that ranges from 50 × up to 500 × magnification) and a digital video camera, represents a method for an early diagnosis and follow-up of nailfold microangiopathy—one of the earliest signs of morphological damage and change in SSc—and is a non-invasive, user-friendly, well-accepted, accessible and portable tool [28].

That is why abnormal nailfold capillaroscopic images, i.e., "scleroderma patterns", were included in the 2013 European League Against Rheumatism and American College of Rheumatology's classification criteria for SSc [103]. Several studies have also demonstrated that NVC is a promising tool for the prediction of clinical complication markers of severity and progression of SSc organ involvement [49–54].

11. The Correlation Between Peripheral Vascular and Pulmonary Involvement

Various studies have demonstrated that NVC alterations are associated with different SSc clinical complications and organ involvement [106–112]. Moreover, other authors reported on the correlation between NVC alterations and SSc-ILD diagnosed by HRCT [110,111]. Caetano et al., made a cross-sectional analysis of 48 SSc-ILD patients with HRCT and the presence of ground-glass opacities and/or fibrosis [111]. The same authors investigated the association between NVC findings, the presence and extent of ILD, as well as functional impairment. Capillary loss and avascular areas were significantly associated with the presence of ILD. The receiver operating characteristic (ROC) curve analysis confirmed the association between capillary loss and ILD (the area under the ROC curve, 90.1%; 95% CI, 81.8–91.4). Avascular areas and capillary loss were associated with a worse pulmonary function. No additional statistically significant difference was observed between ILD and other NVC findings (i.e., capillary dimension (p-value = 0.328), abnormal capillary morphology (p-value = 0.790) or the presence of hemorrhages (p-value = 0.187)) [111]. In another cross-sectional study, Guillen-del-Castillo et al. evaluated 134 SSc patients (58 with ILD on HRCT) with at least eight NVC (200 × magnification) images through both quantitative and qualitative examinations [110]. The SSc ILD patients had a lower median capillary density (4.86/mm vs 5.88/mm, p-value = 0.005) and higher median neoangiogenesis (0.56/mm vs 0.31/mm, p-value = 0.005). Moreover, more neoangiogenesis capillaries were observed in PAH patients (0.70/mm vs 0.33/mm, p-value = 0.008). A multivariate linear regression analysis emphasized a correlation between neoangiogenesis and decreased FVC (p-value < 0.001) and between the number of giant capillaries and reduced DLCO (p-value = 0.016) [110]. Guillen-del-Castillo et al., demonstrated that the late pattern was associated with lower FVC (p-value = 0.018) [110]. Jehangir et al.,'s case-control study made use of a dermascope to study the NVC pattern in 65 subjects: 10 patients with primary Raynaud's phenomenon (RP), 40 with SSc and 15 age- and gender-matched controls. When testing HRCT and NVC patterns, only one patient with the early pattern had ILD, whereas those with an active or late pattern had a higher percentage of 55% and 100%, respectively [108] (Figure 3).

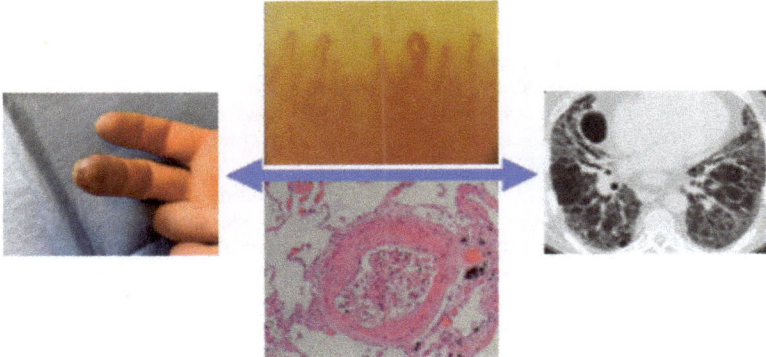

Figure 3. Vasculopathy in systemic sclerosis patients and the link between pulmonary damage and peripheral vascular manifestations.

Markusse et al. performed NVC in 287 SSc patients aimed at assessing whether it could improve the detection of patients at high risk of cardiopulmonary involvement (82). The study population included 51% ILD patients, 59% with a DLCO decrease and 16% with a systolic pulmonary artery pressure (sPAP) of >35 mmHg. The NVC pattern showed a stable association with the presence of ILD or sPAP. The odds ratio (OR) for ILD was 1.3–1.4 (p-value < 0.05 for analyses with anti-RNAPIII, anti-RNP). The OR for DLCO was 1.5 (p-value < 0.05 for analyses with ACA, anti-Scl70, anti-RNAPIII, anti-RNP). The OR for sPAP was 2.2–2.4 (p-value < 0.05 for analyses with anti-RNAPIII, anti-RNP) [82].

It has been demonstrated that SSc-associated PAH is correlated with capillaroscopic changes identified by NVC [112–127]. NVC data are also markers of SSc severity and progression, such as reduced capillary density, which is associated with a high risk of developing PAH [112–123]. Some authors have supported the possibility of an early identification of a subset of patients with severe disease [112–127]. Hofstee et al. studied capillary density and dimensions and their association with pulmonary hemodynamic characteristics in 21 healthy controls, 20 idiopathic PAH patients and 40 SSc patients (21/40 had SSc-PAH, as determined by RHC) [123]. This study reported a significantly lower capillary density in SSc-PAH patients than in those without SSc-PAH (p-value = 0.001), although no statistically significant difference was observed for capillary dimensions (p-value > 0.05) [123].

Similarly, Corrado et al. evaluated 25 healthy subjects, 21 idiopathic PAH patients and 39 SSc patients (19/39 affected by SSc-PAH, determined by RHC, as mPAP $\geq$ 25 mmHg, PCWP $\leq$ 15 mmHg and pulmonary vascular resistance > 3 Wood units) [118]. The authors observed that the presence of PAH had a significantly inverse correlation with capillary density (p-value < 0.05) and correlated with both capillary dimension and giant capillaries (p-value < 0.05), which correlated with abnormal capillary morphology (p-value < 0.01) in SSc patients [118].

Riccieri et al.'s cross-sectional study evaluated NVC alterations in 12 consecutive SSc-PAH patients, confirmed by RHC. They demonstrated that NVC damage is correlated with the grade of PAH.

Indeed, the NVC score (combining a semiquantitative score for density, dimension, presence of hemorrhage and morphology) and avascular area grading had a statistically significant correlation with PAH (p-value = 0.03 and p-value = 0.003, respectively) [121]. Furthermore, they observed that the active/late pattern was more common in SSc-PAH patients than in those without SSc-PAH (73% vs 50%, p-value < 0.05) [121]. This led to two recent meta-analyses confirming that microvascular changes detected by NVC are significantly associated with SSc-PAH, in particular lower capillary density and higher capillary width [112,117].

Kim et al. investigated the relationship between clinical manifestations and quantitative analysis of computerized NVC. They observed a strong correlation between capillary dimension and capillary loss with SSc-PAH (p-value < 0.05) and digital ulceration (p-value < 0.01) [114]. Moreover, a cross-sectional pilot study also assessed sublingual microvasculature by videocapillaroscope. The authors demonstrated that PAH patients had a lower sublingual microvasculature flow index and a higher vascular tortuosity than healthy age- and gender-matched control subjects [128].

In addition to the cross-sectional evidence, Smith et al.'s prospective longitudinal research studied 66 consecutive SSc patients. They defined the NVC pattern according to Cutolo's classification and clinical evaluation was performed according to Medsger's disease severity scale (DSS), with an 18–24 month follow-up [120]. They observed a statistically significant association between the NVC patterns and the development of future severe peripheral vascular or lung involvement. Indeed, the OR for future severe lung involvement, based on simple/multiple regression was 2.54/2.33 (p-value < 0.05) for early patterns, 6.43/5.44 for active patterns and 16.30/12.68 for late patterns.

12. Conclusions

The characteristic features of SSc include extensive fibrosis, fibroproliferative vasculopathy and systemic autoimmunity (autoantibodies and T cell autoantigen reactivity). However, the vascular pathology in SSc is not necessarily an inflammatory process and may be better characterized as a vasculopathy. Some autopsy studies have shown that vasculopathy is a systemic process [128]. One such study is that of D'Angelo et al., who reported that SSc patients had widespread intimal proliferation in the pulmonary arteries [128]. Moreover, complex interactions between endothelial cells, vascular smooth muscle cells, extracellular matrix and circulating mediators contribute to vascular remodeling, vasospasm and vessel occlusion [128].

There is evidence to support the hypothesis that microangiopathy may be an important component of internal organ involvement and that NVC is a candidate biomarker for the assessment of pulmonary damage.

There are numerous reports finding a good correlation between distinctive quantitative and qualitative NVC features and the presence of ILD on HRCT, as well as lung functional parameters such as FVC and DLCO. Therefore, it might well be that microangiopathy is a pivotal process in the establishment and progression of SSc-ILD. Similarly, as NVC is capable of detecting the early microvascular changes associated with the presence of PAH, it may well play a significant role in early prediction of SSc-PAH.

The gold standard with which to diagnose SSc-ILD is still the chest HRCT, whilst RHC is the validated test with which to diagnose PAH. Due to the poor prognosis for SSc patients with organ damage, in particular those with pulmonary manifestations, all these patients should be carefully evaluated from the early disease phase and followed-up. This should hopefully facilitate early identification and the choice of an early appropriate therapeutic regimen.

This review reports on the different clinical manifestations and tests, i.e., clinical, radiological and pulmonary function tests that may be used for the early prediction of lung involvement in SSc patients. It also includes evidence from the literature on how NVC may also be a promising tool for early identification and/or prediction of pulmonary complications. The data herein reported support the possibility that NVC might be incorporated together with other parameters in high-performance algorithms (e.g., DETECT algorithm for SSc-PAH, ILD screening procedures) in the early detection of lung involvement in SSc.

Author Contributions: B.R., C.B. and M.C. contributed to study design. F.S., B.W., E.B. and P.C. contributed to manuscript drafting. P.G., M.B. and M.K. contributed to literature revision. All the authors critically revised the manuscript and approved the final version. All authors have read and agreed to the published version of the manuscript.

Funding: The authors received no financial support for the research, authorship, and/or publication of this article.

Institutional Review Board Statement: Not applicable.

Informed Consent Statement: Not applicable.

Data Availability Statement: Not applicable.

Conflicts of Interest: The authors declare that there are no conflict of interest.

References

1. Varga, J.; Trojanowska, M.; Kuwana, M. Pathogenesis of systemic sclerosis: Recent insights of molecular and cellular mechanisms and therapeutic opportunities. *J. Scleroderma Relat. Disord.* **2017**, *2*, 137–152. [CrossRef]
2. Smith, V.; Scirè, C.A.; Talarico, R.; Airo, P.; Alexander, T.; Allanore, Y.; Bruni, C.; Codullo, V.; Dalm, V.; De Vries-Bouwstra, J.; et al. Systemic sclerosis: State of the art on clinical practice guidelines. *RMD Open* **2018**, *4* (Suppl. 1), e000782. [CrossRef]
3. Hinchcliff, M.; O'Reilly, S. Current and Potential New Targets in Systemic Sclerosis Therapy: A New Hope. *Curr. Rheumatol. Rep* **2020**, *22*, 42. [CrossRef]
4. Ruaro, B.; Soldano, S.; Smith, V.; Paolino, S.; Contini, P.; Montagna, P.; Pizzorni, C.; Casabella, A.; Tardito, S.; Sulli, A.; et al. Correlation between circulating fibrocytes and dermal thickness in limited cutaneous systemic sclerosis patients: A pilot study. *Rheumatol. Int.* **2019**, *39*, 1369–1376. [CrossRef]
5. Bruni, C.; Frech, T.; Manetti, M.; Rossi, F.W.; Furst, D.E.; De Paulis, A.; Rivellese, F.; Guiducci, S.; Matucci-Cerinic, M.; Bellando-Randone, S. Vascular leaking, a pivotal and early pathogenetic event in systemic sclerosis: Should the door be closed? *Front. Immunol.* **2018**, *9*, 2045. [CrossRef]
6. Ruaro, B.; Smith, V.; Sulli, A.; Pizzorni, C.; Tardito, S.; Patané, M.; Paolino, S.; Cutolo, M. Innovations in the Assessment of Primary and Secondary Raynaud's Phenomenon. *Front. Pharmacol.* **2019**, *10*, 360. [CrossRef] [PubMed]
7. Altorok, N.; Nada, S.; Kahaleh, B. The isolation and characterization of systemic sclerosis vascular smooth muscle cells: Enhanced proliferation and apoptosis resistance. *J. Scleroderma Relat. Disord.* **2016**, *1*, 307–315. [CrossRef]
8. Ruaro, B.; Nallino, M.G.; Casabella, A.; Salton, F.; Confalonieri, P.; De Tanti, A.; Bruni, C. Monitoring the microcirculation in the diagnosis and follow-up of systemic sclerosis patients: Focus on pulmonary and peripheral vascular manifestations. *Microcirculation* **2020**, *27*, e12647. [CrossRef] [PubMed]
9. Ruaro, B.; Sulli, A.; Smith, V.; Pizzorni, C.; Paolino, S.; Alessandri, E.; Trombetta, A.C.; Cutolo, M. Advances in nailfold capillaroscopic analysis in systemic sclerosis. *J. Scleroderma Relat. Disord.* **2018**, *3*, 122–131. [CrossRef]
10. Hoffmann-Vold, A.M.; Maher, T.M.; Philpot, E.E.; Ashrafzadeh, A.; Barake, R.; Barsotti, S.; Bruni, C.; Carducci, P.; Carreira, P.E.; Castellví, I.; et al. The identification and management of interstitial lung disease in systemic sclerosis: Evidence-based European consensus statements. *Lancet Rheumatol.* **2020**, *2*, e71–e83. [CrossRef]
11. Hoffmann-Vold, A.M.; Allanore, Y.; Bendstrup, E.; Bruni, C.; Distler, O.; Maher, T.M.; Wijsenbeek, M.; Kreuter, M. The need for a holistic approach for SSc-ILD—Achievements and ambiguity in a devastating disease. *Respir. Res.* **2020**, *21*, 197. [CrossRef]
12. Bruni, C.; Guignabert, C.; Manetti, M.; Cerinic, M.M.; Humbert, M. The multifaceted problem of pulmonary arterial hypertension in systemic sclerosis. *Lancet Rheumatol.* **2021**, *3*, E149–E159. [CrossRef]
13. Bruni, C.; De Luca, G.; Lazzaroni, M.G.; Zanatta, E.; Lepri, G.; Airò, P.; Dagna, L.; Doria, A.; Matucci-Cerinic, M. Screening for pulmonary arterial hypertension in systemic sclerosis: A systematic literature review. *Eur. J. Intern. Med.* **2020**, *78*, 17–25. [CrossRef] [PubMed]
14. Quinn, R.; Koh, D.; Kelly, D.; Beattie, K.A.; Larché, M.J. Pulmonary arterial hypertension screening practices in scleroderma patients among Canadian rheumatologists. *J. Scleroderma Relat. Disord.* **2020**, *5*, 237–241. [CrossRef]
15. Vandecasteele, E.; Melsens, K.; Thevissen, K.; De Pauw, M.; Deschepper, E.; Decuman, S.; Piette, Y.; De Keyser, F.; Brusselle, G.; Smith, V. Prevalence and incidence of pulmonary arterial hypertension: 10-year follow-up of an unselected systemic sclerosis cohort. *J. Scleroderma Relat. Disord.* **2017**, *2*, 196–202. [CrossRef]
16. Hoffmann-Vold, A.-M.; Maher, T.M.; Philpot, E.E.; Ashrafzadeh, A.; Distler, O. Evidence based consensus recommendations for the identification and management of interstitial lung disease in systemic sclerosis. *Ann. Rheum. Dis.* **2019**, *78* (Suppl. 2), 104.
17. Roofeh, D.; Jaafar, S.; Vummidi, D.; Khanna, D. Management of systemic sclerosis-associated interstitial lung disease. *Curr. Opin. Rheumatol.* **2019**, *31*, 241–249. [CrossRef]
18. Khanna, D.; Strek, M.; Southern, B.; Saggar, R.; Hsu, V.; Mayes, M.D.; Silver, R.; Steen, V.D.; Zoz, D.; Rahaghi, F. Expert consensus on the screening, treatment, and management of patients with systemic sclerosis interstitial lung disease, and the potential role of anti-Fibrotics in a treatment paradigm for systemic sclerosis-interstitial lung disease: A Delphi Consensus Study. *Arthritis Rheum.* **2018**, *70*, 12–15.
19. Galie, N.; Humbert, M.; Vachiery, J.L.; Gibbs, S.; Lang, I.; Torbicki, A.; Simonneau, G.; Peacock, A.; Vonk Noordegraaf, A.; Beghetti, M.; et al. 2015 ESC/ERS Guidelines for the diagnosis and treatment of pulmonary hypertension. *Eur. Respir. J.* **2015**, *46*, 903–975. [CrossRef]

20. Humbert, M.; Yaici, A.; de Groote, P.; Montani, D.; Sitbon, O.; Launay, D.; Gressin, V.; Guillevin, L.; Clerson, P.; Simonneau, G.; et al. Screening for pulmonary arterial hypertension in patients with systemic sclerosis: Clinical characteristics at diagnosis and long-term survival. *Arthritis Rheumatol.* **2011**, *63*, 3522–3530. [CrossRef] [PubMed]
21. Hachulla, E.; Launay, D.; Yaici, A.; Berezne, A.; de Groote, P.; Sitbon, O.; Mouthon, L.; Guillevin, L.; Hatron, P.Y.; Simonneau, G.; et al. Pulmonary arterial hypertension associated with systemic sclerosis in patients with functional class II dyspnoea: Mild symptoms but severe outcome. *Rheumatology* **2010**, *49*, 940–944. [CrossRef] [PubMed]
22. Phung, S.; Strange, G.; Chung, L.P.; Leong, J.; Dalton, B.; Roddy, J.; Deague, J.; Playford, D.; Musk, M.; Gabbay, E. Prevalence of pulmonary arterial hypertension in an Australian scleroderma population: Screening allows for earlier diagnosis. *Intern. Med. J.* **2009**, *39*, 682–691. [CrossRef] [PubMed]
23. Vandecasteele, E.; Drieghe, B.; Melsens, K.; Thevissen, K.; De Pauw, M.; Deschepper, E.; Decuman, S.; Bonroy, C.; Piette, Y.; De Keyser, F.; et al. Screening for pulmonary arterial hypertension in an unselected prospective systemic sclerosis cohort. *Eur. Respir. J.* **2017**, *49*, pii1602275. [CrossRef]
24. Coghlan, J.G.; Denton, C.P.; Grunig, E.; Bonderman, D.; Distler, O.; Khanna, D.; Müller-Ladner, U.; Pope, J.E.; Vonk, M.C.; Doelberg, M.; et al. Evidence-based detection of pulmonary arterial hypertension in systemic sclerosis: The DETECT study. *Ann. Rheum. Dis.* **2014**, *73*, 1340–1349. [CrossRef] [PubMed]
25. Humbert, M.; Guignabert, C.; Bonnet, S.; Dorfmuller, P.; Klinger, J.R.; Nicolls, M.R.; Olschewski, A.J.; Pullamsetti, S.S.; Schermuly, R.T.; Stenmark, K.R.; et al. Pathology and pathobiology of pulmonary hypertension: State of the art and research perspectives. *Eur. Respir. J.* **2019**, *53*, pii 1801887. [CrossRef]
26. Lambova, S.N.; Müller-Ladner, U. Nailfold capillaroscopy in systemic sclerosis—State of the art: The evolving knowledge about capillaroscopic abnormalities in systemic sclerosis. *J. Scleroderma Relat. Disord.* **2019**, *4*, 200–211. [CrossRef]
27. Smith, V.; Beeckman, S.; Herrick, A.L.; Decuman, S.; Deschepper, E.; De Keyser, F.; Distler, O.; Foeldvari, I.; Ingegnoli, F.; Müller-Ladner, U.; et al. An EULAR study group pilot study on reliability of simple capillaroscopic definitions to describe capillary morphology in rheumatic diseases. *Rheumatology* **2016**, *55*, 883–890. [CrossRef]
28. Smith, V.; Vanhaecke, A.; Guerra, M.; De Angelis, R.; Deschepper, E.; Denton, C.; De Angelis, R.; Deschepper, E.; Denton, C.; Distler, O.; et al. Fast track algorithm: How to differentiate a scleroderma pattern from a non-scleroderma pattern. *Ann. Rheum. Dis.* **2019**, *78*, 1224–1225.
29. Smith, V.; Riccieri, V.; Pizzorni, C.; Decuman, S.; Deschepper, E.; Bonroy, C.; Sulli, A.; Piette, Y.; De Keyser, F.; Cutolo, M. Nailfold capillaroscopy for prediction of novel future severe organ involvement in systemic sclerosis. *J. Rheumatol.* **2013**, *40*, 2023–2028. [CrossRef] [PubMed]
30. Cutolo, M.; Herrick, A.L.; Distler, O.; Becker, M.O.; Beltran, E.; Carpentier, P.; Ferri, C.; Inanç, M.; Vlachoyiannopoulos, P.; Chadha-Boreham, H.; et al. Nailfold videocapillaroscopic features and other clinical risk factors for digital ulcers in systemic sclerosis: A multicenter, prospective cohort study. *Arthritis Rheum.* **2016**, *68*, 2527–2539. [CrossRef]
31. Smith, V.; De Keyser, F.; Pizzorni, C.; Van Praet, J.T.; Decuman, S.; Sulli, A.; Deschepper, E.; Cutolo, M. Nailfold capillaroscopy for day-to-day clinical use: Construction of a simple scoring modality as a clinical prognostic index for digital trophic lesions. *Ann. Rheum. Dis.* **2011**, *70*, 180–183. [CrossRef]
32. Pavan, T.R.; Bredemeier, M.; Hax, V.; Capobianco, K.G.; da Silva Mendonça Chakr, R. Capillary loss on nailfold capillary microscopy is associated with mortality in systemic sclerosis. *Clin. Rheumatol.* **2018**, *37*, 475–481. [CrossRef] [PubMed]
33. Cutolo, M.; Ruaro, B.; Smith, V. Macrocirculation versus microcirculation and digital ulcers in systemic sclerosis patients. *Rheumatology* **2017**, *56*, 1834–1836. [CrossRef] [PubMed]
34. Trombetta, A.C.; Pizzorni, C.; Ruaro, B.; Paolino, S.; Sulli, A.; Smith, V.; Cutolo, M. Effects of Longterm Treatment with Bosentan and Iloprost on Nailfold Absolute Capillary Number, Fingertip Blood Perfusion, and Clinical Status in Systemic Sclerosis. *J. Rheumatol.* **2016**, *43*, 2033–2041. [CrossRef]
35. Ruaro, B.; Casabella, A.; Paolino, S.; Pizzorni, C.; Ghio, M.; Seriolo, C.; Molfetta, L.; Odetti, P.; Smith, V.; Cutolo, M. Dickkopf-1 (Dkk-1) serum levels in systemic sclerosis and rheumatoid arthritis patients: Correlation with the Trabecular Bone Score (TBS). *Clinic. Rheumatol.* **2018**, *37*, 3057–3062. [CrossRef]
36. Volkmann, E.R.; Fischer, A. Update on morbidity and mortality in systemic sclerosis–related interstitial lung disease. *J. Scleroderma Relat. Disord.* **2021**, *6*, 11–20. [CrossRef]
37. Moore, D.F.; Steen, V.D. Overall mortality. *J. Scleroderma Relat. Disord.* **2021**, *6*, 3–10. [CrossRef]
38. Elhai, M.; Meune, C.; Boubaya, M.; Avouac, J.; Hachulla, E.; Balbir-Gurman, A.; Riemekasten, G.; Airò, P.; Joven, B.; Vettori, S.; et al. Mapping and predicting mortality from systemic sclerosis. *Ann. Rheum. Dis.* **2017**, *76*, 1897–1905. [CrossRef]
39. Walker, U.A.; Tyndall, A.; Czirják, L.; Denton, C.; Farge-Bancel, D.; Kowal-Bielecka, O.; Müller-Ladner, U.; Bocelli-Tyndall, C.; Matucci-Cerinic, M. Clinical risk assessment of organ manifestations in systemic sclerosis: A report from the EULAR Scleroderma Trials and Research group database. *Ann. Rheum. Dis.* **2007**, *66*, 754–763. [CrossRef] [PubMed]
40. Elhai, M.; Meune, C.; Avouac, J.; Kahan, A.; Allanore, Y. Trends in mortality in patients with systemic sclerosis over 40 years: A systematic review and meta-analysis of cohort studies. *Rheumatology* **2012**, *51*, 1017–1026. [CrossRef]
41. Rubio-Rivas, M.; Royo, C.; Simeón, C.P.; Corbella, X.; Fonollosa, V. Mortality and survival in systemic sclerosis: Systematic review and meta-analysis. *Semin. Arthritis Rheum.* **2014**, *44*, 208–219. [CrossRef]

42. Clements, P.J.; Roth, M.D.; Elashoff, R.; Tashkin, D.P.; Goldin, J.; Silver, R.M.; Sterz, M.; Seibold, J.R.; Schraufnagel, D.; Simms, R.W.; et al. Scleroderma Lung Study (SLS): Differences in the presentation and course of patients with limited versus diffuse systemic sclerosis. *Ann. Rheum. Dis.* **2007**, *66*, 1641–1647. [CrossRef] [PubMed]
43. Lescoat, A.; Roofeh, D.; Townsend, W.; Hughes, M.; Sandler, R.D.; Zimmermann, F.; Pauling, J.D.; Buch, M.H.; Khanna, D. Domains and outcome measures for the assessment of limited cutaneous systemic sclerosis: A scoping review protocol. *BMJ Open* **2021**, *11*, e044765. [CrossRef]
44. Mouthon, L.; Berezné, A.; Brauner, M.; Kambouchner, M.; Guillevin, L.; Valeyre, D. Pneumopathie infiltrante diffuse de la sclerodermie systemique [Interstitial lung disease in systemic sclerosis]. *Rev. Mal. Respir.* **2007**, *24*, 1035–1046. [CrossRef]
45. Steen, V.D.; Conte, C.; Owens, G.R.; Medsger, T.A., Jr. Severe restrictive lung disease in systemic sclerosis. *Arthritis Rheumatol.* **1994**, *37*, 1283–1289. [CrossRef]
46. Frauenfelder, T.; Winklehner, A.; Nguyen, T.D.; Dobrota, R.; Baumueller, S.; Maurer, B.; Distler, O. Screening for interstitial lung disease in systemic sclerosis: Performance of high-resolution CT with limited number of slices: A prospective study. *Ann. Rheum. Dis.* **2014**, *73*, 2069–2073. [CrossRef]
47. Hoffmann-Vold, A.M.; Aaløkken, T.M.; Lund, M.B.; Garen, T.; Midtvedt, Ø.; Brunborg, C.; Gran, J.T.; Molberg, Ø. Predictive value of serial high-resolution computed tomography analyses and concurrent lung function tests in systemic sclerosis. *Arthritis Rheumatol.* **2015**, *67*, 2205–2212. [CrossRef] [PubMed]
48. Hoffmann-Vold, A.M.; Allanore, Y.; Alves, M.; Brunborg, C.; Airó, P.; Ananieva, L.P.; Alves, M.; Brunborg, C.; Airó, P.; Ananieva, L.P.; et al. Progressive interstitial lung disease in patients with systemic sclerosis-associated interstitial lung disease in the EUSTAR database. *Ann. Rheum. Dis.* **2021**, *80*, 219–227. [CrossRef] [PubMed]
49. Ruaro, B.; Confalonieri, M.; Matucci-Cerinic, M.; Salton, F.; Confalonieri, P.; Santagiuliana, M.; Citton, G.M.; Baratella, E.; Bruni, C. The treatment of lung involvement in systemic sclerosis. *Pharmaceuticals* **2021**, *14*, 154. [CrossRef]
50. Shah, R.M.; Jimenez, S.; Wechsler, R. Significance of ground-glass opacity on HRCT in long-term follow-up of patients with systemic sclerosis. *J. Thorac. Imaging* **2007**, *22*, 120–124. [CrossRef]
51. Occhipinti, M.; Bruni, C.; Camiciottoli, G.; Bartolucci, M.; Bellando-Randone, S.; Bassetto, A.; Cuomo, G.; Giuggioli, D.; Ciardi, G.; Fabbrizzi, A.; et al. Quantitative analysis of pulmonary vasculature in systemic sclerosis at spirometry-gated chest CT. *Ann. Rheum. Dis.* **2020**, *79*, 1210–1217. [CrossRef]
52. Launay, D.; Remy-Jardin, M.; Michon-Pasturel, U.; Mastora, I.; Hachulla, E.; Lambert, M.; Delannoy, V.; Queyrel, V.; Duhamel, A.; Matran, R.; et al. High resolution computed tomography in fibrosing alveolitis associated with systemic sclerosis. *J. Rheumatol.* **2006**, *33*, 1789–1801. [PubMed]
53. Goldin, J.; Elashoff, R.; Kim, H.J.; Yan, X.; Lynch, D.; Strollo, D.; Roth, M.D.; Clements, P.; Furst, D.E.; Khanna, D.; et al. Treatment of scleroderma-interstitial lung disease with cyclophosphamide is associated with less progressive fibrosis on serial thoracic high-resolution CT scan than placebo: Findings from the Scleroderma Lung Study. *Chest* **2009**, *136*, 1333–1340. [CrossRef]
54. Bouros, D.; Wells, A.U.; Nicholson, A.G.; Colby, T.V.; Polychronopoulos, V.; Pantelidis, P.; Haslam, P.L.; Vassilakis, D.A.; Black, C.M.; du Bois, R.M. Histopathologic subsets of fibrosing alveolitis in patients with systemic sclerosis and their relationship to outcome. *Am. J. Respir. Crit. Care Med.* **2002**, *165*, 1581–1586. [CrossRef] [PubMed]
55. Zamora, F.D.; Kim, H.J.; Wang, Q. Prevalence of pulmonary function test abnormalities and their correlation to high resolution computer tomography in a large scleroderma population. *Am. J. Respir. Crit. Care Med.* **2013**, *187*, A2920.
56. Suliman, Y.A.; Dobrota, R.; Huscher, D.; Nguyen-Kim, T.D.; Maurer, B.; Jordan, S.; Speich, R.; Frauenfelder, T.; Distler, O. Brief Report: Pulmonary Function Tests: High Rate of False-Negative Results in the Early Detection and Screening of Scleroderma-Related Interstitial Lung Disease. *Arthritis Rheumatol.* **2015**, *67*, 3256–3261. [CrossRef] [PubMed]
57. Baratella, E.; Marrocchio, C.; Cifaldi, R.; Santagiuliana, M.; Bozzato, A.M.; Crivelli, P.; Ruaro, B.; Salton, F.; Confalonieri, M.; Cova, M.A. Interstitial lung disease in patients with antisynthetase syndrome: A retrospective case series study. *Jpn. J. Radiol.* **2021**, *39*, 40–46. [CrossRef] [PubMed]
58. Mulkoju, R.; Saka, V.K.; Rajaram, M.; Kumari, R.; Negi, V.S.; Mohanty Mohapatra, M.; Govindaraj, V.; Dwivedi, D.P.; Mahesh Babu, V. Pulmonary Manifestations in Systemic Sclerosis: Hospital-Based Descriptive Study. *Cureus* **2020**, *12*, e8649. [CrossRef] [PubMed]
59. Kang, E.H.; Song, Y.W. Pharmacological Interventions for Pulmonary Involvement in Rheumatic Diseases. *Pharmaceuticals* **2021**, *14*, 251. [CrossRef]
60. Ooi, G.C.; Mok, M.Y.; Tsang, K.W.; Wong, Y.; Khong, P.L.; Fung, P.C.; Chan, S.; Tse, H.F.; Wong, R.W.; Lam, W.K.; et al. Interstitial lung disease in systemic sclerosis. *Acta Radiol.* **2003**, *44*, 258–264.
61. Olson, A.; Hartmann, N.; Patnaik, P.; Wallace, L.; Schlenker-Herceg, R.; Nasser, M.; Richeldi, L.; Hoffmann-Vold, A.M.; Cottin, V. Estimation of the prevalence of progressive fibrosing interstitial lung diseases: Systematic literature review and data from a physician survey. *Adv. Ther.* **2021**, *38*, 854–867. [CrossRef]
62. Spagnolo, P.; Distler, O.; Ryerson, C.J.; Tzouvelekis, A.; Lee, J.S.; Bonella, F.; Bouros, D.; Hoffmann-Vold, A.M.; Crestani, B.; Matteson, E.L. Mechanisms of progressive fibrosis in connective tissue disease (CTD)-associated interstitial lung diseases (ILDs). *Ann. Rheum. Dis.* **2021**, *80*, 143–150. [CrossRef]
63. Ruaro, B.; Salton, F.; Braga, L.; Wade, B.; Confalonieri, P.; Volpe, M.C.; Baratella, E.; Maiocchi, S.; Confalonieri, M. The History and Mystery of Alveolar Epithelial Type II Cells: Focus on Their Physiologic and Pathologic Role in Lung. *Int. J. Mol. Sci.* **2021**, *22*, 2566. [CrossRef] [PubMed]

64. Goh, N.S.; Desai, S.R.; Veeraraghavan, S.; Hansell, D.M.; Copley, S.J.; Maher, T.M.; Corte, T.J.; Sander, C.R.; Ratoff, J.; Devaraj, A.; et al. Interstitial lung disease in systemic sclerosis: A simple staging system. *Am. J. Respir. Crit. Care Med.* **2008**, *177*, 1248–1254.
65. Saldana, D.C.; Hague, C.J.; Murphy, D.; Coxson, H.O.; Tschirren, J.; Peterson, S.; Sieren, J.P.; Kirby, M.; Ryerson, C.J. Association of Computed Tomography Densitometry with Disease Severity, Functional Decline, and Survival in Systemic Sclerosis-associated Interstitial Lung Disease. *Ann. Am. Thorac. Soc.* **2020**, *17*, 813–820. [CrossRef] [PubMed]
66. Colaci, M.; Giuggioli, D.; Sebastiani, M.; Manfredi, A.; Lumetti, F.; Luppi, F.; Cerri, S.; Ferri, C. Predictive value of isolated DLCO reduction in systemic sclerosis patients without cardio-pulmonary involvement at baseline. *Reumatismo* **2015**, *85*, 149–155. [CrossRef] [PubMed]
67. Tashkin, D.P.; Volkmann, E.R.; Tseng, C.H.; Kim, H.J.; Goldin, J.; Clements, P.; Furst, D.; Khanna, D.; Kleerup, E.; Roth, M.D.; et al. Relationship between quantitative radiographic assessments of interstitial lung disease and physiological and clinical features of systemic sclerosis. *Ann. Rheum. Dis.* **2016**, *75*, 374–381. [CrossRef] [PubMed]
68. Gargani, L.; Bruni, C.; De Marchi, D.; Romei, C.; Guiducci, S.; Bellando-Randone, S.; Aquaro, G.D.; Pepe, A.; Neri, E.; Colagrande, S.; et al. Lung magnetic resonance imaging in systemic sclerosis: A new promising approach to evaluate pulmonary involvement and progression. *Clin. Rheumatol.* **2020**, *7*. [CrossRef]
69. Barskova, T.; Gargani, L.; Guiducci, S.; Randone, S.B.; Bruni, C.; Carnesecchi, G.; Conforti, M.L.; Porta, F.; Pignone, A.; Caramella, D.; et al. Lung ultrasound for the screening of interstitial lung disease in very early systemic sclerosis. *Ann. Rheum. Dis.* **2013**, *72*, 390–395. [CrossRef]
70. Hughes, M.; Bruni, C.; Cuomo, G.; Delle Sedie, A.; Gargani, L.; Gutierrez, M.; Lepri, G.; Ruaro, B.; Santiago, T.; Suliman, Y.; et al. The role of ultrasound in systemic sclerosis: On the cutting edge to foster clinical and research advancement. *J. Scleroderma Relat. Disord.* **2020**. [CrossRef]
71. Gargani, L.; Bruni, C.; Romei, C.; Frumento, P.; Moreo, A.; Agoston, G.; Guiducci, S.; Bellando-Randone, S.; Lepri, G.; Belloli, L.; et al. Prognostic Value of Lung Ultrasound B-Lines in Systemic Sclerosis. *Chest* **2020**, *158*, 1515–1525. [CrossRef]
72. Behr, J.; Furst, D.E. Pulmonary function tests. *Rheumatology* **2008**, *47* (Suppl. 5), v65–v67. [CrossRef]
73. Roofeh, D.; Lin, C.J.F.; Goldin, J.; Kim, G.H.; Furst, D.E.; Denton, C.P.; Huang, S.; Khanna, D. focuSSced investigators. Tocilizumab Prevents Progression of Early Systemic Sclerosis Associated Interstitial Lung Disease. *Arthritis Rheumatol.* **2021**, *3*. [CrossRef]
74. Rubio-Rivas, M.; Corbella, X.; Pestaña-Fernández, M.; Tolosa-Vilella, C.; Guillen-Del Castillo, A.; Colunga-Argüelles, D.; Trapiella-Martínez, L.; Iniesta-Arandia, N.; Castillo-Palma, M.J.; Sáez-Comet, L.; et al. First clinical symptom as a prognostic factor in systemic sclerosis: Results of a retrospective nationwide cohort study. *Clin. Rheumatol.* **2018**, *37*, 999–1009. [CrossRef] [PubMed]
75. Kennedy, B.; Branagan, P.; Moloney, F.; Haroon, M.; O'Connell, O.J.; O'Connor, T.M.; O'Regan, K.; Harney, S.; Henry, M.T. Biomarkers to identify ILD and predict lung function decline in scleroderma lung disease or idiopathic pulmonary fibrosis. *Sarcoidosis Vasc. Diffus. Lung Dis.* **2015**, *32*, 228–236.
76. Bernstein, E.J.; Jaafar, S.; Assassi, S.; Domsic, R.T.; Frech, T.M.; Gordon, J.K.; Broderick, R.J.; Hant, F.N.; Hinchcliff, M.E.; Shah, A.A.; et al. Performance Characteristics of Pulmonary Function Tests for the Detection of Interstitial Lung Disease in Adults With Early Diffuse Cutaneous Systemic Sclerosis. *Arthritis Rheum.* **2020**, *72*, 1892–1896. [CrossRef] [PubMed]
77. Steen, V.D.; Graham, G.; Conte, C.; Owens, G.; Medsger, T.A., Jr. Isolated diffusing capacity reduction in systemic sclerosis. *Arthritis Rheum.* **1992**, *35*, 765–770. [CrossRef]
78. Galiè, N.; McLaughlin, V.V.; Rubin, L.J.; Simonneau, G. An overview of the 6th World Symposium on Pulmonary Hypertension. *Eur. Respir. J.* **2019**, *53*, 1802148. [CrossRef]
79. Thakkar, V.; Stevens, W.; Prior, D.; Youssef, P.; Liew, D.; Gabbay, E.; Roddy, J.; Walker, J.G.; Zochling, J.; Sahhar, J.; et al. The inclusion of N-terminal pro-brain natriuretic peptide in a sensitive screening strategy for systemic sclerosis-related pulmonary arterial hypertension: A cohort study. *Arthritis Res. Ther.* **2013**, *15*, R193. [CrossRef] [PubMed]
80. Denton, C.P.; Cailes, J.B.; Phillips, G.D.; Wells, A.U.; Black, C.M.; Bois, R.M. Comparison of Doppler echocardiography and right heart catheterization to assess pulmonary hypertension in systemic sclerosis. *Br. J. Rheumatol.* **1997**, *36*, 239–243. [CrossRef] [PubMed]
81. Voilliot, D.; Magne, J.; Dulgheru, R.; Kou, S.; Henri, C.; Caballero, L.; De Sousa, C.; Sprynger, M.; Andre, B.; Pierard, L.A.; et al. Cardiovascular outcome in systemic sclerosis. *Acta Cardiol.* **2015**, *70*, 554–563. [CrossRef] [PubMed]
82. Markusse, I.M.; Meijs, J.; de Boer, B.; Bakker, J.A.; Schippers, H.P.C.; Schouffoer, A.A.; Bakker, J.A.; Schippers, H.; Schouffoer, A.A.; Ajmone Marsan, N.; et al. Predicting cardiopulmonary involvement in patients with systemic sclerosis: Complementary value of nailfold videocapillaroscopy patterns and disease-specific autoantibodies. *Rheumatology* **2017**, *56*, 1081–1088. [CrossRef]
83. De Scordilli, M.; Pinamonti, B.; Albani, S.; Gregorio, C.; Barbati, G.; Daneluzzi, C.; Korcova, R.; Perkan, A.; Fabris, E.; Geri, P.; et al. Reliability of noninvasive hemodynamic assessment with Doppler echocardiography: Comparison with the invasive evaluation. *J. Cardiovasc. Med.* **2019**, *20*, 682–690. [CrossRef]
84. Oudiz, R.; Langleben, D. Cardiac catheterization in pulmonary arterial hypertension: An updated guide to proper use. *Adv. Pulm. Hypertens. J.* **2005**, *4*, 15–25. [CrossRef]
85. Herrick, A.L. Raynaud's phenomenon. *J. Scleroderma Relat. Disord.* **2019**, *4*, 89–101. [CrossRef]
86. Pauling, J.D.; Frech, T.M.; Hughes, M.; Gordon, J.K.; Domsic, R.T.; Anderson, M.E.; Ingegnoli, F.; McHugh, N.J.; Johnson, S.R.; Hudson, M.; et al. Patient-reported outcome instruments for assessing Raynaud's phenomenon in systemic sclerosis: A SCTC vascular working group report. *J. Scleroderma Relat. Disord.* **2018**, *3*, 249–252. [CrossRef]

87. Ruaro, B.; Pizzorni, C.; Paolino, S.; Alessandri, E.; Sulli, A. Aminaphtone Efficacy in Primary and Secondary Raynaud's Phenomenon: A Feasibility Study. *Front. Pharmacol.* **2019**, *10*, 293. [CrossRef] [PubMed]
88. Smith, V.; Thevissen, K.; Trombetta, A.C.; Pizzorni, C.; Ruaro, B.; Piette, Y.; Paolino, S.; De Keyser, F.; Sulli, A.; Melsens, K.; et al. Nailfold Capillaroscopy and clinical applications in Systemic Sclerosis. *Microcirculation* **2016**, *105*, 119–124. [CrossRef] [PubMed]
89. Hughes, M.; Bruni, C.; Ruaro, B.; Confalonieri, M.; Matucci-Cerinic, M.; Randone, S.B. Digital Ulcers in Systemic Sclerosis. *Presse Med.* **2021**, *3*, 104064. [CrossRef]
90. Amanzi, L.; Braschi, F.; Fiori, G.; Galluccio, F.; Miniati, I.; Guiducci, S.; Conforti, M.L.; Kaloudi, O.; Nacci, F.; Sacu, O.; et al. Digital ulcers in scleroderma: Staging, characteristics and sub-setting through observation of 1614 digital lesions. *Rheumatology* **2010**, *49*, 1374–1382. [CrossRef]
91. Minier, T.; Guiducci, S.; Bellando-Randone, S.; Bruni, C.; Lepri, G.; Czirják, L.; Distler, O.; Walker, U.A.; Fransen, J.; Allanore, Y.; et al. Preliminary analysis of the very early diagnosis of systemic sclerosis (VEDOSS) EUSTAR multicentre study: Evidence for puffy fingers as a pivotal sign for suspicion of systemic sclerosis. *Ann. Rheum. Dis.* **2014**, *73*, 2087–2093. [CrossRef] [PubMed]
92. Vasile, M.; Avouac, J.; Sciarra, I.; Stefanantoni, K.; Iannace, N.; Cravotto, E.; Valesini, G.; Allanore, Y.; Riccieri, V. From VEDOSS to established systemic sclerosis diagnosis according to ACR/EULAR 2013 classification criteria: A French-Italian capillaroscopic survey. *Clin. Exp. Rheumatol.* **2018**, *36*, 82–87. [CrossRef] [PubMed]
93. Bernero, E.; Sulli, A.; Ferrari, G.; Ravera, F.; Pizzorni, C.; Ruaro, B.; Zampogna, G.; Alessandri, E.; Cutolo, M. Prospective capillaroscopy-based study on transition from primary to secondary Raynaud's phenomenon: Preliminary results. *Reumatismo* **2013**, *65*, 186–191. [CrossRef]
94. Cutolo, M.; Grassi, W.; Matucci Cerinic, M. Raynaud's phenomenon and the role of capillaroscopy. *Arthr. Rheum.* **2003**, *48*, 3023–3030. [CrossRef] [PubMed]
95. Pizzorni, C.; Sulli, A.; Smith, V.; Ruaro, B.; Trombetta, A.C.; Cutolo, M.; Paolino, S. Primary Raynaud's phenomenon and nailfold videocapillaroscopy: Age-related changes in capillary morphology. *Clin. Rheumatol.* **2017**, *36*, 1637–1642. [CrossRef] [PubMed]
96. Herrick, A.L.; Murray, A. The role of capillaroscopy and thermography in the assessment and management of Raynaud's phenomenon. *Autoimmun. Rev.* **2018**, *17*, 465–472. [CrossRef] [PubMed]
97. Cutolo, M.; Trombetta, A.C.; Melsens, K.; Pizzorni, C.; Sulli, A.; Ruaro, B.; Paolino, S.; Deschepper, E.; Smith, V. Automated assessment of absolute nailfold capillary number on videocapillaroscopic images: Proof of principle and validation in systemic sclerosis. *Microcirculation* **2018**, *25*, e12447. [CrossRef]
98. Cutolo, M.; Melsens, K.; Herrick, A.L.; Foeldvari, I.; Deschepper, E.; De Keyser, F.; Distler, O.; Ingegnoli, F.; Mostmans, Y.; Müller-Ladner, U.; et al. EULAR Study Group on Microcirculation in Rheumatic Diseases. Reliability of simple capillaroscopic definitions in describing capillary morphology in rheumatic diseases. *Rheumatology* **2018**, *57*, 757–759. [CrossRef]
99. Ruaro, B.; Sulli, A.; Pizzorni, C.; Smith, V.; Gotelli, E.; Alsheyyab, J.; Trombetta, A.C.; Cutolo, M. Longitudinal assessment of nailfold capillary number, peripheral blood perfusion and dermal thickness in systemic sclerosispatients over a period of 5 years. *Ann. Rheum. Dis.* **2018**, *77*, 1508.
100. Ruaro, B.; Pizzorni, C.; Paolino, S.; Smith, V.; Ghio, M.; Casabella, A.; Alessandri, E.; Patané, M.; Sulli, A.; Cutolo, M. Correlations between nailfold microvascular damage and skin involvement in systemic sclerosis patients. *Microvasc. Res.* **2019**, *125*, 103874. [CrossRef] [PubMed]
101. Ruaro, B.; Casabella, A.; Paolino, S.; Pizzorni, C.; Alessandri, E.; Seriolo, C.; Botticella, G.; Molfetta, L.; Odetti, P.; Smith, V.; et al. Correlation between bone quality and microvascular damage in systemic sclerosis patients. *Rheumatology* **2018**, *57*, 1548–1554. [CrossRef]
102. Bruni, C.; Guiducci, S.; Bellando-Randone, S.; Lepri, G.; Braschi, F.; Fiori, G.; Bartoli, F.; Peruzzi, F.; Blagojevic, J.; Matucci-Cerinic, M. Digital ulcers as a sentinel sign for early internal organ involvement in very early systemic sclerosis. *Rheumatology* **2015**, *54*, 72–76. [CrossRef]
103. Van den Hoogen, F.; Khanna, D.; Fransen, J.; Johnson, S.R.; Baron, M.; Tyndall, A.; Matucci-Cerinic, M.; Naden, R.P.; Medsger, T.A., Jr.; Carreira, P.E.; et al. 2013 classification criteria for systemic sclerosis: An American college of rheumatology/European league against rheumatism collaborative initiative. *Ann. Rheum. Dis.* **2013**, *72*, 1747–1755. [CrossRef] [PubMed]
104. Ghizzoni, C.; Sebastiani, M.; Manfredi, A.; Campomori, F.; Colaci, M.; Giuggioli, D.; Ferri, C. Prevalence and evolution of scleroderma pattern at nailfold videocapillaroscopy in sistemic sclerosis patients: Clinical and prognostic implications. *Microvasc. Res.* **2015**, *99*, 92–95. [CrossRef] [PubMed]
105. Sulli, A.; Secchi, M.E.; Pizzorni, C.; Cutolo, M. Scoring the nailfold microvascular changes during the capillaroscopic analysis in systemic sclerosis patients. *Arthritis Rheum.* **2012**, *64*, 821–825. [CrossRef]
106. Medsger, T.A., Jr.; Silman, A.J.; Steen, V.D.; Black, C.M.; Akesson, A.; Bacon, P.A.; Harris, C.A.; Jablonska, S.; Jayson, M.I.; Jimenez, S.A.; et al. A disease severity scale for systemic sclerosis: Development and testing. *J. Rheumatol.* **1999**, *26*, 2159–2167. [PubMed]
107. Smith, V.; Vanhaecke, A.; Guerra, M.; Ruaro, B.; Sulli, A.; Vandecasteele, E. Capillaroscopy in systemic sclerosis related pulmonary arterial hypertension. *Ann. Rheum. Dis.* **2019**, *78*, 854–855.
108. Jehangir, M.; Qayoom, S.; Jeelani, S.; Yousuf, R. Nailfold capillaroscopy in patients of systemic sclerosis and its association with disease severity as evidenced by high resolution computed tomography lung: A hospital based cross sectional study. *Int. J. Res. Med. Sci.* **2017**, *3*, 5.

109. Pizzorni, C.; Ruaro, B.; Paolino, S.; Camellino, D.; Cimmino, M.A.; Cutolo, M.; Sulli, A. Twelve year follow-up on progression of nailfold microangiopathy detected through transition between different capillaroscopic patterns of microvascular damage in systemic sclerosis. *Ann. Rheum. Dis.* **2016**, *75*, 746. [CrossRef]
110. Guillen-Del-Castillo, A.; Simeon-Aznar, C.P.; Callejas-Moraga, E.L.; Tolosa-Vilella, C.; Alonso-Vila, S.; Fonollosa-Pla, V.; Selva-O'Callaghan, A. Quantitative videocapillaroscopy correlates with functional respiratory parameters: A clue for vasculopathy as a pathogenic mechanism for lung injury in systemic sclerosis. *Arthritis Res. Ther.* **2018**, *20*, 281. [CrossRef] [PubMed]
111. Caetano, J.; Paula, F.S.; Amaral, M.; Oliveira, S.; Alves, J.D. Nailfold videocapillaroscopy changes are associated with the presence and severity of systemic sclerosis-related interstitial lung disease. *J. Clin. Rheumatol.* **2019**, *25*, e12–e15. [CrossRef]
112. Xia, Z.; Wang, G.; Xiao, H.; Guo, S.; Liu, Y.; Meng, F.; Liu, D.; Li, G.; Zong, L. Diagnostic value of nailfold videocapillaroscopy in systemic sclerosis secondary pulmonary arterial hypertension: A meta-analysis. *Intern. Med. J.* **2018**, *48*, 1355–1359. [CrossRef]
113. Meier, F.; Geyer, M.; Tiede, H.; Rieth, A.; Ghofrani, H.A.; Müller-Ladner, U.; Zong, L. Is nailfold videocapillaroscopy a valuable diagnostic tool in pulmonary hypertension? *Eur. Respir. J.* **2012**, *40*, 972. [CrossRef]
114. Kim, H.S.; Park, M.K.; Kim, H.Y.; Park, S.H. Capillary dimension measured by computer-based digitalized image correlated with plasma endothelin-1 levels in patients with systemic sclerosis. *Clin. Rheumatol.* **2010**, *29*, 247–254. [CrossRef]
115. Avouac, J.; Lepri, G.; Smith, V.; Toniolo, E.; Hurabielle, C.; Vallet, A.; Amrouche, F.; Kahan, A.; Cutolo, M.; Allanore, Y. Sequential nailfold videocapillaroscopy examinations have responsiveness to detect organ progression in systemic sclerosis. *Semin. Arthritis Rheum.* **2017**, *47*, 86–94. [CrossRef] [PubMed]
116. Hofstee, H.M.; Vonk Noordegraaf, A.; Voskuyl, A.E.; Dijkmans, B.A.; Postmus, P.E.; Smulders, Y.M.; Serné, E.H. Nailfold capillary density is associated with the presence and severity of pulmonary arterial hypertension in systemic sclerosis. *Ann. Rheum. Dis.* **2009**, *68*, 191–195. [CrossRef]
117. Pizzorni, C.; Sulli, A.; Smith, V.; Lladó, A.; Paolino, S.; Cutolo, M.; Ruaro, B. Capillaroscopy 2016: New perspectives in systemic sclerosis. *Acta Reumatol. Port.* **2016**, *41*, 8–14. [PubMed]
118. Corrado, A.; Correale, M.; Mansueto, N.; Monaco, I.; Carriero, A.; Mele, A.; Colia, R.; Di Biase, M.; Cantatore, F.P. Nailfold capillaroscopic changes in patients with idiopathic pulmonary arterial hypertension and systemic sclerosis-related pulmonary arterial hypertension. *Microvasc. Res.* **2017**, *114*, 46–51. [CrossRef] [PubMed]
119. Anderson, M.E.; Allen, P.D.; Moore, T.; Hillier, V.; Taylor, C.J.; Herrick, A.L. Computerized nailfold video capillaroscopy—A new tool for assessment of Raynaud's phenomenon. *J. Rheumatol.* **2005**, *32*, 841–848. [PubMed]
120. Smith, V.; Decuman, S.; Sulli, A.; Bonroy, C.; Piettte, Y.; Deschepper, E.; de Keyser, F.; Cutolo, M. Do worsening scleroderma capillaroscopic patterns predict future severe organ involvement? A pilot study. *Ann. Rheum. Dis.* **2012**, *71*, 1636–1639. [CrossRef] [PubMed]
121. Riccieri, V.; Vasile, M.; Iannace, N.; Stefanantoni, K.; Sciarra, I.; Vizza, C.D.; Badagliacca, R.; Poscia, R.; Papa, S.; Mezzapesa, M.; et al. Systemic sclerosis patients with and without pulmonary arterial hypertension: A nailfold capillaroscopy study. *Rheumatology* **2013**, *52*, 1525–1528. [CrossRef] [PubMed]
122. Chaisson, N.F.; Hassoun, P.M. Systemic sclerosis-associated pulmonary arterial hypertension. *Chest* **2013**, *144*, 1346–1356. [CrossRef]
123. Hax, V.; Bredemeier, M.; Didonet Moro, A.L.; Pavan, T.R.; Vieira, M.V.; Pitrez, E.H.; da Silva Chakr, R.M.; Xavier, R.M. Clinical algorithms for the diagnosis and prognosis of interstitial lung disease in systemic sclerosis. *Semin. Arthritis Rheum.* **2017**, *47*, 228–234. [CrossRef] [PubMed]
124. Karayusuf, L.; Akdoğan, A.; Kılıç, L.; Karadağ, Ö.; Kalyoncu, U.; Bilgen, Ş.A.; Ertenli, I.; Kiraz, S. Evaluation of association between capillaroscopic findings and organ involvements in Turkish systemic sclerosis patients. *RAED Derg.* **2014**, *6*, 43–52. [CrossRef]
125. Ong, Y.Y.; Nikoloutsopoulos, T.; Bond, C.P.; Smith, M.D.; Ahern, M.J.; Roberts-Thomson, P.J. Decreased nailfold capillary density in limited scleroderma with pulmonary hypertension. *Asian Pac. J. Allergy Immunol.* **1998**, *16*, 81–86.
126. Hurabielle, C.; Avouac, J.; Lepri, G.; de Risi, T.; Kahan, A.; Allanore, Y. Skin Telangiectasia and the Identification of a Subset of Systemic Sclerosis Patients with Severe Vascular Disease. *Arthritis Care Res.* **2016**, *68*, 1021–1027. [CrossRef] [PubMed]
127. Dababneh, L.; Cikach, F.; Alkukhun, L.; Dweik, R.A.; Tonelli, A.R. Sublingual microcirculation in pulmonary arterial hypertension. *Ann. Am. Thorac. Soc.* **2014**, *11*, 504–512. [CrossRef]
128. D'Angelo, W.A.; Fries, J.F.; Masi, A.T.; Shulman, L.E. Pathologic observations in systemic sclerosis (scleroderma). A study of fifty-eight autopsy cases and fifty-eight matched controls. *Am. J. Med.* **1969**, *46*, 428–440.

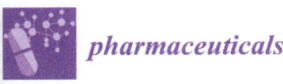

Review

The Treatment of Lung Involvement in Systemic Sclerosis

Barbara Ruaro [1],*, Marco Confalonieri [1], Marco Matucci-Cerinic [2], Francesco Salton [1], Paola Confalonieri [1], Mario Santagiuliana [1], Gloria Maria Citton [1], Elisa Baratella [3] and Cosimo Bruni [2]

[1] Department of Pulmonology, University Hospital of Cattinara, 34149 Trieste TS, Italy; marco.confalonieri@asugi.sanita.fvg.it (M.C.); francesco.salton@gmail.com (F.S.); paola.confalonieri.24@gmail.com (P.C.); mario@marionline.it (M.S.); gloriacitton@gmail.com (G.M.C.)

[2] Department of Experimental and Clinical Medicine, Division of Rheumatology, University of Firenze, 50121 Firenze FI, Italy; marco.matuccicerinic@unifi.it (M.M.-C.); cosimobruni85@gmail.com (C.B.)

[3] Department of Radiology, Cattinara Hospital, University of Trieste, 34127 Trieste TS, Italy; elisa.baratella@gmail.com

* Correspondence: barbara.ruaro@yahoo.it; Tel.: +39-3470502394

Abstract: Systemic sclerosis (SSc) patients are often affected by interstitial lung disease (ILD) and, although there have been recent treatment advances, it remains the leading cause of death among SSc, with a 10-year mortality up to 40%. African Americans and subjects with diffuse cutaneous SSc or anti-topoisomerase 1 antibodies are most commonly affected. Currently, early ILD diagnosis can be made, and it is pivotal to improve the prognosis. The diagnostic mainstay test for SSc-ILD is high-resolution computed tomography for the morphology and pulmonary function tests for the functional aspects. Treatment planning and intensity are guided by the disease severity and risk of progression. Traditionally, therapy has depended on combinations of immunosuppressants, particularly cyclophosphamide and mycophenolate mofetil, which can be supplemented by targeted biological and antifibrotic therapies. Benefits have been observed in trials on hematopoietic autologous stem cell transplantation for patients with progressive SSc, whilst lung transplantation is reserved for refractory SSc-ILD cases. Herein, recent advances in SSc-ILD treatment will be explored.

Keywords: systemic sclerosis; scleroderma; interstitial lung disease; pulmonary function tests; high-resolution computed tomography

1. Introduction

Scleroderma or Systemic Sclerosis (SSc), a disease characterized by fibrosis, vasculopathy, and inflammation, may affect different organ and systems, with severe prognostic implications [1,2]. When SSc pathogenetic processes manifest at lung level [3], pulmonary disease may manifest both as interstitial lung disease (ILD) and/or pulmonary arterial hypertension (PAH) [4,5]. The European Scleroderma Trials and Research (EUSTAR) group reported that 53% of cases with diffuse cutaneous SSc (dcSSc) have ILD, as do 35% of cases with limited cutaneous SSc [6]. Moreover, high-resolution computed tomography (HRCT) evidences interstitial abnormalities in 90% of SSc patients [7], and pulmonary function tests (PFT) showed alterations in 40–75% [8]. There has been no significant change in SSc mortality rate over the past 40 years [9,10], although an increase in mortality due to ILD and PAH [11,12] is significant, a decrease in deaths due to renal crisis has been recorded [13]. Nowadays, ILD and PAH are the two leading causes of death in SSc, accounting for 33% and 28% of deaths, respectively [10–12]. The survival of systemic sclerosis-related interstitial lung disease (SSc-ILD) patients is reported to be 29–69% at 10 years [9,12]. Early autopsy studies demonstrated that up to 100% of patients had parenchymal involvement [14]. Considering the frequency and the prognosis of SSc-ILD patients, it is essential to attempt to identify pulmonary disease early, at a potentially reversible stage [15].

Unfortunately, there are limited treatment options for this manifestation, given that the paucity of high-quality, randomized, controlled trials specifically targeting SSc-ILD are scanty, and, historically, studies have favored cyclophosphamide (CYC) for the treatment of SSc-ILD, as also suggested in the most recent European League against Rheumatism (EULAR) recommendations [16–19]. The most recent and supportive data showed the positive effect of nintedanib, a multi-tyrosine kinase inhibitor, as a significant inhibitor of progressive functional decline [20]. Innovative proposals have also recently been made on the basis of clinical and preclinical evidence for rituximab (RTX), tocilizumab (TCZ), and pirfenidone (PIRF), as well as hematopoietic stem cell transplantation and lung transplantation [21]. However, the safety and efficacy of emerging experimental therapies for SSc-ILD require further investigation. The aim of this review is to summarize the state-of-the art in SSc-ILD treatments.

2. Management Principles

As SSc-ILD is a very heterogeneous disease, management tends to differ according to the profile of the patient. Furthermore, with the advent of the new aforementioned treatment options, it is pivotal to detect ILD [22–24] as early as possible and also to assign the right treatment as early as possible [7,19]. Toward this aim, precise and objective ILD classification tools that allow for patient stratification at ILD detection and diagnosis play a major role [25]. Indeed, patients must be classified by a severity assessment of ILD at diagnosis, performed by HRCT and PFT, and then by the evaluation of the risk of ILD progression [25,26].

The HRCT variables predictive of mortality and ILD progression in SSc–ILD were studied and reported in a recent meta-analysis of 27 studies, which concluded that the extent of disease on HRCT was an independent predictor of both mortality and ILD progression [27].

It is a must to detect the subset of clinical ILD patients with progressive disease, defined as a decline in Forced Vital Capacity (FVC) levels of >10% from baseline or a ≥ 5% to < 10% relative decline in FVC and a ≥ 15% relative decline in Diffusion Lung Capacity of Carbon monoxide (DLCO) over 12 months [28]. Despite this cut-off being proposed for clinical trials and applied also in clinical practice, smaller changes may also be of clinical importance, in particular worsening symptoms attributable to ILD [25,26,29]. DLCO alone was also one of the most consistent predictors of mortality, a finding that may well help in the identification of patients with a poor prognosis, even if these preliminary findings should be confirmed and expanded by further rigorous studies [25–27]. The likelihood of progression, comorbidities, and toxicity risks and current data on efficacy are often the basis for decisions taken to initiate or advance treatment [30]. The goal of treating clinical SSc-ILD is the stabilization or prevention of progressive disease.

3. Treatment Options

The 2017 EULAR recommendations for the treatment of SSc state that the physician's assessment of symptoms, disease severity, and/or disease progression form the basis for decisions to initiate SSc-ILD treatment, with a tailored risk–benefit evaluation especially in progressive SSc-ILD patients [18]. There was also a recommendation for the use of CYC and hematopoietic stem-cell transplantation for SSc-ILD patients. After the release of this recommendations, evidences for a positive effect of mycophenolate mofetil (MMF) and nintedanib have also become available [17,20]. Several studies have also been reported that tocilizumab and rituximab might be able to slow down ILD progression [21]. A summary of the treatment options further discussed is presented in Table 1.

Table 1. Summary of current treatment options for systemic sclerosis related interstitial lung disease.

Drug	Study Designs	Pulmonary Parameters Tested
Cyclophosphamide [16,17,31–39]	RCT, OS	FVC, DLCO, ILD progression, HRCT disease extent, PROs
Mycophenolate Mofetil [17,33,40–42]	RCT, OS	FVC, DLCO, ILD progression, HRCT disease extent, PROs
Azathioprine [31,34–36]	RCT, CS/CR	FVC, DLCO, PROs
Autologous Haematopoietic Stem Cell Transplantation [38,39,43–47]	RCT, CS/CR	FVC, DLCO, Total Lung capacity, Vital Capacity, HRCT disease extent
Tocilizumab [48–51]	RCT, CS/CR	FVC, DLCO, HRCT disease extent, PROs
Rituximab [37,52–55]	RCT, OS, CS/CR	FVC, DLCO, PROs
Abatacept [51,56,57]	RCT, CS/CR	FVC, DLCO, PROs
Nintedanib [20,58,59]	RCT	FVC, DLCO, PROs
Pirfenidone [60–63]	RCT, CS/CR	FVC, DLCO, PROs

DLCO = diffusion lung capacity of carbone monoxyde; FVC = forced vital capacity; HRCT = high resolution computed tomography; ILD = interstitial lung disease; OS = observational study; PROs = patient reported outcomes; RCT = randomized clinical trial; CR/CS = case report/case series.

4. Conventional and Biologic Immunosuppressants

SSc is a connective tissue disease where inflammation and immune abnormalities play a central role [64–67]. The immune system, especially B and T lymphocytes, is involved in fibroblast activation and fibrogenesis as they secrete proinflammatory and profibrotic cytokines and growth factors [64–67]. That is why traditional immunosuppressant, e.g., CYC, MMF and azathioprine (AZA) have been so far considered the milestones of SSc-ILD treatment.

4.1. Cyclophosphamide

CYC is the most commonly used immunosuppressant, and it has been tested in numerous open-label studies, as well as in a few randomized control trials (RCT) [68]. CYC is recommended as first-line therapy in SSc–ILD patients in the EULAR guidelines [18].

In the Scleroderma Lung Study (SLS) I, 1-year course of oral CYC up to 2 mg/kg/day showed a statistically significant but small improvement in FVC (2.5% improvement) vs. placebo and little sustained benefit after discontinuation [16]. Similar results were not confirmed in the Fibrosing Alveolitis in Scleroderma Trial (FAST), which reported no statistically significant difference between the placebo and CYC group [31]. The clinical significance of this is modest, yet real improvement in FVC is still under debate and it seems that there will be decades of pros and cons. Noteworthy is the fact that the SLS I patients most likely had a stable SSc-ILD, as only 15% of them needed to restart an immunosuppressive treatment after the end of the study [16].

The SLS II (head-to-head comparison of oral CYC up to 2 mg/kg/day for 1 year plus 1 year of placebo versus MMF at up to 1.5 g twice daily for 2 years) showed that the benefits of MMF on FVC and on improvement in dyspnea were similar to those obtained with oral CYC at 2 years (MMF 2.2%, CYC 2.9%), with a safety profile favoring MMF [17].

In conclusion, it seems that CYC can either stabilize worsening SSc-ILD or modestly improve stable SSc-ILD; these data were also confirmed in a recent comparison between intravenous and oral CYC administration analyzing patients derived from the SLS1, SLS2, and EUSTAR cohorts. These results showed non-different effect on FVC change and ILD progression for the two routes of administration, despite a significantly lower CYC dosages in the intravenous group and a significantly different safety profile [32].

4.2. Mycophenolate Mofetil

MMF inhibits lymphocyte proliferation and is a safer, less toxic alternative to CYC for the treatment of SSc–ILD. Indeed, the safety and efficacy of MMF in SSc–ILD patients has been reported in several case series, uncontrolled studies, and, more recently, 2 meta-analyses [17,33,40,41]. Recently, the SLS II study, which reported on SSc–ILD patients treated with MMF for 2 years or CYC for 1 year followed by one year of placebo, showed that both treatment regimens led to a significant improvement in the pre-specified measurements of lung function over the 2-year study period. However, even if MMF was better tolerated and had lower toxicity levels, the hypothesis that it would be more efficacious at 24 months than CYC was not confirmed [17]. Although these data support the potential clinical efficacy of both CYC and MMF for progressive SSc–ILD, there is a possible preference for MMF due to its better tolerability and toxicity profile [17]. Lastly, Owen et al. demonstrated that MMF therapy was associated with a clinical stability for up to 36 months and lower frequency of early adverse events compared to AZA for SSc–ILD patients with a decline in pulmonary function [42].

4.3. Azathioprine

Although some small case series and retrospective studies suggested that AZA could be used as maintenance immunosuppressive treatment for SSc–ILD [34,35], a randomized unblinded clinical trial comparing the use of CYC and AZA (a purine analog) as first-line treatment did not evidence the efficacy of AZA in the treatment of SSc–ILD [36]. In addition, the very recent study by Owen et al. showed the better efficacy and tolerability of MMF versus AZA in the management of SSc–ILD [42].

4.4. Rituximab

A few case reports and open-label uncontrolled studies reported an improvement in SSc–ILD with RTX. Indeed, RTX therapy in SSc has gained favor after reports on its promising effects on both ILD and skin thickening [52,53,69]. The largest observational study available so far was published by the EUSTAR group and included 254 SSc patients treated with RTX, showing a good safety profile, steroid sparing agent potential and good efficacy profile on the skin but not on the lung. At pulmonary level, the combination of RTX + MMF determined a significant reduction in FVC decline over time, compared to monotherapy, therefore hypothesizing a higher promising potential for the combination treatment [54]. A similar safety profile and potential beneficial effect was also confirmed in an observational cohort receiving biosimilar RTX [55].

A recent open-label, randomized, controlled trial of head-to-head RTX vs. monthly pulse CYC reported on a population of 60 early, treatment naïve, anti-SCL-70+, dcSSc with ILD patients receiving either CYC or RTX. At the end of 6 months, the authors observed that FVC improved from 61.3% to 67.5% in the RTX group, whilst it did not in the CYC group (59.3% to 58.1%) [37]. The currently ongoing Rituximab versus Cyclophosphamide in Connective Tissue Disease-ILD (RECITAL) study (NCT01862926) is investigating the same topic in a larger cohort of connective tissue diseases related ILD, with a longer follow-up (48 weeks) [70].

4.5. Tocilizumab

The first two studies on TCZ, an anti-IL-6 soluble receptor monoclonal antibody, reported inconclusive results [48,49]. TCZ was administered in a phase 2 study (FaSScinate), and the data suggested this drug played a role in the IL-6 pathway in SSc–ILD and treatment of early SSc with elevated C-Reactive protein (CRP) and that it led to the stabilization of the FVC% in the tocilizumab group vs. a clinically meaningful decline in the placebo group over 48 weeks [48]. In this view, the phase 3 double-blind randomized placebo-controlled study (FocuSSced) of TCZ enrolled 210 early dcSSc patients. Similarly, a reduced FVC decline was seen in the TCZ group (difference between groups 4.2 (95% CI 2.0–6.4) favoring TCZ;

$p = 0.0002$), with a trend for a lower rate of patients requiring rescue immunosuppressive therapy for ILD indication ($p = 0.08$) [49].

Although the primary (skin) endpoint was not met, both trials showed some efficacy and a good safety profile for using TCZ in SSc and evidenced a potential benefit of treating subclinical ILD patients with high risk features (early dcSSc, and elevated CRP) [50].

4.6. Abatacept

Abatacept is a recombinant fusion protein that inhibits T cell activation. An observational study was carried out on 20 patients with SSc-associated polyarthritis and myopathy to evaluate the safety and efficacy of TCZ. However, despite having a good safety profile, there was no change in lung fibrosis in patients treated with abatacept [51]. A similar, more recent, observational experiment from the EUSTAR group, which included 27 SSc patients (15 with ILD), confirmed the good safety profile of the drug as well as a beneficial effect on joint and muscle disease. In addition, a possible positive effect was also seen for skin fibrosis (despite the lack of a control group), while no significant change in lung function was detected [56]. Finally, a recent phase II multicentre double-blind placebo-controlled trial of abatacept in early dcSSc showed a trend for a significant lower decline of FVC% predicted (mean difference 2.79, 95% CI −0,69–6,27, $p = 0{,}11$ favouring Abatacept), although the change in skin fibrosis as a primary endpoint was, again, not met [57]. Despite this, there is a promising potential for Abatacept in SSc, which could be investigated in a phase III study.

5. Other Treatment Options

5.1. Immunoglobulins

A randomized control trial assessing the change in skin fibrosis as primary endpoint failed to demonstrate a significant beneficial reduction of modified Rodnan skin score in Intravenous immunoglobulin (IVIg) administration versus placebo [71]. Different authors have shown the beneficial effect of the use of IVIg in SSc patients with arthritis [72] and inflammatory myopathy [73], and they have demonstrated some potential benefit on early-stage ILD, with the authors reporting a regression in ground glass opacity, septal thickening, and a full recovery of lung function [74]. A randomized phase II trial (NCT04137224) is currently testing a possible similar effect and the safety of subcutaneous immunoglobulins and IVIg [75].

5.2. Autologous Hematopoietic Stem Cell Transplant

Hematopoietic stem cell transplant (HSCT) is an emerging treatment option, aimed at regenerating the patient's immune system [43,76]. It is based on the use of high-intensity immunosuppression (conditioning regimen) aimed at a strong reduction/eradication of the "auto-reactive" immune system, followed by a re-population with antigen-naïve T cells previously isolated from the same individual [76]. It has been proposed for patients with dcSSc (with or without SSc-ILD) that is severe and refractory to standard therapy, who will probably benefit from the procedure but are more unlikely to develop post-transplant complications [44,77]. Indeed, improved survival compared to CYC has been reported by three trials, i.e., Autologous Stem Cell Systemic Sclerosis Immune Suppression Trial (ASSIST), Autologous Stem Cell Transplantation International Scleroderma trial for (ASTIS), and Scleroderma: Cyclophosphamide Or Transplantation trial (SCOT). Moreover, there was an improvement in skin thickening and FVC, as well as quality of life [38,39,45]. In addition to these results, an observational analysis of ILD extent in SSc patients receiving HSCT versus CYC was recently published, showing significant reduction in total ILD extent and, in particular, in the extent of ground glass opacifications, which were not seen in the CYC group [46]. With this promising background, a phase III randomized clinical trial (NCT044644) is currently testing upfront HSCT versus intravenous CYC induction followed by maintenance with MMF in early dcSSc, including pulmonary endpoints [78].

5.3. Lung Transplant

Lung Transplant is a life-saving option and remains a therapy for appropriately selected candidates with treatment-refractory lung disease [47,79]. An early referral should be made for advancing disease so as to provide these patients with a multi-disciplinary evaluation before transplant is considered an option. A few recent studies have demonstrated an increase in survival after lung transplantation [47,79].

5.4. Non-Pharmacologic Therapy

SSc-ILD should be managed by a multidisciplinary team [80]. Among non-pharmacologic options, pulmonary rehabilitation is aimed at improving lung function [81]; in particular, when an SSc-ILD patient is being considered for a transplant, pulmonary rehabilitation is a necessary step in their evaluation [81]. Furthermore, supplemental oxygen should be given whenever deemed necessary.

6. Anti-Fibrotic Therapies

Nintedanib is an intracellular tyrosine kinase inhibitor approved for the first time for the treatment of idiopathic pulmonary fibrosis (IPF) [82,83]. Its pharmacological effect covers numerous pathophysiological pathways, such as fibroblast activation, myofibroblast accumulation, and fibrogenic cytokine and growth factor expression. The increasing number of national and international authorities giving approval for treatment with the antifibrotic agent nintedanib to slow down the rate of decline of pulmonary function in SSc-ILD patients is opening up a new era [84]. The results of the recently published Safety and Efficacy of Nintedanib in Systemic Sclerosis (SENSCIS) trial supported the decision [20]. The SENSCIS trial, a double blind, randomized, placebo-controlled trial, evaluated the efficacy and safety of oral nintenadib (150 mg bid) treatment in patients with SSc-ILD for at least 52 weeks [20]. It reported that almost 50% of the subjects had dcSSc; a similar percentage was on a stable dose of MMF and HRCT evidenced fibrosis in at least 10% of the lungs (the latter as per study inclusion criteria). In this trial, patients with SSc-ILD treated with nintedanib showed a significantly lower rate of annual FVC decline than those receiving placebo, despite no significant improvement or benefit in any of the other organ manifestations. Although the change in FVC was small (absolute mean decline mean −52.4 mL per year in the nintedanib versus −93.3 mL per year in the placebo group), the mean decline reached a previously shown value of minimal clinically important difference (MCID) in the placebo group, but not in the nintedanib treated population [85]. This beneficial effect on FVC preservation was seen both in MMF and non-MMF co-treated patients, with a numerically lower decline in patients receiving the combination treatment [58]. In the SENSCIS study, Nintedanib showed a safety profile similar to the side effects seen in IPF, particularly affecting the gastrointestinal tract (75.7% of treated patients manifested diarrhea) and requiring dose-adjustment/temporary interruption in almost half of the treated patients [59]. Interestingly, the safety profile was similar in patients receiving or not receiving co-treatment with MMF, which itself carries a gastro-intestinal burden in terms of adverse events [58].

With a similar multi-target pathogenetic activity, pirfenidone (a pyridone showing both anti-inflammatory and anti-fibrotic effects) is another antifibrotic agents approved for the management of IPF patients [86]. The initial compassionate use in selected patients with SSc–ILD showed that the drug was well tolerated and, although it did not improve survival, it did stabilize the effects of progressive pulmonary fibrosis [60,61]. Recently, the Safety and Tolerability of Pirfenidone in Participants with Systemic Sclerosis-related Interstitial Lung Disease (LOTUSS) study, a phase II, open-label, randomized, 16-week study, assessed the safety and tolerability of pirfenidone in SSc–ILD patients. The drug was reported to have an acceptable tolerability profile that was not affected by concomitant treatment with MMF, although data as to its efficacy is not yet available [62]. Indeed, pirfenidone can be associated with adverse events of the gastrointestinal system and the skin in patients with IPF, two organs very frequently involved in SSc-ILD. Sometimes these adverse events can lead to drug discontinuation [63]. Given the promising effect in the stabilization of SSc-ILD, the drug is now tested versus placebo in SSc-ILD patients receiving MMF as a background immunosuppressive therapy in a placebo-controlled multi-center double blind randomized SLS study III [87].

7. Conclusions

Although ILD is a common finding in SSc, currently there is a paucity of detailed data to help in predicting which subsets of patients will or will not develop organ and potentially life-threatening disease. Despite this, the potential risk of morbidity and mortality supports the need for a thorough and early monitoring of the signs and symptoms of the development and progression of ILD.

At time of writing, the standard of care includes the use of CYC and MMF (which have only provided modest improvements in FVC) and Nintedanib (which is not available worldwide). Preliminary data on newer therapies, like biologics, stem cell transplant, and other anti-fibrotics suggest improved efficacy and safety profiles compared to those obtained with conventional immunosuppressive therapy.

Following the SLS II trial, a Delphi consensus treatment algorithm advocated MMF as first-line treatment of SSc-ILD and suggested that second-line treatment should include CYC or rituximab as an induction therapy, followed by MMF as a maintenance therapy [88].

A more recently published European consensus on SSc-ILD identification and management stressed the importance of different factors guiding treatment initiation, including speed of disease progression, survival rate, response rate after previous treatment, prolongation of time to progression, speed of improvement of patients' symptoms, safety and tolerability, scientific evidence of efficacy, and impact on quality of life [15].

In addition, disease severity and speed of progression could be the main drivers of treatment escalation [15]. Although consensus and recommendations are nowadays available, these do not fully cover the different clinical scenarios, in particular regarding time to initiation and a possibly more effective treatment protocol. In this context, SSc experts still relay on their clinical experience and take into account the different abovementioned factors to guide their decision in a patient-tailored, customized treatment regimen [89], possibly informed also by molecular biomarkers [90].

Although a substantial amount of evidences in SSc-ILD management resemble IPF, SSc-ILD is not IPF, as patients with SSc-ILD have a systemic disease. It has been hypothesized that future therapeutic options may be provided by targeting the self-perpetuating fibrosis [91], although whether an early (immunosuppressive) aggressive treatment will lead to a modification of disease progression and prevention of irreversible lung damage remains a question of debate. In this context, limiting fibrogenesis by the use of antifibrotic therapy and controlling inflammation/immunological abnormalities through immunosuppressants could well become the new paradigm of treatment in SSc-ILD. If available and well-tolerated, a combination regimen with immunosuppression and anti-fibrotic may allow a multi-target treatment and, potentially, a multiple organ/system benefit. Specifically, immunosuppression could also be personalized according to non-ILD organ complications such as cutaneous involvement, arthritis, myositis, and cardiomyopathy.

Clearly, there is a need for guidance in the new treatment regimens, in particular regarding the use of upfront or add-on combination treatment with immunosuppressants/antifibrotic, which could be the possible second/third level option in case of treatment failure. Hopefully, our understanding of the pathogenesis of SSc-ILD will evolve, along with the development of specific therapies for the organ systems affected by this disease, thus improving patients' survival, function, and quality of life [92,93].

Author Contributions: B.R. and M.M.-C. contributed to the study design; B.R., C.B., and M.C. contributed to manuscript drafting; F.S., M.S., G.M.C., E.B. and P.C. contributed to literature revision. All authors have critically revised the manuscript and approved the final version. All authors have read and agreed to the published version of the manuscript.

Funding: The authors received no financial support for the research, authorship, and/or publication of this article.

Acknowledgments: The authors would like to express their appreciation to Barbara Wade for her language assistance.

Conflicts of Interest: The authors declare that there is no conflict of interest.

References

1. Varga, J.; Trojanowska, M.; Kuwana, M. Pathogenesis of systemic sclerosis: Recent insights of molecular and cellular mechanisms and therapeutic opportunities. *J. Scleroderma Relat. Disord.* **2017**, *2*, 137–152. [CrossRef]
2. Ruaro, B.; Nallino, M.G.; Casabella, A.; Salton, F.; Confalonieri, P.; de Tanti, A.; Bruni, C. Monitoring the microcirculation in the diagnosis and follow-up of systemic sclerosis patients: Focus on pulmonary and peripheral vascular manifestations. *Microcirculation* **2020**, *27*, e12647. [CrossRef]
3. Nihtyanova, S.I.; Denton, C.P. Pathogenesis of systemic sclerosis associated interstitial lung disease. *J. Scleroderma Relat. Disord.* **2020**, *5*, 6–16. [CrossRef]
4. Bruni, C.; de Luca, G.; Lazzaroni, M.G.; Zanatta, E.; Lepri, G.; Airo, P.; Dagna, L.; Doria, A.; Matucci-Cerinic, M. Screening for pulmonary arterial hypertension in systemic sclerosis: A systematic literature review. *Eur. J. Intern. Med.* **2020**, *78*, 17–25. [CrossRef]
5. Occhipinti, M.; Bruni, C.; Camiciottoli, G.; Bartolucci, M.; Bellando-Randone, S.; Bassetto, A.; Cuomo, G.; Giuggioli, D.; Ciardi, G.; Fabbrizzi, A.; et al. Quantitative analysis of pulmonary vasculature in systemic sclerosis at spirometry-gated chest CT. *Ann. Rheum. Dis.* **2020**, *79*, 1210–1217. [CrossRef]
6. Walker, U.A.; Tyndall, A.; Czirjak, L.; Denton, C.; Farge-Bancel, D.; Kowal-Bielecka, O.; Muller-Ladner, U.; Bocelli-Tyndall, C.; Matucci-Cerinic, M. Clinical risk assessment of organ manifestations in systemic sclerosis: A report from the EULAR Scleroderma Trials And Research group database. *Ann. Rheum. Dis.* **2007**, *66*, 754–763. [CrossRef] [PubMed]
7. Volkmann, E.R.; Chung, A.; Tashkin, D.P. Managing Systemic Sclerosis-Related Interstitial Lung Disease in the Modern Treatment Era. *J. Scleroderma Relat. Disord.* **2017**, *2*, 72–83. [CrossRef]
8. Steen, V.D.; Conte, C.; Owens, G.R.; Medsger, T.A., Jr. Severe restrictive lung disease in systemic sclerosis. *Arthritis Rheumatol.* **1994**, *37*, 1283–1289. [CrossRef]
9. Elhai, M.; Meune, C.; Boubaya, M.; Avouac, J.; Hachulla, E.; Balbir-Gurman, A.; Riemekasten, G.; Airò, P.; Joven, B.; Vettori, S.; et al. Mapping and predicting mortality from systemic sclerosis. *Ann. Rheum. Dis.* **2017**, *76*, 1897–1905. [CrossRef] [PubMed]
10. Moore, D.F.; Steen, V.D. Overall mortality. *J. Scleroderma Relat. Disord.* **2020**, 2397198320924873. [CrossRef]
11. Bruni, C.; Guignabert, C.; Manetti, M.; Cerinic, M.M.; Humbert, M. The multifaceted problem of pulmonary arterial hypertension in systemic sclerosis. *Lancet Rheumatol.* **2020**, *3*, e149–e159. [CrossRef]
12. Volkmann, E.R.; Fischer, A. Update on morbidity and mortality in systemic sclerosis–related interstitial lung disease. *J. Scleroderma Relat. Disord.* **2020**. [CrossRef]
13. Bruni, C.; Cuomo, G.; Rossi, F.W.; Praino, E.; Bellando-Randone, S. Kidney involvement in systemic sclerosis: From pathogenesis to treatment. *J. Scleroderma Relat. Disord.* **2018**, *3*, 43–52. [CrossRef]
14. Bouros, D.; Wells, A.U.; Nicholson, A.G.; Colby, T.V.; Polychronopoulos, V.; Pantelidis, P.; Haslam, P.L.; Vassilakis, D.A.; Black, C.M.; du Bois, R.M. Histopathologic subsets of fibrosing alveolitis in patients with systemic sclerosis and their relationship to outcome. *Am. J. Respir. Crit. Care Med.* **2002**, *165*, 1581–1586. [CrossRef] [PubMed]
15. Hoffmann-Vold, A.-M.; Maher, T.M.; Philpot, E.E.; Ashrafzadeh, A.; Barake, R.; Barsotti, S.; Bruni, C.; Carducci, P.; Carreira, P.E.; Castellví, I.; et al. The identification and management of interstitial lung disease in systemic sclerosis: Evidence-based European consensus statements. *Lancet Rheumatol.* **2020**, *2*, e71–e83. [CrossRef]
16. Tashkin, D.P.; Elashoff, R.; Clements, P.J.; Goldin, J.; Roth, M.D.; Furst, D.E.; Arriola, E.; Silver, R.; Strange, C.; Bolster, M.; et al. Cyclophosphamide versus placebo in scleroderma lung disease. *N. Engl. J. Med.* **2006**, *354*, 2655–2666. [CrossRef]
17. Tashkin, D.P.; Roth, M.D.; Clements, P.J.; Furst, D.E.; Khanna, D.; Kleerup, E.C.; Goldin, J.; Arriola, E.; Volkmann, E.R.; Kafaja, S.; et al. Mycophenolate mofetil versus oral cyclophosphamide in scleroderma-related interstitial lung disease (SLS II): A randomised controlled, double-blind, parallel group trial. *Lancet Respir. Med.* **2016**, *4*, 708–719. [CrossRef]
18. Kowal-Bielecka, O.; Fransen, J.; Avouac, J.; Becker, M.; Kulak, A.; Allanore, Y.; Distler, O.; Clements, P.; Cutolo, M.; Czirjak, L.; et al. Update of EULAR recommendations for the treatment of systemic sclerosis. *Ann. Rheum. Dis.* **2017**, *76*, 1327–1339. [CrossRef] [PubMed]
19. Kuwana, M.; Distler, O. Recent progress and missing gaps to achieve goal in the care of systemic sclerosis–associated interstitial lung disease. *J. Scleroderma Relat. Disord.* **2020**, *5*, 3–5. [CrossRef]
20. Distler, O.; Highland, K.B.; Gahlemann, M.; Azuma, A.; Fischer, A.; Mayes, M.D.; Raghu, G.; Sauter, W.; Girard, M.; Alves, M.; et al. Nintedanib for Systemic Sclerosis-Associated Interstitial Lung Disease. *N. Engl. J. Med.* **2019**, *380*, 2518–2528. [CrossRef]
21. Bruni, C.; Praino, E.; Allanore, Y.; Distler, O.; Gabrielli, A.; Iannone, F.; Matucci-Cerinic, M. Use of biologics and other novel therapies for the treatment of systemic sclerosis. *Expert Rev. Clin. Immunol.* **2017**, *13*, 469–482. [CrossRef] [PubMed]

22. Barskova, T.; Gargani, L.; Guiducci, S.; Randone, S.B.; Bruni, C.; Carnesecchi, G.; Conforti, M.L.; Porta, F.; Pignone, A.; Caramella, D.; et al. Lung ultrasound for the screening of interstitial lung disease in very early systemic sclerosis. *Ann. Rheum. Dis.* **2013**, *72*, 390–395. [CrossRef]
23. Bernstein, E.J.; Khanna, D.; Lederer, D.J. Screening High-Resolution Computed Tomography of the Chest to Detect Interstitial Lung Disease in Systemic Sclerosis: A Global Survey of Rheumatologists. *Arthritis Rheumatol.* **2013**, *70*, 971–972. [CrossRef] [PubMed]
24. Suliman, Y.A.; Dobrota, R.; Huscher, D.; Nguyen-Kim, T.D.; Maurer, B.; Jordan, S.; Speich, R.; Frauenfelder, T.; Distler, O. Brief Report: Pulmonary Function Tests: High Rate of False-Negative Results in the Early Detection and Screening of Scleroderma-Related Interstitial Lung Disease. *Arthritis Rheumatol.* **2015**, *67*, 3256–3261. [CrossRef] [PubMed]
25. Volkmann, E.R.; Tashkin, D.P.; Sim, M.; Kim, G.H.; Goldin, J.; Clements, P.J. Determining progression of scleroderma-related interstitial lung disease. *J. Scleroderma Relat. Disord.* **2019**, *4*, 62–70. [CrossRef]
26. Distler, O.; Assassi, S.; Cottin, V.; Cutolo, M.; Danoff, S.K.; Denton, C.P.; Distler, J.H.W.; Hoffmann-Vold, A.M.; Johnson, S.R.; Muller Ladner, U.; et al. Predictors of progression in systemic sclerosis patients with interstitial lung disease. *Eur. Respir. J.* **2020**, *55*, 1902026. [CrossRef]
27. Winstone, T.A.; Assayag, D.; Wilcox, P.G.; Dunne, J.V.; Hague, C.J.; Leipsic, J.; Collard, H.R.; Ryerson, C.J. Predictors of mortality and progression in scleroderma-associated interstitial lung disease: A systematic review. *Chest* **2014**, *146*, 422–436. [CrossRef]
28. Goh, N.S.; Hoyles, R.K.; Denton, C.P.; Hansell, D.M.; Renzoni, E.A.; Maher, T.M.; Nicholson, A.G.; Wells, A.U. Short-Term Pulmonary Function Trends Are Predictive of Mortality in Interstitial Lung Disease Associated With Systemic Sclerosis. *Arthritis Rheumatol.* **2017**, *69*, 1670–1678. [CrossRef]
29. Caron, M.; Hoa, S.; Hudson, M.; Schwartzman, K.; Steele, R. Pulmonary function tests as outcomes for systemic sclerosis interstitial lung disease. *Eur. Respir. Rev.* **2018**, *27*, 170102. [CrossRef]
30. Bruni, C.; Furst, D.E. The burning question: To use or not to use cyclophosphamide in systemic sclerosis. *Eur. J. Rheumatol.* **2020**, *7*, S237–S241. [CrossRef]
31. Hoyles, R.K.; Ellis, R.W.; Wellsbury, J.; Lees, B.; Newlands, P.; Goh, N.S.; Roberts, C.; Desai, S.; Herrick, A.L.; McHugh, N.J.; et al. A multicenter, prospective, randomized, double-blind, placebo-controlled trial of corticosteroids and intravenous cyclophosphamide followed by oral azathioprine for the treatment of pulmonary fibrosis in scleroderma. *Arthritis Rheumatol.* **2006**, *54*, 3962–3970. [CrossRef]
32. Bruni, C.; Tashkin, D.P.; Steen, V.; Allanore, Y.; Distler, O.; Grotts, J.; Matucci-Cerinic, M.; Furst, D.E.; Eustar, S.I.; collaborators, S.I.c. Intravenous versus oral cyclophosphamide for lung and/or skin fibrosis in systemic sclerosis: An indirect comparison from EUSTAR and randomised controlled trials. *Clin. Exp. Rheumatol.* **2020**, *38* (Suppl. 125), 161–168. [PubMed]
33. Panopoulos, S.T.; Bournia, V.K.; Trakada, G.; Giavri, I.; Kostopoulos, C.; Sfikakis, P.P. Mycophenolate versus cyclophosphamide for progressive interstitial lung disease associated with systemic sclerosis: A 2-year case control study. *Lung* **2013**, *191*, 483–489. [CrossRef] [PubMed]
34. Paone, C.; Chiarolanza, I.; Cuomo, G.; Ruocco, L.; Vettori, S.; Menegozzo, M.; La Montagna, G.; Valentini, G. Twelve-month azathioprine as maintenance therapy in early diffuse systemic sclerosis patients treated for 1-year with low dose cyclophosphamide pulse therapy. *Clin. Exp. Rheumatol.* **2007**, *25*, 613–616. [PubMed]
35. Berezne, A.; Ranque, B.; Valeyre, D.; Brauner, M.; Allanore, Y.; Launay, D.; Le Guern, V.; Kahn, J.E.; Couderc, L.J.; Constans, J.; et al. Therapeutic strategy combining intravenous cyclophosphamide followed by oral azathioprine to treat worsening interstitial lung disease associated with systemic sclerosis: A retrospective multicenter open-label study. *J. Rheumatol.* **2008**, *35*, 1064–1072.
36. Nadashkevich, O.; Davis, P.; Fritzler, M.; Kovalenko, W. A randomized unblinded trial of cyclophosphamide versus azathioprine in the treatment of systemic sclerosis. *Clin. Rheumatol.* **2006**, *25*, 205–212. [CrossRef]
37. Sircar, G.; Goswami, R.P.; Sircar, D.; Ghosh, A.; Ghosh, P. Intravenous cyclophosphamide vs rituximab for the treatment of early diffuse scleroderma lung disease: Open label, randomized, controlled trial. *Rheumatology* **2018**, *57*, 2106–2113. [CrossRef]
38. van Laar, J.M.; Farge, D.; Sont, J.K.; Naraghi, K.; Marjanovic, Z.; Larghero, J.; Schuerwegh, A.J.; Marijt, E.W.; Vonk, M.C.; Schattenberg, A.V.; et al. Autologous hematopoietic stem cell transplantation vs intravenous pulse cyclophosphamide in diffuse cutaneous systemic sclerosis: A randomized clinical trial. *JAMA* **2014**, *311*, 2490–2498. [CrossRef]
39. Burt, R.K.; Shah, S.J.; Dill, K.; Grant, T.; Gheorghiade, M.; Schroeder, J.; Craig, R.; Hirano, I.; Marshall, K.; Ruderman, E.; et al. Autologous non-myeloablative haemopoietic stem-cell transplantation compared with pulse cyclophosphamide once per month for systemic sclerosis (ASSIST): An open-label, randomised phase 2 trial. *Lancet* **2011**, *378*, 498–506. [CrossRef]
40. Yilmaz, N.; Can, M.; Kocakaya, D.; Karakurt, S.; Yavuz, S. Two-year experience with mycophenolate mofetil in patients with scleroderma lung disease: A case series. *Int. J. Rheum. Dis.* **2014**, *17*, 923–928. [CrossRef]
41. Omair, M.A.; Alahmadi, A.; Johnson, S.R. Safety and effectiveness of mycophenolate in systemic sclerosis. A systematic review. *PLoS ONE* **2015**, *10*, e0124205. [CrossRef] [PubMed]
42. Owen, C.; Ngian, G.S.; Elford, K.; Moore, O.; Stevens, W.; Nikpour, M.; Rabusa, C.; Proudman, S.; Roddy, J.; Zochling, J.; et al. Mycophenolate mofetil is an effective and safe option for the management of systemic sclerosis-associated interstitial lung disease: Results from the Australian Scleroderma Cohort Study. *Clin. Exp. Rheumatol.* **2016**, *34* (Suppl. 100), 170–176. [PubMed]
43. Spierings, J.; de Bresser, C.J.; van Rhijn-Brouwer, F.C.; Pieterse, A.; Vonk, M.C.; Voskuyl, A.E.; de Vries-Bouwstra, J.K.; van Laar, J.M.; Kars, M.C. From "being at war" to "getting back on your feet": A qualitative study on experiences of patients with systemic sclerosis treated with hematopoietic stem cell transplantation. *J. Scleroderma Relat. Disord.* **2020**, *5*, 202–209. [CrossRef]

44. Shah, A.; Spierings, J.; van Laar, J.; Sullivan, K.M. Re-evaluating inclusion criteria for autologous hematopoietic stem cell transplantation in advanced systemic sclerosis: Three successful cases and review of the literature. *J. Scleroderma Relat. Disord.* **2021**, 2397198320985766. [CrossRef]
45. Sullivan, K.M.; Goldmuntz, E.A.; Keyes-Elstein, L.; McSweeney, P.A.; Pinckney, A.; Welch, B.; Mayes, M.D.; Nash, R.A.; Crofford, L.J.; Eggleston, B.; et al. Myeloablative Autologous Stem-Cell Transplantation for Severe Scleroderma. *N. Engl. J. Med.* **2018**, *378*, 35–47. [CrossRef] [PubMed]
46. Ciaffi, J.; van Leeuwen, N.M.; Boonstra, M.; Kroft, L.J.M.; Schouffoer, A.A.; Ninaber, M.K.; Huizinga, T.W.J.; de Vries-Bouwstra, J.K. Evolution of interstitial lung disease one year after hematopoietic stem cell transplantation or cyclophosphamide for systemic sclerosis. *Arthritis Care Res.* **2020**, 24451. [CrossRef]
47. Bernstein, E.J.; Peterson, E.R.; Sell, J.L.; D'Ovidio, F.; Arcasoy, S.M.; Bathon, J.M.; Lederer, D.J. Survival of adults with systemic sclerosis following lung transplantation: A nationwide cohort study. *Arthritis Rheumatol.* **2015**, *67*, 1314–1322. [CrossRef]
48. Khanna, D.; Denton, C.P.; Jahreis, A.; van Laar, J.M.; Frech, T.M.; Anderson, M.E.; Baron, M.; Chung, L.; Fierlbeck, G.; Lakshminarayanan, S.; et al. Safety and efficacy of subcutaneous tocilizumab in adults with systemic sclerosis (faSScinate): A phase 2, randomised, controlled trial. *Lancet* **2016**, *387*, 2630–2640. [CrossRef]
49. Khanna, D.; Lin, C.J.F.; Furst, D.E.; Goldin, J.; Kim, G.; Kuwana, M.; Allanore, Y.; Matucci-Cerinic, M.; Distler, O.; Shima, Y.; et al. Tocilizumab in systemic sclerosis: A randomised, double-blind, placebo-controlled, phase 3 trial. *Lancet Respir. Med.* **2020**, *8*, 963–974. [CrossRef]
50. Khanna, D.; Jahreis, A.; Furst, D.E. Tocilizumab Treatment of Patients with Systemic Sclerosis: Clinical Data. *J. Scleroderma Relat. Disord.* **2017**, *2*, S29–S35. [CrossRef]
51. Elhai, M.; Meunier, M.; Matucci-Cerinic, M.; Maurer, B.; Riemekasten, G.; Leturcq, T.; Pellerito, R.; von Muhlen, C.A.; Vacca, A.; Airo, P.; et al. Outcomes of patients with systemic sclerosis-associated polyarthritis and myopathy treated with tocilizumab or abatacept: A EUSTAR observational study. *Ann. Rheum. Dis.* **2013**, *72*, 1217–1220. [CrossRef]
52. Yoo, W.H. Successful treatment of steroid and cyclophosphamide-resistant diffuse scleroderma-associated interstitial lung disease with rituximab. *Rheumatol. Int.* **2012**, *32*, 795–798. [CrossRef]
53. Jordan, S.; Distler, J.H.; Maurer, B.; Huscher, D.; van Laar, J.M.; Allanore, Y.; Distler, O.; on behalf of the EUSTAR Rituximab study group. Effects and safety of rituximab in systemic sclerosis: An analysis from the European Scleroderma Trial and Research (EUSTAR) group. *Ann. Rheum. Dis.* **2015**, *74*, 1188–1194. [CrossRef] [PubMed]
54. Elhai, M.; Boubaya, M.; Distler, O.; Smith, V.; Matucci-Cerinic, M.; Alegre Sancho, J.J.; Truchetet, M.E.; Braun-Moscovici, Y.; Iannone, F.; Novikov, P.I.; et al. Outcomes of patients with systemic sclerosis treated with rituximab in contemporary practice: A prospective cohort study. *Ann. Rheum. Dis.* **2019**, *78*, 979–987. [CrossRef] [PubMed]
55. Campochiaro, C.; de Luca, G.; Lazzaroni, M.G.; Zanatta, E.; Bosello, S.L.; de Santis, M.; Cariddi, A.; Bruni, C.; Selmi, C.; Gremese, E.; et al. Safety and efficacy of rituximab biosimilar (CT-P10) in systemic sclerosis: An Italian multicentre study. *Rheumatology* **2020**, *59*, 3731–3736. [CrossRef] [PubMed]
56. Castellvi, I.; Elhai, M.; Bruni, C.; Airo, P.; Jordan, S.; Beretta, L.; Codullo, V.; Montecucco, C.M.; Bokarewa, M.; Iannonne, F.; et al. Safety and effectiveness of abatacept in systemic sclerosis: The EUSTAR experience. *Semin. Arthritis Rheum.* **2020**, *50*, 1489–1493. [CrossRef]
57. Khanna, D.; Spino, C.; Johnson, S.; Chung, L.; Whitfield, M.L.; Denton, C.P.; Berrocal, V.; Franks, J.; Mehta, B.; Molitor, J.; et al. Abatacept in Early Diffuse Cutaneous Systemic Sclerosis: Results of a Phase II Investigator-Initiated, Multicenter, Double-Blind, Randomized, Placebo-Controlled Trial. *Arthritis Rheumatol.* **2020**, *72*, 125–136. [CrossRef]
58. Highland, K.B.; Distler, O.; Kuwana, M.; Allanore, Y.; Assassi, S.; Azuma, A.; Bourdin, A.; Denton, C.P.; Distler, J.H.W.; Hoffmann-Vold, A.M.; et al. Efficacy and safety of nintedanib in patients with systemic sclerosis-associated interstitial lung disease treated with mycophenolate: A subgroup analysis of the SENSCIS trial. *Lancet Respir. Med.* **2021**, *9*, 96–106. [CrossRef]
59. Seibold, J.R.; Maher, T.M.; Highland, K.B.; Assassi, S.; Azuma, A.; Hummers, L.K.; Costabel, U.; von Wangenheim, U.; Kohlbrenner, V.; Gahlemann, M.; et al. Safety and tolerability of nintedanib in patients with systemic sclerosis-associated interstitial lung disease: Data from the SENSCIS trial. *Ann. Rheum. Dis.* **2020**, *79*, 1478–1484. [CrossRef]
60. Nagai, S.; Hamada, K.; Shigematsu, M.; Taniyama, M.; Yamauchi, S.; Izumi, T. Open-label compassionate use one year-treatment with pirfenidone to patients with chronic pulmonary fibrosis. *Intern. Med.* **2002**, *41*, 1118–1123. [CrossRef] [PubMed]
61. Udwadia, Z.F.; Mullerpattan, J.B.; Balakrishnan, C.; Richeldi, L. Improved pulmonary function following pirfenidone treatment in a patient with progressive interstitial lung disease associated with systemic sclerosis. *Lung India* **2015**, *32*, 50–52. [CrossRef] [PubMed]
62. Khanna, D.; Albera, C.; Fischer, A.; Khalidi, N.; Raghu, G.; Chung, L.; Chen, D.; Schiopu, E.; Tagliaferri, M.; Seibold, J.R.; et al. An Open-label, Phase II Study of the Safety and Tolerability of Pirfenidone in Patients with Scleroderma-associated Interstitial Lung Disease: The LOTUSS Trial. *J. Rheumatol.* **2016**, *43*, 1672–1679. [CrossRef] [PubMed]
63. Miura, Y.; Saito, T.; Fujita, K.; Tsunoda, Y.; Tanaka, T.; Takoi, H.; Yatagai, Y.; Rin, S.; Sekine, A.; Hayashihara, K.; et al. Clinical experience with pirfenidone in five patients with scleroderma-related interstitial lung disease. *Sarcoidosis Vasc. Diffus. Lung Dis.* **2014**, *31*, 235–238.
64. Ruaro, B.; Soldano, S.; Smith, V.; Paolino, S.; Contini, P.; Montagna, P.; Pizzorni, C.; Casabella, A.; Tardito, S.; Sulli, A.; et al. Correlation between circulating fibrocytes and dermal thickness in limited cutaneous systemic sclerosis patients: A pilot study. *Rheumatol. Int.* **2019**, *39*, 1369–1376. [CrossRef] [PubMed]

65. Trombetta, A.C.; Soldano, S.; Contini, P.; Tomatis, V.; Ruaro, B.; Paolino, S.; Brizzolara, R.; Montagna, P.; Sulli, A.; Pizzorni, C.; et al. A circulating cell population showing both M1 and M2 monocyte/macrophage surface markers characterizes systemic sclerosis patients with lung involvement. *Respir. Res.* **2018**, *19*, 186. [CrossRef]
66. Bruni, C.; Frech, T.; Manetti, M.; Rossi, F.W.; Furst, D.E.; de Paulis, A.; Rivellese, F.; Guiducci, S.; Matucci-Cerinic, M.; Bellando-Randone, S. Vascular Leaking, a Pivotal and Early Pathogenetic Event in Systemic Sclerosis: Should the Door Be Closed? *Front. Immunol.* **2018**, *9*, 2045. [CrossRef]
67. O'Reilly, S.; Hügle, T.; van Laar, J.M. T cells in systemic sclerosis: A reappraisal. *Rheumatology* **2012**, *51*, 1540–1549. [CrossRef]
68. Bruni, C.; Shirai, Y.; Kuwana, M.; Matucci-Cerinic, M. Cyclophosphamide: Similarities and differences in the treatment of SSc and SLE. *Lupus* **2019**, *28*, 571–574. [CrossRef]
69. Bosello, S.L.; de Luca, G.; Rucco, M.; Berardi, G.; Falcione, M.; Danza, F.M.; Pirronti, T.; Ferraccioli, G. Long-term efficacy of B cell depletion therapy on lung and skin involvement in diffuse systemic sclerosis. *Semin. Arthritis Rheum.* **2015**, *44*, 428–436. [CrossRef]
70. Rituximab Versus Cyclophosphamide in Connective Tissue Disease-ILD (RECITAL). Available online: https://clinicaltrials.gov/ct2/show/record/NCT01862926?term=RECITAL&draw=2&rank=2 (accessed on 18 January 2021).
71. Takehara, K.; Ihn, H.; Sato, S. A randomized, double-blind, placebo-controlled trial: Intravenous immunoglobulin treatment in patients with diffuse cutaneous systemic sclerosis. *Clin. Exp. Rheumatol.* **2013**, *31*, 151–156.
72. Nacci, F.; Righi, A.; Conforti, M.L.; Miniati, I.; Fiori, G.; Martinovic, D.; Melchiorre, D.; Sapir, T.; Blank, M.; Shoenfeld, Y.; et al. Intravenous immunoglobulins improve the function and ameliorate joint involvement in systemic sclerosis: A pilot study. *Ann. Rheum. Dis.* **2007**, *66*, 977–979. [CrossRef]
73. Chaigne, B.; Rodeia, S.; Benmostefa, N.; Berezne, A.; Authier, J.; Cohen, P.; Regent, A.; Terrier, B.; Costedoat-Chalumeau, N.; Guillevin, L.; et al. Corticosteroid-sparing benefit of intravenous immunoglobulin in systemic sclerosis-associated myopathy: A comparative study in 52 patients. *Autoimmun. Rev.* **2020**, *19*, 102431. [CrossRef]
74. Mauhin, W.; Riviere, S.; Cabane, J.; Tiev, K.P. Improvement in lung fibrosis using intravenous immunoglobulin in systemic sclerosis with myositis. *Scand. J. Rheumatol.* **2014**, *43*, 170–171. [CrossRef]
75. Safety and Pharmacokinetics of IgPro20 and IgPro10 in Adults With Systemic Sclerosis (SSc). Available online: https://clinicaltrials.gov/ct2/show/NCT04137224 (accessed on 18 January 2021).
76. Burt, R.K.; Kallunian, K.; Patel, D.; Thomas, J.; Yeager, A.; Traynor, A.; Heipe, F.; Arnold, R.; Marmont, A.; Collier, D.; et al. The rationale behind autologous autoimmune hematopoietic stem cell transplant conditioning regimens: Concerns over the use of total-body irradiation in systemic sclerosis. *Bone Marrow Transplant.* **2004**, *34*, 745–751. [CrossRef]
77. AlOdhaibi, K.A.; Varga, J.; Furst, D.E. Hematopoietic stem cell transplantation in systemic sclerosis: Yes!! BUT. *J. Scleroderma Relat. Disord.* **2020**, 2397198320971967. [CrossRef]
78. Upfront Autologous HSCT Versus Immunosuppression in Early Diffuse Cutaneous Systemic Sclerosis (UPSIDE). Available online: https://clinicaltrials.gov/ct2/show/record/NCT04464434?term=stem+cell&recrs=abd&ccnd=systemic+sclerosis+OR+scleroderma&draw=2&rank=6 (accessed on 18 January 2021).
79. Miele, C.H.; Schwab, K.; Saggar, R.; Duffy, E.; Elashoff, D.; Tseng, C.H.; Weigt, S.; Charan, D.; Abtin, F.; Johannes, J.; et al. Lung Transplant Outcomes in Systemic Sclerosis with Significant Esophageal Dysfunction. A Comprehensive Single-Center Experience. *Ann. Am. Thorac. Soc.* **2016**, *13*, 793–802. [CrossRef]
80. Hoffmann-Vold, A.M.; Allanore, Y.; Bendstrup, E.; Bruni, C.; Distler, O.; Maher, T.M.; Wijsenbeek, M.; Kreuter, M. The need for a holistic approach for SSc-ILD—Achievements and ambiguity in a devastating disease. *Respir. Res.* **2020**, *21*, 197. [CrossRef]
81. Dowman, L.M.; McDonald, C.F.; Hill, C.J.; Lee, A.L.; Barker, K.; Boote, C.; Glaspole, I.; Goh, N.S.L.; Southcott, A.M.; Burge, A.T.; et al. The evidence of benefits of exercise training in interstitial lung disease: A randomised controlled trial. *Thorax* **2017**, *72*, 610–619. [CrossRef]
82. Wollin, L.; Wex, E.; Pautsch, A.; Schnapp, G.; Hostettler, K.E.; Stowasser, S.; Kolb, M. Mode of action of nintedanib in the treatment of idiopathic pulmonary fibrosis. *Eur. Respir. J.* **2015**, *45*, 1434–1445. [CrossRef]
83. Richeldi, L.; Cottin, V.; du Bois, R.M.; Selman, M.; Kimura, T.; Bailes, Z.; Schlenker-Herceg, R.; Stowasser, S.; Brown, K.K. Nintedanib in patients with idiopathic pulmonary fibrosis: Combined evidence from the TOMORROW and INPULSIS((R)) trials. *Respir. Med.* **2016**, *113*, 74–79. [CrossRef]
84. Wollin, L.; Distler, J.H.; Denton, C.P.; Gahlemann, M. Rationale for the evaluation of nintedanib as a treatment for systemic sclerosis–associated interstitial lung disease. *J. Scleroderma Relat. Disord.* **2019**, *4*, 212–218. [CrossRef]
85. Kafaja, S.; Clements, P.J.; Wilhalme, H.; Tseng, C.H.; Furst, D.E.; Kim, G.H.; Goldin, J.; Volkmann, E.R.; Roth, M.D.; Tashkin, D.P.; et al. Reliability and minimal clinically important differences of forced vital capacity: Results from the Scleroderma Lung Studies (SLS-I and SLS-II). *Am. J. Respir. Crit. Care Med.* **2018**, *197*, 644–652. [CrossRef]
86. King, T.E., Jr.; Bradford, W.Z.; Castro-Bernardini, S.; Fagan, E.A.; Glaspole, I.; Glassberg, M.K.; Gorina, E.; Hopkins, P.M.; Kardatzke, D.; Lancaster, L.; et al. A phase 3 trial of pirfenidone in patients with idiopathic pulmonary fibrosis. *N. Engl. J. Med.* **2014**, *370*, 2083–2092. [CrossRef]
87. Scleroderma Lung Study III-Combining Pirfenidone With Mycophenolate (SLSIII). Available online: https://clinicaltrials.gov/ct2/show/NCT03221257?term=pirfenidone&cond=Systemic+Sclerosis&draw=2&rank=4 (accessed on 18 January 2021).
88. Fernández-Codina, A.; Walker, K.M.; Pope, J.E. Treatment Algorithms for Systemic Sclerosis According to Experts. *Arthritis Rheumatol.* **2018**, *70*, 1820–1828. [CrossRef] [PubMed]

89. Lepri, G.; Hughes, M.; Bruni, C.; Cerinic, M.M.; Randone, S.B. Recent advances steer the future of systemic sclerosis toward precision medicine. *Clin. Rheumatol.* **2020**, *39*, 1–4. [CrossRef]
90. Hoffmann-Vold, A.-M.; Fretheim, H.; Meier, C.; Maurer, B. Circulating biomarkers of systemic sclerosis—Interstitial lung disease. *J. Scleroderma Relat. Disord.* **2020**, *5*, 41–47. [CrossRef]
91. Roofeh, D.; Distler, O.; Allanore, Y.; Denton, C.P.; Khanna, D. Treatment of systemic sclerosis–associated interstitial lung disease: Lessons from clinical trials. *J. Scleroderma Relat. Disord.* **2020**, *5*, 61–71. [CrossRef]
92. Saketkoo, L.A.; Scholand, M.B.; Lammi, M.R.; Russell, A.-M. Patient-reported outcome measures in systemic sclerosis–related interstitial lung disease for clinical practice and clinical trials. *J. Scleroderma Relat. Disord.* **2020**, *5*, 48–60. [CrossRef] [PubMed]
93. Hinchcliff, M.; O'Reilly, S. Current and Potential New Targets in Systemic Sclerosis Therapy: A New Hope. *Curr. Rheumatol. Rep.* **2020**, *22*, 42. [CrossRef]

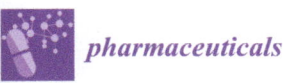

Review

Pharmacological Interactions of Nintedanib and Pirfenidone in Patients with Idiopathic Pulmonary Fibrosis in Times of COVID-19 Pandemic

José M. Serra López-Matencio [1], Manuel Gómez [2], Esther F. Vicente-Rabaneda [3], Miguel A. González-Gay [4], Julio Ancochea [5,6] and Santos Castañeda [3,6,*]

1. Hospital Pharmacy Service, Princesa Hospital, IIS-Princesa, c/Diego de León 62, 28006 Madrid, Spain; josemaria.serra@salud.madrid.org
2. Methodology Unit, Health Research Institute Princesa (IIS-IP), c/Diego de León 62, 28006 Madrid, Spain; mgomezgutierrez@salud.madrid.org
3. Rheumatology Service, Princesa Hospital, IIS-Princesa, c/Diego de León 62, 28006 Madrid, Spain; efvicenter@gmail.com
4. Rheumatology Service, Marqués de Valdecilla University Hospital, University of Cantabria, Av. de Valdecilla 25, 39008 Santander, Spain; miguelaggay@hotmail.com
5. Pneumology Service, Princesa Hospital, Autonomous University of Madrid (UAM), IIS-Princesa, c/Diego de León 62, 28006 Madrid, Spain; j.ancochea@separ.es
6. Department of Medicine, Autonomous University of Madrid (UAM), 28029 Madrid, Spain
* Correspondence: scastas@gmail.com or santos.castaneda@salud.madrid.org; Tel.: +34-915-202-473; Fax: +34-914-018-752

Abstract: The discovery of antifibrotic agents have resulted in advances in the therapeutic management of idiopathic pulmonary fibrosis (IPF). Currently, nintedanib and pirfenidone have become the basis of IPF therapy based on the results of large randomized clinical trials showing their safety and efficacy in reducing disease advancement. However, the goal of completely halting disease progress has not been reached yet. Administering nintedanib with add-on pirfenidone is supposed to enhance the therapeutic benefit by simultaneously acting on two different pathogenic pathways. All this becomes more important in the context of the ongoing global pandemic of coronavirus disease 2019 (COVID-19) because of the fibrotic consequences following SARS-CoV-2 infection in some patients. However, little information is available about their drug–drug interaction, which is important mainly in polymedicated patients. The aim of this review is to describe the current management of progressive fibrosing interstitial lung diseases (PF-ILDs) in general and of IPF in particular, focusing on the pharmacokinetic drug-drug interactions between these two drugs and their relationship with other medications in patients with IPF.

Keywords: antifibrotic agents; COVID-19; interstitial lung disease; IPF; progressive fibrosing ILD; UIP; pharmacological interactions

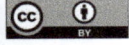

1. Background

Interstitial lung diseases (ILD) are a heterogeneous group of pulmonary disorders characterized by varying degrees of inflammation and fibrosis resulting in the loss of alveolar function and impairment of gas exchange [1]. Idiopathic pulmonary fibrosis (IPF) is an entity that is included in the group of interstitial lung diseases of unknown etiology, being a severe form of pulmonary fibrosis that is associated with high morbidity and mortality [1–3].

IPF has a variable incidence depending on the population under study. Thus, in the United Kingdom, IPF has an incidence of around 7.44 cases per 100,000 inhabitants, while in the United States some series show an incidence of 16.3 cases per 100,000 inhabitants or even 93.7 cases per 100,000 people as described in a systematic review conducted by Hutchinson [4] covering the decade from 2001 to 2011. Overall, it is estimated that the worldwide prevalence may be close to 60 cases per 100,000 inhabitants. This entity predominantly affects males over 65 years of age [2–4].

Since its appearance, the coronavirus disease 2019 (COVID-19) pandemic has affected millions of people worldwide causing more than three million deaths. The available data indicate that a significant percentage of individuals suffering from severe acute respiratory syndrome caused by severe acute respiratory syndrome coronavirus-2 (SARS-CoV-2) develop acute lung injury/acute respiratory distress syndromes (ALI/ARDS), which can become severe. Pulmonary fibrosis is a recognized sequel of ARDS. Currently, there is evidence of fibrotic changes in radiographic images of patients recovered from COVID-19 [5–7].

Although IPF is the most widely studied and most common fibrosing ILD, there are also other progressive fibrosing (PF)-ILDs such as certain connective tissue disease-associated ILDs, which evolve towards pulmonary fibrosis and present a similar behavior to IPF, characterized by worsening of respiratory symptoms, decline in lung function and early mortality despite standard of care treatment [1–3]. In the same line, the PROGRESS study showed data on patients with other chronic PF-ILDs who were admitted to a hospital in Lyon, France, between 2010 and 2017. This study showed that those patients who had a loss of a quarter of their lung function or a loss of forced vital capacity (FVC) $\geq$ 10%, had 3 year survival rates of 83% and 5 year survival rates of 72%. In addition, some factors were shown to be associated with worse evolution, such as age > 70 years; FVC < 70% and/or diffusing capacity of the lungs for carbon monoxide (DLCO) < 40% at diagnosis; reduction in FVC $\geq$ 10% from the estimated value or decrease in DLCO $\geq$ 15% from the estimated value within 6–12 months of follow-up; and decrease > 50 m in the 6 min walking test at 6 months [8].

Indeed, much of the information given in this review is applicable to both IPF and other non-IPF ILDs with a fibrosing phenotype [1,2].

Regarding the pathophysiology of IPF and of other PF-ILDs, it is multifactorial and results in a progressive deterioration of lung function. Some risk factors for progression have been described, including environmental factors, microbial agents or some previous pathologies such as gastroesophageal reflux, which have a probable genetic basis that confers the patient a certain susceptibility to the disease [9].

IPF is the most common idiopathic interstitial pneumonia in the world. It is characterized by a heterogeneous, irreversible, progressive and unpredictable course associated with significant morbidity and poor prognosis after diagnosis [1–3]. There is growing evidence supporting that the disease originates from the interaction between the variable expression of genetic polymorphisms, changes related to cellular aging and exposure to certain environmental factors, such as smoking, industrial powders, chronic gastric microaspiration, viral infections and possibly alterations in the lung microbiome [1,3]. The lesions produced by repetitive exposures aberrantly activate the alveolar epithelial cells of genetically susceptible individuals, promoting apoptosis of the epithelium, recruitment of mesenchymal cells and increased vascular permeability. Unregulated epithelial/mesenchymal interaction results in the secretion of a variety of profibrotic cytokines, metalloproteinases and procoagulant mediators, which promote uncontrolled migration and proliferation, and differentiation in fibroblasts to myofibroblasts as well as fibrosis in the extracellular matrix. The main pro-inflammatory cytokines involved in fibrosis are tumour necrosis factor (TNF)-α and interleukin (IL)-1, as well as some fibrous factors such as transforming growth factor (TGF)-β and platelet-derived growth factor (PDGF) [1–5].

Patients present a nonspecific symptomatology, which is the fundamental cause of the delay in diagnosis. Accordingly, in order to reach a definitive diagnosis, it is essential to combine a detailed medical history with the realization of radiological imaging studies and sometimes with histopathological studies obtained through a pulmonary biopsy (PB). Currently, the gold standard for diagnosis of IPF and other non-IPF PF-ILDs is multidisciplinary discussions that can improve the precision of diagnosis, avoiding unnecessary tests such as pulmonary biopsy and optimizing patient management. The multidisciplinary team should include a pulmonologist, a radiologist, a pathologist, a thoracic surgeon, a rheumatologist and a specialist nurse [10].

Patients with IPF present with dyspnea, cough and asthenia, which are symptoms that cause a reduction in daily physical activity and muscle strength leading to a precarious quality of life and often result in social isolation with increased levels of dependence and immobility as the disease progresses and causing a significant number of cardiopulmonary complications. In addition, these patients experience depressive and anxiety disorders, creating a situation that is difficult to manage for both patients and their caregivers [11].

Another cause for the delay in the diagnosis of IPF is that this is an entity that can be easily confused with other respiratory pathologies requiring multidisciplinary assessment by the pulmonology, radiology and pathological anatomy services, thereby using more healthcare resources [10,12].

Lung transplantation is the only therapeutic option that appears to increase the life expectancy of patients with IPF. This procedure would be indicated when there is a higher probability of accelerated decrease in FVC and, therefore, a poor prognosis in the short term. As the knowledge of IPF has deepened and several technical advances have been achieved, especially in the area of transplant immunology and surgical procedures (involving both means and technique), the average age of recipients undergoing lung transplantation has increased in recent decades from 45 to 55 years. However, this therapeutic option has been extended in recent years to patients up to 65 years of age in specialized centers. Nevertheless, despite these advances, pulmonary recipients with IPF have an overall survival rate upon single transplantation between 4 and 5.5 years, depending on the series, and may exceed 10 years for bilateral pulmonary transplantation [10–12].

Traditionally, IPF treatment was based on immunosuppressants, glucocorticoids, oxygen therapy and palliative measures. However, the PANTHER-IPF study showed that treatment with azathioprine, N-acetyl cysteine and prednisone was associated with increased hospitalizations and mortality [13]. Currently, there are two drugs approved for this pathology that have been shown to delay lung deterioration associated with the disease with satisfactory safety and tolerability profiles. These two drugs are nintedanib and pirfenidone [14,15]. However, there is little information on the pharmacological interactions of these two agents in IPF patients who are usually polymedicated.

The group of COVID-19 patients most affected by severe disease present clinical characteristics highly similar to patients suffering from PF-ILD, rendering PF-ILD management more important than ever [5–7].

Below we review the main pharmacological interactions of the two currently available antifibrotic drugs, used individually or in combination, as well as some practical aspects of their therapeutic management, which have become more complex in this pandemic.

2. COVID-19 and ILD

SARS-CoV (Severe Acute Respiratory Syndrome Coronavirus) and MERS-CoV (Middle East Respiratory Syndrome Coronavirus) are genetically similar to SARS-CoV-2 and cause lung syndromes similar to COVID-19. At the end of the SARS pandemic on June 2003, 8422 people were affected and 916 died. On the other hand, MERS, which began in April 2012, infected 2519 recognized subjects out of which 866 died. Tomographic abnormalities in SARS included the following: rapidly progressive ground-glass opacities, some of them with consolidation of some regions of the lung; and apparent reticular changes approximately two weeks after the onset of symptoms, which persisted in half of the patients for about 4 weeks. A 15 year follow-up study of 71 patients with SARS showed that interstitial and functional abnormalities progressively decreased, resulting in recovery after the first 2 years following infection and then remained stable; at 15 years, only one patient had obstructive pulmonary disease and none had restrictive respiratory dysfunction, while 4–6% showed interstitial abnormalities [6]. Similar to the findings in SARS, ILD with a fibrosing phenotype has been reported in MERS [7].

Several cases of patients with severe pneumonia of unknown cause appeared in Hubei province, China, in December 2019. Almost one month later, these cases were reported to the World Health Organization (WHO). They started an outbreak that was later declared a pandemic by WHO. The causative agent of this disease was identified as a betacoronavirus RNA, similar to SARS-CoV, which was thus called SARS-CoV-2. This coronavirus causes lung, gastrointestinal and neurological disease. It has a diameter between 60 and 140 nanometers and is covered by an envelope formed by different spicules, which gives it a solar corona appearance. By genetic recombination, coronaviruses acquire the capacity to infect any host, including bats and humans. SARS-CoV-2 is able to infect the nasal and bronchial epithelia, as well as pneumocytes, through the binding of the spike (S) protein of viral spicules to its receptor on the cell surface, which is the angiotensin-converting enzyme-2 (ACE-2); this interaction triggers an inflammatory response and, subsequently, the clinical picture of pneumonia and/or respiratory failure [1,6]. In one of the first studies conducted in China during the pandemic, the characteristics of 1099 patients were reported. Out of these, 173 cases were severe, with an average age of 49 years; 57% were male; 28% were smokers; and 23.7% (over 70 years) presented comorbidities such as diabetes, hypertension and chronic obstructive pulmonary disease (COPD); 5% of the cases were in intensive care; 2.3% on mechanical ventilation; and 1.4% of patients died [16]. As of June 2021, 180,569,000 infections and 3,912,200 deaths have been reported worldwide [17].

Fibrotic changes have been found in chest computerized tomography (CT) in patients with COVID-19. Available data indicate that one-third of the recovered patients develop fibrotic abnormalities, 47% have impaired DLCO and 25% have decreased total lung capacity. In a study by Huang et al., all patients who survived had varying degrees of fibrotic damage ranging from subtle linear opacities to diffuse distribution of crazy paving pattern, with extensive fibrosis evidenced in 52% of patients. In another study by Zhou et al. including 62 patients, 21 (33.9%) had fibrotic changes, which were more likely to occur in advanced stages of the disease (8 to 14 days from onset of symptoms) than in earlier stages (less than 7 days). Similarly, Pan et al. reported fibrotic changes in chest CT in 11 out of 63 patients during acute illness. These reshapings are supported by autopsy reports. Early fibrotic changes in the course of the disease suggest repair attempts following lung damage; all this results in pulmonary sequelae, which include impaired exercise capacity, fibrotic lung tissue and impaired diffusing capacity. However, although pulmonary function can be improved over time, moderate fibrosis could be irreversible in some patients [18,19]. Thus, it would make sense to apply the same strategy as in other non-IPF PF-ILDs in these patients and antifibrotic agents could play a relevant role.

The early identification of subpopulations of patients developing PF-ILD phenotype after COVID-19 infection is important since it is presumed that, by acting early in the course of ARDS, the development of lung damage could be avoided, delayed or decreased [18]. Several markers associated with mortality risk including age, disease severity, time of Intensive Care Unit (ICU) stay, mechanical ventilation and hyperinflammatory markers may be potential predictors of PF-ILD. Other factors such as male sex, smoking and underlying diseases have also been described. In addition, prolonged fever prior to hospital admission, tachypnea and eosinopenia at admission may be useful as a combination of early risk indicators [19].

Age: Pulmonary fibrosis is most often reported in elderly individuals. The exact reason for this association is unknown; however, older individuals are more susceptible to SARS, MERS and SARS-CoV-2 and are more likely to possess severe symptoms [17].

Disease severity: According to the WHO, 80% of COVID-19 cases are mild, 14% develop severe symptoms and 6% are very severe. Comorbidities such as high blood pressure, diabetes and coronary artery disease are factors associated with increased severity. Laboratory findings that correlate with increased severity are as follows: lymphocytopenia, leukocytosis and lactate dehydrogenase (LDH) increase. Serum LDH levels have been used as a marker of disease severity following acute lung damage. LDH is an indicator of lung tissue destruction and correlates with mortality risk. Peak LDH levels were significantly correlated with the risk of pulmonary fibrosis after infection in MERS and SARS [17]. In a meta-analysis, Chen et al. reported that elevated LDH values were associated with a 12-fold increase in the risk for severe COVID-19 and concluded that LDH levels can be used to predict severe disease [20].

Time of hospitalization at the ICU and mechanical ventilation: Five percent to twelve percent of COVID-19 patients required ICU admission. Although disease severity is closely related to the time of hospitalization at the ICU, mechanical ventilation provides an additional risk of ventilator-induced lung damage. Ventilator-associated lung damage is an acute damage that is initiated or exacerbated by mechanical ventilation and is associated with increased mortality in ARDS. Pressure and volume abnormalities induce this damage, resulting in the release of proinflammatory modulators, worsening of acute lung damage, increased mortality and pulmonary fibrosis in survivors. In a follow-up study of 27 patients with ARDS who received mechanical ventilation, 23 (87%) had pulmonary fibrosis between 110 and 267 days after extubation [17].

Smoking: It is associated with chronic oxidative stress, increased expression of inflammatory cytokines and pulmonary fibrosis. The harm associated with smoking continues even after smoking cessation. A systematic review by Vardavas and Nikitara showed that smokers are 1.4 times more likely to have more severe symptoms of COVID-19 and 2.4 times more likely to need the ICU, mechanical ventilation or die than non-smokers [17].

Chronic Alcoholism: Alcohol abuse is associated with recurrent pneumonia due to the aspiration of gastric contents. Clinical and experimental studies show that alcoholism causes glutathione depletion, chronic oxidative stress, inflammation and induction of TGF-B in the lungs, thereby increasing the risk of acute lung injury and pulmonary fibrosis [17].

Patients should be advised not to leave the house and to use non-face-to-face methods for consultations (telemedicine), to obtain medicine stocks (they can be formulated for 3 months) and, if required, to ask for help in order to avoid leaving the house (from family or friends). They should also take into account the different recommendations on fever, odynophagia, dry cough and dyspnoea for 1 week and consult for suspected COVID-19. A management strategy should be established with patients and family members, if possible, with recommendations on how to proceed during a mild exacerbation at home, including indications about warning signs for them to attend emergencies or to contact their physician and reminding them that they may not necessarily be infected with COVID-19. Medications for interstitial lung disease should be maintained at the dose recommended by the attending physician but should be discontinued at the time of acute COVID-19 infection in order to avoid drug interaction or side effects. The patient's immune response appears to play an important role in the pathophysiology of both acute lung injury and ARDS. Patients with COVID-19, particularly those with pneumonia and ARDS have elevated levels of proinflammatory cytokines and other inflammatory biomarkers. Currently, the most commonly used drugs for the acute phase of COVID-19 are glucocorticoids. In fact, in the RECOVERY trial, dexamethasone has shown a moderate but significant reduction in mortality among those patients who were receiving either invasive mechanical ventilation or oxygen alone at randomization but not among those receiving no respiratory support. However, despite this clinical trial being one of the most robust studies regarding the use of glucocorticoids in COVID-19, its methodology is somehow questionable among other reasons because no severity markers were recorded. Furthermore, several routes of administration of dexamethasone, oral or intravenous, were used [21]. Notwithstanding the need of further evidence, glucocorticoids seem to be the cornerstone of the treatment of the acute phase of COVID-19 to date. Additionally, the combination of supportive therapy along with antiviral treatment, oxygen therapy and anticoagulation must be emphasized [22]. In order to clarify the role of anti-inflammatory and immunomodulatory treatment of the acute phases of COVID-19 on the occurrence of long-COVID and post-ARDS interstitial lung disease, further research is needed. Finally, pulmonary rehabilitation in the acute and inflammatory phases is essential for the full recovery of lung function in these patients.

3. Pharmacovigilance

According to the WHO, pharmacovigilance is defined as "the science and activities related to the detection, assessment, understanding and prevention of adverse drug effects or any other possible drug-related problem". The safety system covers adverse drug reactions (ADR) produced by medications, dosing errors, falsified medicinal products, their lack of effectiveness and misuse and/or abuse and drug interactions, among others. It also involves monitoring the safety of natural and traditional medicines, blood products, radioactive substances, contrast media, biological products, vaccines and even medical devices [23]. The main purpose of pharmacovigilance is to determine the cause, frequency and severity of ADRs in such a manner that the necessary preventive measures can be put in place in order to preserve patient safety and achieve the rational use of medicinal products optimizing the benefit/risk ratio. Therefore, it is considered a key piece for ensuring the efficiency and effectiveness of the pharmaceutical regulatory systems, clinical practice and the programmes implemented in healthcare [24].

Drug Interactions

When a medicine is administered, it undergoes a series of processes that contribute in inducing its therapeutics and toxic effects in the organism and are summarized under the acronym LADME (liberation, absorption, distribution, metabolism and excretion). A drug interaction occurs when the concomitant administration of two drugs alters any of the aforementioned processes [25]. There are several scenarios resulting from a drug–drug interaction: drug absorption can be delayed, decreased or increased; the distribution within the body and the pharmacological effect for which the drugs were designed may be altered; or their metabolism and/or excretion can be significantly modified [26].

The understanding of the mechanism involved in a given drug interaction is essential for its interpretation, prevention and treatment. However, it is not easy to establish a clear mechanism for each interaction since they usually involve more than one drug acting simultaneously through different mechanisms [27]. Two main groups of drug interactions can be considered:

1. Pharmacodynamic: They take place at biologically active sites, such as receptors, and produce changes in pharmacological activity. They do not usually affect pharmacokinetic parameters, but they alter the patient's response to the drug. These interactions are as clinically important as pharmacokinetic interactions but much more difficult to study systematically since they usually take place affecting pairs of medications, which makes it difficult to establish common mechanisms explaining the effects on both drugs. Two types of pharmacodynamic interactions can be defined [26]:
    - Synergistic: Two drugs with the same pharmacological effect are administered together;
    - Antagonistic: Two drugs that are administered together have opposite actions.
2. Pharmacokinetic: They affect different drug kinetic processes, resulting in modifications in plasma drug concentration. There are different types of pharmacokinetic interactions depending on whether they occur at the level of absorption, distribution, metabolism or excretion [26,28].

Absorption: They can affect both the speed and magnitude of absorption. In general, these interactions have little clinical relevance and can be avoided by separating the administration of the two drugs.

Distribution: Displacement of plasma protein binding. They occur when two drugs compete for the same binding site in plasma proteins; in this case, the drug with the lowest affinity for the protein is displaced by the one with the highest affinity. The result is an increase in the concentration of free (active) drug, which is usually compensated by an increase in its excretion. These interactions are only clinically important for drugs in which the percentage of plasma protein binding is greater than 90%.

Metabolism: The interactions at this level are the most important from a clinical point of view. Cytochrome P-450 is the main responsible for the metabolism of drugs, as well as other exogenous substances (polycyclic aromatic hydrocarbons, etc.) and endogenous compounds (steroids, hormones, prostaglandins, lipids and fatty acids), through mono-oxidation reactions.

The term cytochrome P-450 refers to a group of numerous isoenzymes located in the membrane of the smooth endoplasmic reticulum of hepatocytes. They are also present at high concentrations in small intestine enterocytes and in small amounts in extra-hepatic tissues, such as kidney, lung and brain. Cytochrome P-450 enzymes form a genetic super-family that can be divided into families and subfamilies. To date, more than 30 different isoenzymes have been identified in humans, but 90% of oxidation reactions can be attributed to the six main families: CYP1A2, CYP2C9, CYP2C19, CYP2D6, CYP2E1 and CYP3A4.

Interactions affecting the metabolism are caused by the induction or inhibition of cytochrome P-450 isoenzymes. Enzymatic induction is a gradual process since it requires the synthesis of new enzymes and produces a decrease in the plasma level of the drug being metabolized. Enzymatic inhibition, on the other hand, takes place more quickly and results in an increase in the plasma concentration of the affected drug. A drug can be metabolized simultaneously by more than one isoenzyme. In addition, a drug does not need to be a substrate of this enzyme to behave as an inducer or inhibitor of a specific isoenzyme.

Excretion: Those drugs that alter the renal excretion of other drugs can affect their plasma levels. The two most common mechanisms of interaction at the renal level are competition for active tubular secretion and the modification of urinary pH. The clinical impact of these types of interactions depends on the percentage of renal elimination of a drug or its metabolites, but these mechanisms are not as important as those involving the metabolism in general.

It should be emphasized that the probability of drug interactions increases substantially with the number drugs administered simultaneously to a patient. Accordingly, drug interactions are expected to be greater in the polymedicated patient. Therefore, drug interactions go hand-in-hand with polymedication [29,30]. The WHO defines chronic diseases as "diseases of long duration and usually of slow progression" [31]. Heart disease, stroke, respiratory diseases, cancer and diabetes are good examples of chronic diseases. Between 60% and 70% of deaths worldwide are attributed to these diseases. In turn, 80% of these deaths occur in low-income and middle-income countries inhabited by a large part of the global population, affecting important aspects of the lives of both men and women. Other examples of chronic diseases include hearing and visual impairments, oral diseases, osteoarticular diseases, gene and mental disorders. The main risk factors for the development of chronic disease are smoking, an unhealthy diet, physical inactivity and alcoholism [31].

4. Pirfenidone

Pirfenidone (5 methyl-1-phenyl-2-[1H] pyridone) is an agent that combines anti-inflammatory and antifibrotic effects acting on the regulation of TGF-5 activity, TNF-α and β pathways, as well as cellular oxidation. Pirfenidone is indicated for the treatment of mild to moderate IPF [15]. Pirfenidone was approved for IPF based mainly on the two CAPACITY trials [32] (Table 1). Moreover, in order to confirm the beneficial effect of pirfenidone on disease progression, another trial was performed showing positive outcomes [33] (Table 1). According to the RELIEF study, inpatients with fibrotic ILDs other than IPF (such as connective tissue disease-associated ILDs, fibrotic non-specific interstitial pneumonia, chronic hypersensitivity pneumonitis and pneumoconiosis) attended in 17 centers specialized in ILD in Germany deteriorated despite conventional therapy. However, with the addition of pirfenidone to the existing treatment there was an attenuation of disease progression, as measured by decline in FVC [34]. Nevertheless, more studies for assessing the efficacy and safety of pirfenidone in this kind of patients are needed.

Table 1. Main clinical trials on pirfenidone and nintedanib in idiopathic pulmonary fibrosis (IPF).

Study (References)	Design	Treatment	Main Endpoints	Patients
CAPACITY 004 [32]	Phase 3 Randomized Parallel Assignment Double-Blind	Pirfenidone (2403 mg or 1197 mg) versus Placebo	Absolute Change in Percentage of predicted FVC Mean Change in Percent Predicted FVC as measured from baseline to week 72	435
CAPACITY 006 [32]	Phase 3 Randomized Parallel Assigment Double-Blind	Pirfenidone (2403 mg) versus Placebo	Change in percentage of predicted FVC at week 72	344
ASCEND [33]	Phase 3 Randomized Parallel Assigment Double-Blind	Pirfenidone (2403 mg) versus Placebo	Change in FVC or death at week 52	555
RELIEF [34]	Phase 2 Randomized Parallel assignment Double blinded	Pirfenidone (267 mg or 534 mg or 801 mg) versus placebo	Absolute change in percentage of predicted FVC at week 48	127
TOMORROW [35]	Phase 2 Randomized Parallel assignment Double blinded	Nintedanib (50 mg, 100 mg, 200 mg or 300 mg) versus Placebo	Annual rate of decline in FVC over 52 weeks	432
INPULSIS 1-INPULSIS 2 [36]	Phase 3 Randomized Parallel assignment Double blinded	Nintedanib (200 mg or 300 mg) versus Placebo	Annual rate of decline in FVC over 52 weeks	1066
SENSCIS [37]	Phase 3 Randomized Parallel assigment Double blinded	Nintedanib (150 mg) versus placebo	Annual rate of decline in FVC over 52 weeks	576
INBUILD [38]	Phase 3 Randomized Parallel assigment Double blinded	Nintedanib (150 mg) versus placebo	Annual rate of decline in FVC over 52 weeks	663
INJOURNEY [39]	Phase 4 Randomized Parallel assignment Open-label	Nintedanib (150 mg) versus Pirfenidone (2403 mg)	Percentage of patients with on-treatment gastrointestinal AEs from baseline to week 12	105

Abbreviations: FVC: forced vital capacity. AE: Adverse Events.

Pharmacologically, pirfenidone belongs to the group of immunosuppressive agents. It was approved by the US Food and Drug Administration (FDA) and the European Medicines Agency (EMA) in 2011, becoming the first drug authorized for the treatment of IPF. Pirfenidone has antifibrotic and anti-inflammatory properties both in vitro and in animal models of pulmonary fibrosis [15]. In addition, pirfenidone reduces the accumulation of inflammatory cells and attenuates the proliferation of fibroblasts, the production of cytokines and proteins related to fibrosis and the increased synthesis and accumulation of extracellular matrix [15].

Treatment of mild to moderate IPF with pirfenidone in adults begins with 800 mg/day and is increased up to 2400 mg/day over the course of 3 weeks. The most common adverse reactions are observed at the gastrointestinal, skin and liver level (Table 2). It is worth highlighting that polymedicated patients should be closely monitored, as pirfenidone metabolism can be influenced in these patients by inhibition or induction of liver enzyme systems such as cytochrome P450 1A2 (CYP1A2), CYP3A4 and P-glycoprotein (P-gp) [15]. Table 2 shows a list of drugs that should be avoided when initiating pirfenidone treatment because the risk/gravity of their adverse effects outweighs the benefit from treatment (major interactions).

Table 2. Pharmacological characteristics of nintedanib and pirfenidone.

	Pirfenidone	Nintedanib
Pharmaceutical form (orally)	Capsules Tablets	Capsules
Half-life (hours)	3	9.5
Side effects	Bloating, dizziness, diarrhoea, dyspepsia, gastroesophageal reflux, nausea, vomiting, fatigue, weight loss, photosensitivity reactions and rash	Increased liver enzymes, abdominal pain, diarrhoea, nausea, vomiting weight loss
Major pharmacological Interactions *	Aminolevulinic acid, amiodarone, enoxacin, fluvoxamine, leflunomide, mibefradil, mipomersen, rucaparib, teriflunomide, vemurafenib	Carbamazepine, dexamethasone, drotrecogin alfa, phenytoin, leflunomide, lomitapide, mipomersen, mitotane, phenobarbital, primidone, rifampicin, St. John's wort, tripanavir, teriflunomide
Contraindications	Smoking Kidney failure Liver failure	Thromboembolic disease Lung toxicity Gastric perforation Smoking Kidney failure Liver failure
Pregnancy Category (FDA)	C	D

Abbreviations: Pregnancy category C: Animal reproduction studies have shown adverse effects on the foetus or its safety could not be demonstrated. There are no adequate and well-controlled studies in humans. Drugs included in this category should only be used when the potential benefits justify the potential risks to the foetus. Pregnancy category D: There is evidence of risk to the foetus based on research data, post-marketing data, adverse reaction records or human studies. However, the potential benefits of its use in pregnant women may be acceptable despite the likely risks in some situations. FDA: Food and Drug Administration. * Major interactions: Highly relevant at the clinical level. Combinations causing this type of interactions should be avoided since their risk exceeds the potential benefit.

Various analyses of cumulative information from several studies have provided several important conclusions [40,41]. For instance, in a single-dose drug interaction study involving 27 volunteers, co-administration of 800 mg pirfenidone and 750 mg ciprofloxacin (moderate CYP1A2 inhibitor) two times daily for 6 days increased exposure to pirfenidone by 81% [15] (Table 1). Consequently, in the case of strong CYP1A2 inhibitors such as fluvoxamine or enoxacin, the dose of pirfenidone should be reduced to one-third of the usual dose, while for moderate inhibitors such as ciprofloxacin, it should be reduced to 66% of the commonly used dose [15].

For P450 1A2 inducers, a study in which a single pirfenidone dose of 801 mg was administered to 25 healthy non-smoking patients and 25 smokers without concomitant therapy at the time of the study showed less exposure to the drug in smoking subjects (area under the curve (AUC) 46% in smokers and 68% in non-smokers) (Table 1) [40].

Pirfenidone has been shown to exert low inhibition (10% to 30%) of P-gp-mediated digoxin (5.0 μM) efflux at concentrations of 100 M and higher [8]. The inhibitory activity of pirfenidone for CYP2C9 and 2C19 or 1A2, 2D6 and 3A4 was evaluated in vitro at a concentration of 1000 μM (approximately 10 times the average of the maximum concentration (Cmax) in humans). The activity of these enzymes was reduced by 30.4%, 27.5%, 34.1%, 21% and 9.6%, respectively; this effect has great clinical relevance, as it increases Cmax and AUC values proportionally to the dose used [41].

5. Nintedanib

Nintedanib is an intracellular tyrosine kinase inhibitor developed for the treatment of various types of cancer (lung, ovary, renal, colo-rectal and liver), as well as an antifibrotic agent. The first clinical trial that confirmed the effects of nintedanib slowing the progression of idiopathic pulmonary fibrosis was the phase II TOMORROW [35], which was confirmed in the phase III INPULSIS-1 and INPULSIS-2 [36].

In 2014, it was approved for the treatment of IPF in the USA and Europe, and it received a new indication for systemic sclerosis (SSc)-associated ILD (SSc-ILD) therapy in

2019 [37]. More recently, this drug has been approved for the treatment of other progressive fibrosing interstitial lung diseases (PF-ILD) [38].

Nintedanib is a potent oral inhibitor of the tyrosine-kinase activity of several pro-angiogenic receptors: vascular endothelial growth factor receptors (VEGFR) 1–3, fibroblast growth factor receptors (FGFR) 1–3 and platelet-derived growth factor receptors (PDGFR) α and β. Additionally, it inhibits the kinase activity of RET receptors, FLT3 and the Src family of tyrosine kinases. Overall, more than 12 tyrosine-kinase receptors and signalling molecules are inhibited by nintedanib, suggesting potential effects on multiple signalling pathways [14].

Nintedanib displays linear pharmacokinetics for a dose of 350 mg twice daily. The maximum plasma concentrations are normally reached 2–4 h after oral administration with food. Its half-life is 9.5 h (Table 2), and the average concentration in the steady state is normally reached in one week, with low concentrations remaining stable for a period longer than 1 year. The absolute bioavailability of nintedanib 100 mg is 4.7%. This pharmacokinetic profile is due to the quick metabolization of the molecule by methylesterases [14,35,36].

The main metabolic pathway of nintedanib is esterase-mediated hydrolysis followed by glucuronidation. CYP450, primarily CYP3A4, plays a minor role in nintedanib biotransformation. The main route of nintedanib elimination is the bile/faecal pathway (which accounts for about 93% of the administered dose). The contribution of renal excretion to total clearance is low at about 0.65% [14]. The co-administration of nintedanib with ketoconazole, a CYP3A4 and P-gp inhibitor, increases nintedanib exposure by 60%; patients receiving nintedanib concomitantly with P-gp and CYP3A4 inhibitors should be closely monitored. The co-administration of nintedanib and rifampicin, a P-gp and CYP3A4 inducer, decreases nintedanib exposure by 50%. Therefore, concomitant administration of nintedanib with P-gp or CYP3A4 inducers should be avoided [14,35,36]. Table 2 shows a list of drugs that should be taken into account when treating patients with nintedanib due to the risk of major drug interactions.

6. Managing the Adverse Effects of Antifibrotic Therapy

The most common adverse events (AEs) of antifibrotic therapy occur at the gastrointestinal tract [14,15] (Table 2). Grouped data from TOMORROW and INPULSIS trials (Table 1) showed that the AE most commonly associated with daily nintedanib 300 mg was diarrhoea, reported in 61.5% of cases (17.9% with placebo) [13,42]. In most patients, nintedanib-associated gastrointestinal AEs can be managed by reducing the dose (200 mg/day), discontinuing treatment and applying symptomatic measures with loperamide or similar [14]. The most common AE associated with pirfenidone in the CAPACITY and ASCEND studies was nausea, which appeared in 35.5% of patients vs. 15.1% in patients treated with placebo [43]. Gastrointestinal toxicity associated with pirfenidone is managed by reducing the dose or interrupting treatment [14]. Taking treatment after meals can also be helpful [43]. Photosensitivity and rash associated with pirfenidone appear mostly in the first months of treatment. In CAPACITY and ASCEND trials, rash was reported in 29.2% of patients treated with pirfenidone compared to 9% in patients treated with placebo [43]. This AE can be reduced by the use of photoprotective creams [14]. Table 3 shows recommended strategies for the prevention and treatment of the most common AEs associated with antifibrotic agents.

In addition, nintedanib and pirfenidone may cause an increase in liver enzymes. Therefore, it is necessary to perform control analyses at the start of treatment as well as periodically during treatment for the early detection of potential liver damage [14,15,44,45]. Dose adjustments made to manage AEs do not reduce the effectiveness of nintedanib or pirfenidone decreasing FVC [46–49].

Table 3. Strategy for the prevention and management of adverse events related to antifibrotic therapy.

Type of AE	Pirfenidone			Nintedanib	
	Gastrointestinal	Cutaneous	Hepatic	Gastrointestinal	Hepatic
AE prevention	Take pirfenidone with plenty of food. Titration for 4 weeks instead of 2.	Avoid exposure to sunlight or intense artificial light. Applications of complete protection cream every 2 h. Use of sunglasses and protective clothing. Avoid use of phototoxic drugs.	Monitor liver bio-chemistry (ALT, AST and bilirubin) at baseline, monthly for 6 months and then every 3 months.	Take nintedanib with food.	Monitor liver biochemistry (ALT, AST, bilirubin) at baseline, monthly for the first 3 months and then periodically.
AE treatment	Prokinetics and proton pump inhibitors.	Steroids or sulphadiazine if severe phototoxicity.		Antidiarrheal (loperamide). Antiemetics. Proper hydration.	
Dose reduction	Reduce doses to 1–2 capsules 2–3 times daily. Make the reduction at the time point in which the AE is most pronounced.	Reduce dose to 1 capsule every 8 h for one week.	If AST and ALT are increased (>3 to 5× ULN) or there are symptoms or hyperbilirubine-mia, reduce doses until values recovery.	Reduce to 100 mg/12 h if persistent diarrhoea.	If AST/ALT are increased (>3 to 5× ULN) reduce dosage until values recovery. Then, re-scale doses up to max tolerated.
Dose interruption	If AE persists, temporarily discontinue therapy until symptom resolution.	Discontinue doses for 14 days if rash persists and subsequently re-escalate. Do not re-escalate if the rash does not subside.	Permanently discontinue if the elevations of AST and ALT are accompanied by symptoms of hyperbilirubinemia or if the elevations are >5× ULN.	Stop doses if severe diarrhoea for one week. Discontinue permanently if there is no improvement.	Permanently stop doses if elevations are accompanied by severe symptoms of liver damage.

Abbreviations: AE: adverse events; ALT: alanine amino-transferase; AST: aspartate amino transferase; max.: maximum; ULN: upper limit of normality.

Results from a study of 186 patients from a single centre in the United States showed that the percentage of patients who had to discontinue treatment with pirfenidone or nintedanib due to AEs was similar to that observed in clinical trials (20.9% and 26.3%, respectively), with gastrointestinal AEs being primarily responsible for discontinuation [49]. Moreover, several studies have shown that efficacy and safety data in clinical practice are similar to those described in clinical trials [50–54].

7. Concomitant Administration of Nintedanib and Pirfenidone

AUC and Cmax values obtained for nintedanib administration in conjunction with pirfenidone in IPF patients, indicate that there are no clinically relevant interactions between these two agents. Although exposure to nintedanib in these studies decreased when administered with pirfenidone compared to monotherapy, this fact lacks clinical relevance and can be attributed to the great inter-individual variability among patients, as it is also observed when nintedanib is administered as monotherapy [55,56].

Regarding pharmacokinetics of pirfenidone, the AUC and Cmax values are similar when this drug is used alone or in combination with nintedanib [55,56]. This information was more consistent in the INJOURNEY study, which evaluated the safety, efficacy and pharmacokinetic profile of nintedanib alone or in combination with pirfenidone. Interestingly, combined treatment reduced FVC less than nintedanib in monotherapy, although these data should be interpreted with caution [39].

As both drugs produce similar AEs [4,5], a negative additive effect could be expected when they are administered together. However, the AEs of the combined administration were similar to those of individual treatments [57,58].

The data analysed until now suggest the absence of relevant clinical interactions between these two drugs. Although there is a lot of information regarding long-term individual administration of pirfenidone and nintedanib [57,58], information about their combined administration is very limited. There is only a small Phase IV study in 20 patients with IPF under long-term treatment with both drugs (Table 1), in which no added AEs were observed [39].

Cost-effectiveness remains to be improved, as the association of two antifibrotic agents considerably increases the cost of treatment per patient and year, thereby increasing the economic burden on healthcare providers. In recent years, inhaled administration of new antifibrotic agents has been explored; this new administration route could improve adherence to treatment in polymedicated patients [59].

8. Final Considerations

In December 2019, reports emerged from Wuhan, China, of a new severe acute respiratory disease caused by SARS-CoV-2. COVID-19 pneumonia presents as an acute respiratory infection, with fever, dry cough, dyspnoea, arthralgia and other symptoms, which may be similar to some interstitial lung diseases. Therefore, history, epidemiological link, physical examination and clinical examination of the patient should be taken into account for a correct differential diagnosis. In this manner, when a physician faces a patient with this type of interstitial lung disease, it is important to define the complete medical history in order to determine whether the interstitial disease is acute or chronic and to consider the diagnosis of infection by COVID-19, which is, perhaps, the greatest challenge [5–7].

Data from previous coronavirus-induced diseases such as SARS and MERS, as well as emerging data from the COVID-19 pandemic, suggest there could be substantial fibrotic consequences following SARS-CoV-2 infection. Nintedanib and pirfenidone might have a role in preventing severe lung fibrosis after SARS-CoV-2 infection, especially in patients with the PF-ILD phenotype [5–7,60]. Furthermore, we must take into account that these drugs do not produce immunosuppression, which is an advantage over the use of corticosteroids in the acute phase of the disease. This becomes particularly important in patients at high risk of contracting any type of infection during COVID treatment. Thus, switching to antifibrotic therapy is an option to be considered in some patients.

In addition, chronic diseases are a growing threat capable of triggering serious repercussions ranging from negatively affecting health-related quality of life and being an underestimated cause of poverty for both families and society in general to being the leading cause of premature deaths worldwide [60]. It is important to note that these population groups are especially susceptible to interactions, mainly because of polypharmacy. Polymedication is a frequent phenomenon in chronic diseases and, in the majority of cases, is associated with non-compliance with treatment, inappropriate use and/or abuse of drugs, dosing mistakes or inadequate medication, among others. Its prevalence is an imminent alarm in the health sector as it has undergone significant growth in the last years [60].

IPF and PF-ILDs are chronic diseases affecting patients who often take at least four different kinds of drugs [61]. In these patients, the risk of a harmful and unwanted response increases exponentially, resulting in new requirements for dealing with conditions wrongly interpreted as "new pathological processes", which give rise to a therapeutic cascade. Moreover, drug interactions are more frequent in the polymedicated patient [62].

Although not all drug interactions are clinically significant, it is important to remain vigilant for those that are relevant. It is impossible to keep in mind all the relevant interactions described, but knowledge of the main types of drugs most frequently involved in interactions can be crucial for establishing an alert system that contributes to improving prescription of drug therapy. Several methods that allow the reduction in the risks associated with interactions and thus improve the therapeutic risk/benefit ratio have been described, including among others the reduction in the number of drugs administered, avoiding unnecessary polymedication, the selection of alternative drugs with low AE rate, an adequate dosing regimen adjusted to the individualized characteristics of every patient, pharmacokinetic monitoring of serum concentrations of drugs in those cases in which this is possible and constant clinical observations in order to detect the consequences of an interaction as quickly as possible [62–65].

Nintedanib and pirfenidone have represented a breakthrough in the treatment of IPF in recent years. Their different mechanisms of action open the possibility of using them in combination, thus providing an interesting therapeutic option, especially for those cases with worse prognosis. However, little information is currently available on the possible pharmacological interactions that could occur in the case of combined administration and on the additive effects that this interaction could exert on the effectiveness and safety of both drugs.

Author Contributions: Conception and design of the manuscript: J.M.S.L.-M., J.A. and S.C.; data collection: not applicable; analysis and interpretation of data: J.M.S.L.-M., M.G., E.F.V.-R., M.A.G.-G., J.A. and S.C.; drafting, revision and approval of the manuscript: J.M.S.L.-M., M.G., E.F.V.-R., M.A.G.-G., J.A. and S.C. All authors have read and agreed to the published version of the manuscript.

Funding: This research has not received specific funding from public, commercial or for-profit agencies.

Institutional Review Board Statement: Not applicable.

Informed Consent Statement: Not applicable.

Data Availability Statement: Data sharing not applicable.

Acknowledgments: We thank our colleagues of the hospital Pharmacy and Pneumology services for their advice and constant help and Francisco Abad, Head of Clinical Pharmacology Service at the Princesa University Hospital, for his critical reading and constructive comments.

Conflicts of Interest: S. Castañeda is an assisstant professor at the UAM-Roche EPID Future cathedra at the Autonomous University of Madrid (UAM). J. Ancochea is Head of that department. The rest of the authors have no conflict of interest in relation to this work.

References

1. Brown, K.K.; Martinez, F.J.; Walsh, S.L.; Thannickal, V.J.; Prasse, A.; Schlenker-Herceg, R.; Goeldner, R.-G.; Clerisme-Beaty, E.; Tetzlaff, K.; Cottin, V.; et al. The natural history of progressive fibrosing interstitial lung diseases. *Eur. Respir. J.* **2020**, *55*, 2000085. [CrossRef] [PubMed]
2. Wijsenbeek, M.; Cottin, V. Spectrum of Fibrotic Lung Diseases. *N. Engl. J. Med.* **2020**, *383*, 958–968. [CrossRef]
3. Raghu, G.; Collard, H.R.; Egan, J.J.; Martinez, F.J.; Behr, J.; Brown, K.K.; Colby, T.V.; Cordier, J.-F.; Flaherty, K.R.; Lasky, J.A.; et al. An Official ATS/ERS/JRS/ALAT Statement: Idiopathic Pulmonary Fibrosis: Evidence-based Guidelines for Diagnosis and Management. *Am. J. Respir. Crit. Care Med.* **2011**, *183*, 788–824. [CrossRef]
4. Hutchinson, J.P.; Fogarty, A.; Hubbard, R.B.; McKeever, T. Global incidence and mortality of idiopathic pulmonary fibrosis: A systematic review. *Eur. Respir. J.* **2015**, *46*, 795–806. [CrossRef]
5. Vasarmidi, E.; Tsitoura, E.; Spandidos, D.A.; Tzanakis, N.; Antoniou, K.M. Pulmonary fibrosis in the aftermath of the Covid-19 era (Review). *Exp. Ther. Med.* **2020**, *20*, 2557–2560. [CrossRef] [PubMed]
6. Spagnolo, P.; Balestro, E.; Aliberti, S.; Cocconcelli, E.; Biondini, D.; Della Casa, G.; Sverzellati, N.; Maher, T. Pulmonary fibrosis secondary to COVID-19: A call to arms? *Lancet Respir. Med.* **2020**, *8*, 750–752. [CrossRef]
7. Ojo, A.S.; Balogun, S.A.; Williams, O.T.; Ojo, O.S. Pulmonary Fibrosis in COVID-19 Survivors: Predictive Factors and Risk Reduction Strategies. *Pulm. Med.* **2020**, *2020*, 6175964. [CrossRef] [PubMed]
8. Nasser, M.; Larrieu, S.; Si-Mohamed, S.; Ahmad, K.; Boussel, L.; Brevet, M.; Chalabreysse, L.; Fabre, C.; Marque, S.; Revel, D.; et al. Progressive fibrosing interstitial lung disease: A clinical cohort (the PROGRESS study). *Eur. Respir. J.* **2021**, *57*, 2002718. [CrossRef] [PubMed]
9. Caminati, A.; Madotto, F.; Conti, S.; Cesana, G.; Mantovani, L.; Harari, S. The natural history of idiopathic pulmonary fibrosis in a large European population: The role of age, sex and comorbidities. *Intern. Emerg. Med.* **2021**, 1–10. [CrossRef]

10. Snyder, L.D.; Mosher, C.; Holtze, C.H.; Lancaster, L.H.; Flaherty, K.R.; Noth, I.; Neely, M.L.; Hellkamp, A.S.; Bender, S.; Conoscenti, C.S.; et al. Time to diagnosis of idiopathic pulmonary fibrosis in the IPF-PRO Registry. *BMJ Open Respir. Res.* **2020**, *7*, e000567. [CrossRef]
11. Kaunisto, J.; Salomaa, E.-R.; Hodgson, U.; Kaarteenaho, R.; Kankaanranta, H.; Koli, K.; Vahlberg, T.; Myllärniemi, M. Demographics and survival of patients with idiopathic pulmonary fibrosis in the FinnishIPF registry. *ERJ Open Res.* **2019**, *5*, 00170–02018. [CrossRef]
12. Raghu, G.; Remy-Jardin, M.; Myers, J.L.; Richeldi, L.; Ryerson, C.J.; Lederer, D.J.; Behr, J.; Cottin, V.; Danoff, S.K.; Morell, F.; et al. Diagnosis of Idiopathic Pulmonary Fibrosis. An Official ATS/ERS/JRS/ALAT Clinical Practice Guideline. *Am. J. Respir. Crit. Care Med.* **2018**, *198*, e44–e68. [CrossRef]
13. The Idiopathic Pulmonary Fibrosis Clinical Research Network Prednisone, Azathioprine, and N-Acetylcysteine for Pulmonary Fibrosis. *N. Engl. J. Med.* **2012**, *366*, 1968–1977. [CrossRef] [PubMed]
14. OFEV (Nintedanib) Summary of Product Characteristics. Available online: https://ec.europa.eu/health/documents/communityregister/2015/20150115130436/anx_130436_en.pdf (accessed on 16 April 2021).
15. ESBRIET (Pirfenidone) Summary of Product Characteristics. Available online: https://www.ema.europa.eu/en/documents/product-information/esbriet-epar-product-information_en.pdf (accessed on 16 April 2021).
16. Li, Q.; Guan, X.; Wu, P.; Wang, X.; Zhou, L.; Tong, Y.; Ren, R.; Leung, K.S.; Lau, E.H.; Wong, J.Y.; et al. Early Transmission Dynamics in Wuhan, China, of Novel Coronavirus-Infected Pneumonia. *N. Engl. J. Med.* **2020**, *382*, 1199–1207. [CrossRef]
17. John Hopkins University of Medicine Coronavirus Resource Center. Available online: https://coronavirus.jhu.edu/ (accessed on 25 February 2021).
18. Eapen, M.S.; Lu, W.; Gaikwad, A.V.; Bhattarai, P.; Chia, C.; Hardikar, A.; Haug, G.; Sohal, S.S. Endothelial to mesenchymal transition: A precursor to post-COVID-19 interstitial pulmonary fibrosis and vascular obliteration? *Eur. Respir. J.* **2020**, *56*, 2003167. [CrossRef] [PubMed]
19. Huang, W.; Wu, Q.; Chen, Z.; Xiong, Z.; Wang, K.; Tian, J.; Zhang, S. The potential indicators for pulmonary fibrosis in survivors of severe COVID-19. *J. Infect.* **2021**, *82*, e5–e7. [CrossRef] [PubMed]
20. Chen, X.-Y.; Huang, M.-Y.; Xiao, Z.-W.; Yang, S.; Chen, X.-Q. Lactate dehydrogenase elevations is associated with severity of COVID-19: A meta-analysis. *Crit. Care* **2020**, *24*, 1–3. [CrossRef] [PubMed]
21. The RECOVERY Collaborative Group. Dexamethasone in Hospitalized Patients with Covid-19—Preliminary Report. *N. Engl. J. Med.* **2021**, *384*, 693–704. [CrossRef] [PubMed]
22. Alunno, A.; Najm, A.; Machado, P.M.; Bertheussen, H.; Burmester, G.R.; Carubbi, F.; De Marco, G.; Giacomelli, R.; Hermine, O.; Isaacs, J.D.; et al. EULAR points to consider on pathophysiology and use of immunomodulatory therapies in COVID-19. *Ann. Rheum. Dis.* **2021**, *80*, 698–706. [CrossRef] [PubMed]
23. Khouri, C.; Petit, C.; Tod, M.; Lepelley, M.; Revol, B.; Roustit, M.; Cracowski, J.-L. Adverse drug reaction risks obtained from meta-analyses and pharmacovigilance disproportionality analyses are correlated in most cases. *J. Clin. Epidemiol.* **2021**, *134*, 14–21. [CrossRef] [PubMed]
24. Khalil, H.; Huang, C. Adverse drug reactions in primary care: A scoping review. *BMC Health Serv. Res.* **2020**, *20*, 1–13. [CrossRef] [PubMed]
25. Insani, W.N.; Whittlesea, C.; Alwafi, H.; Man, K.K.C.; Chapman, S.; Wei, L. Prevalence of adverse drug reactions in the primary care setting: A systematic review and meta-analysis. *PLoS ONE* **2021**, *16*, e0252161. [CrossRef]
26. Cascorbi, I. Drug Interactions. *Dtsch. Aerzteblatt Online* **2012**, *109*, 546–556. [CrossRef]
27. Zheng, W.Y.; Richardson, L.C.; Li, L.; Day, R.; Westbrook, J.; Baysari, M. Drug-drug interactions and their harmful effects in hospitalised patients: A systematic review and meta-analysis. *Eur. J. Clin. Pharmacol.* **2018**, *74*, 15–27. [CrossRef]
28. Klomp, F.; Wenzel, C.; Drozdzik, M.; Oswald, S. Drug–Drug Interactions Involving Intestinal and Hepatic CYP1A Enzymes. *Pharmaceutics* **2020**, *12*, 1201. [CrossRef] [PubMed]
29. Davies, L.E.; Spiers, G.; Kingston, A.; Todd, A.; Adamson, J.; Hanratty, B. Adverse Outcomes of Polypharmacy in Older People: Systematic Review of Reviews. *J. Am. Med. Dir. Assoc.* **2020**, *21*, 181–187. [CrossRef]
30. Khezrian, M.; McNeil, C.J.; Murray, A.; Myint, P.K. An overview of prevalence, determinants and health outcomes of polypharmacy. *Ther. Adv. Drug Saf.* **2020**, *11*, 2042098620933741. [CrossRef]
31. Fried, T.R.; Street, R.L.; Cohen, A.B. Chronic Disease Decision Making and "What Matters Most". *J. Am. Geriatr. Soc.* **2020**, *68*, 474–477. [CrossRef]
32. Noble, P.W.; Albera, C.; Bradford, W.Z.; Costabel, U.; Glassberg, M.K.; Kardatzke, D.; King, T.E.; Lancaster, L.; Sahn, S.A.; Szwarcberg, J.; et al. Pirfenidone in patients with idiopathic pulmonary fibrosis (CAPACITY): Two randomised trials. *Lancet* **2011**, *377*, 1760–1769. [CrossRef]
33. King, T.E.; Bradford, W.Z.; Castro-Bernardini, S.; Fagan, E.A.; Glaspole, I.; Glassberg, M.K.; Gorina, E.; Hopkins, P.M.; Kardatzke, D.; Lancaster, L.; et al. A Phase 3 Trial of Pirfenidone in Patients with Idiopathic Pulmonary Fibrosis. *N. Engl. J. Med.* **2014**, *370*, 2083–2092. [CrossRef] [PubMed]
34. Behr, J.; Prasse, A.; Kreuter, M.; Johow, J.; Rabe, K.F.; Bonella, F.; Bonnet, R.; Grohe, C.; Held, M.; Wilkens, H.; et al. Pirfenidone in patients with progressive fibrotic interstitial lung diseases other than idiopathic pulmonary fibrosis (RELIEF): A double-blind, randomised, placebo-controlled, phase 2b trial. *Lancet Respir. Med.* **2021**, *9*, 476–486. [CrossRef]

35. Richeldi, L.; Costabel, U.; Selman, M.; Kim, D.S.; Hansell, D.M.; Nicholson, A.G.; Brown, K.K.; Flaherty, K.R.; Noble, P.W.; Raghu, G.; et al. Efficacy of a Tyrosine Kinase Inhibitor in Idiopathic Pulmonary Fibrosis. *N. Engl. J. Med.* **2011**, *365*, 1079–1087. [CrossRef] [PubMed]
36. Richeldi, L.; Du Bois, R.M.; Raghu, G.; Azuma, A.; Brown, K.K.; Costabel, U.; Cottin, V.; Flaherty, K.R.; Hansell, D.M.; Inoue, Y.; et al. Efficacy and Safety of Nintedanib in Idiopathic Pulmonary Fibrosis. *N. Engl. J. Med.* **2014**, *370*, 2071–2082. [CrossRef] [PubMed]
37. Distler, O.; Highland, K.B.; Gahlemann, M.; Azuma, A.; Fischer, A.; Mayes, M.D.; Raghu, G.; Sauter, W.; Girard, M.; Alves, M.; et al. Nintedanib for Systemic Sclerosis–Associated Interstitial Lung Disease. *N. Engl. J. Med.* **2019**, *380*, 2518–2528. [CrossRef] [PubMed]
38. Clinical Trials. Efficacy and Safety of Nintedanib in Patients with Progressive Fibrosing Interstitial Lung Disease (PF-ILD) (INBUILD®). Available online: https://clinicaltrials.gov/ct2/show/record/NCT02999178 (accessed on 20 July 2021).
39. Vancheri, C.; Kreuter, M.; Richeldi, L.; Ryerson, C.J.; Valeyre, D.; Grutters, J.C.; Wiebe, S.; Stansen, W.; Quaresma, M.; Stowasser, S.; et al. Nintedanib with Add-on Pirfenidone in Idiopathic Pulmonary Fibrosis. Results of the INJOURNEY Trial. *Am. J. Respir. Crit. Care Med.* **2018**, *197*, 356–363. [CrossRef]
40. Albera, C.; Costabel, U.; Fagan, E.A.; Glassberg, M.K.; Gorina, E.; Lancaster, L.; Lederer, D.; Nathan, S.D.; Spirig, D.; Swigris, J.J. Efficacy of pirfenidone in patients with idiopathic pulmonary fibrosis with more preserved lung function. *Eur. Respir. J.* **2016**, *48*, 843–851. [CrossRef]
41. Shi, S.; Wu, J.; Chen, H.; Chen, H.; Wu, J.; Zeng, F. Single- and Multiple-Dose Pharmacokinetics of Pirfenidone, an Antifibrotic Agent, in Healthy Chinese Volunteers. *J. Clin. Pharmacol.* **2007**, *47*, 1268–1276. [CrossRef]
42. Richeldi, L.; Cottin, V.; du Bois, R.M.; Selman, M.; Kimura, T.; Bailes, Z.; Schlenker-Herceg, R.; Stowasser, S.; Brown, K.K. Nintedanib in patients with idiopathic pulmonary fibrosis: Combined evidence from the TOMORROW and INPULSIS® trials. *Respir. Med.* **2016**, *113*, 74–79. [CrossRef]
43. Noble, P.W.; Albera, C.; Bradford, W.Z.; Costabel, U.; Du Bois, R.M.; Fagan, E.A.; Fishman, R.S.; Glaspole, I.; Glassberg, M.K.; Lancaster, L.; et al. Pirfenidone for idiopathic pulmonary fibrosis: Analysis of pooled data from three multinational phase 3 trials. *Eur. Respir. J.* **2015**, *47*, 243–253. [CrossRef]
44. Verma, N.; Kumar, P.; Mitra, S.; Taneja, S.; Dhooria, S.; Das, A.; Duseja, A.; Dhiman, R.K.; Chawla, Y. Drug idiosyncrasy due to pirfenidone presenting as acute liver failure: Case report and mini-review of the literature. *Hepatol Commun.* **2018**, *2*, 142–147. [CrossRef]
45. Corte, T.J.; Bonella, F.; Crestani, B.; Demedts, M.G.; Richeldi, L.; Coeck, C.; Pelling, K.; Quaresma, M.; Lasky, J.A. Safety, tolerability and appropriate use of nintedanib in idiopathic pulmonary fibrosis. *Respir. Res.* **2015**, *16*, 1–10. [CrossRef] [PubMed]
46. Nathan, S.D.; Lancaster, L.H.; Albera, C.; Glassberg, M.K.; Swigris, J.J.; Gilberg, F.; Kirchgaessler, K.-U.; Limb, S.L.; Petzinger, U.; Noble, P.W. Dose modification and dose intensity during treatment with pirfenidone: Analysis of pooled data from three multinational phase III trials. *BMJ Open Respir. Res.* **2018**, *5*, e000323. [CrossRef] [PubMed]
47. Toellner, H.; Hughes, G.; Beswick, W.; Crooks, M.G.; Donaldson, C.; Forrest, I.; Hart, S.P.; Leonard, C.; Major, M.; Simpson, A.J.; et al. Early clinical experiences with nintedanib in three UK tertiary interstitial lung disease centres. *Clin. Transl. Med.* **2017**, *6*, 41. [CrossRef]
48. Noth, I.; Oelberg, D.; Kaul, M.; Conoscenti, C.S.; Raghu, G. Safety and tolerability of nintedanib in patients with idiopathic pulmonary fibrosis in the USA. *Eur. Respir. J.* **2018**, *52*, 1702106. [CrossRef]
49. Cottin, V.; Koschel, D.; Günther, A.; Albera, C.; Azuma, A.; Sköld, C.M.; Tomassetti, S.; Hormel, P.; Stauffer, J.L.; Strombom, I.; et al. Long-term safety of pirfenidone: Results of the prospective, observational PASSPORT study. *ERJ Open Res.* **2018**, *4*. [CrossRef] [PubMed]
50. Galli, J.A.; Pandya, A.; Vega-Olivo, M.; Dass, C.; Zhao, H.; Criner, G.J. Pirfenidone and nintedanib for pulmonary fibrosis in clinical practice: Tolerability and adverse drug reactions. *Respirology* **2017**, *22*, 1171–1178. [CrossRef]
51. Hughes, G.; Toellner, H.; Morris, H.; Leonard, C.; Chaudhuri, N. Real World Experiences: Pirfenidone and Nintedanib are Effective and Well Tolerated Treatments for Idiopathic Pulmonary Fibrosis. *J. Clin. Med.* **2016**, *5*, 78. [CrossRef] [PubMed]
52. Tzouvelekis, A.; Karampitsakos, T.; Ntolios, P.; Tzilas, V.; Bouros, E.; Markozannes, E.; Malliou, I.; Anagnostopoulos, A.; Granitsas, A.; Steiropoulos, P.; et al. Longitudinal "Real-World" Outcomes of Pirfenidone in Idiopathic Pulmonary Fibrosis in Greece. *Front. Med.* **2017**, *4*, 213. [CrossRef]
53. Tzouvelekis, A.; Karampitsakos, T.; Kontou, M.; Granitsas, A.; Malliou, I.; Anagnostopoulos, A.; Ntolios, P.; Tzilas, V.; Bouros, E.; Steiropoulos, P.; et al. Safety and efficacy of nintedanib in idiopathic pulmonary fibrosis: A real-life observational study in Greece. *Pulm. Pharmacol. Ther.* **2018**, *49*, 61–66. [CrossRef]
54. Ogura, T.; Taniguchi, H.; Azuma, A.; Inoue, Y.; Kondoh, Y.; Hasegawa, Y.; Bando, M.; Abe, S.; Mochizuki, Y.; Chida, K.; et al. Safety and pharmacokinetics of nintedanib and pirfenidone in idiopathic pulmonary fibrosis. *Eur. Respir. J.* **2015**, *45*, 1382–1392. [CrossRef]
55. Richeldi, L.; Fletcher, S.; Adamali, H.; Chaudhuri, N.; Wiebe, S.; Wind, S.; Hohl, K.; Baker, A.; Schlenker-Herceg, R.; Stowasser, S.; et al. No relevant pharmacokinetic drug–drug interaction between nintedanib and pirfenidone. *Eur. Respir. J.* **2019**, *53*, 1801060. [CrossRef] [PubMed]
56. Dallinger, C.; Trommeshauser, D.; Marzin, K.; Liesener, A.; Kaiser, R.; Stopfer, P. Pharmacokinetic Properties of Nintedanib in Healthy Volunteers and Patients with Advanced Cancer. *J. Clin. Pharmacol.* **2016**, *56*, 1387–1394. [CrossRef] [PubMed]

57. Cottin, V.; Maher, T. Long-term clinical and real-world experience with pirfenidone in the treatment of idiopathic pulmonary fibrosis. *Eur. Respir. Rev.* **2015**, *24*, 58–64. [CrossRef]
58. Brunnemer, E.; Wälscher, J.; Tenenbaum, S.; Hausmanns, J.; Schulze, K.; Seiter, M.; Heussel, C.P.; Warth, A.; Herth, F.J.; Kreuter, M. Real-World Experience with Nintedanib in Patients with Idiopathic Pulmonary Fibrosis. *Respiration* **2018**, *95*, 301–309. [CrossRef]
59. Sgalla, G.; Lerede, M.; Richeldi, L. Emerging drugs for the treatment of idiopathic pulmonary fibrosis: 2020 phase II clinical trials. *Expert Opin. Emerg. Drugs* **2021**, *26*, 93–101. [CrossRef]
60. Ali, I.; Alharbi, O.M. COVID-19: Disease, management, treatment, and social impact. *Sci. Total Environ.* **2020**, *728*, 138861. [CrossRef]
61. Van der Sar-van der Brugge, S.; Talman, S.; Winter, L.B.-D.; de Mol, M.; Hoefman, E.; van Etten, R.W.; De Backer, I.C. Pulmonary function and health-related quality of life after COVID-19 pneumonia. *Respir. Med.* **2020**, *176*, 106272. [CrossRef] [PubMed]
62. Powell, P.; Saggu, R.; Jones, S.; Clari, M.; Saraiva, I.; Hardavella, G.; Hansen, K.; Pinnock, H. Discussing treatment burden. *Breathe* **2021**, *17*, 200284. [CrossRef]
63. García-Caballero, T.M.; Lojo, J.; Menéndez, C.; Fernández-Álvarez, R.; Mateos, R.; Garcia-Caballero, A. Polimedication: Applicability of a computer tool to reduce polypharmacy in nursing homes. *Int. Psychogeriatr.* **2018**, *30*, 1001–1008. [CrossRef] [PubMed]
64. Gentizon, J.; Büla, C.; Mabire, C. Medication literacy in older patients: Skills needed for self-management of medications. *Rev. Med. Suisse* **2020**, *16*, 2165–2168. [PubMed]
65. McFarland, M.S.; Buck, M.L.; Crannage, E.; Armistead, L.T.; Ourth, H.; Finks, S.W.; McClurg, M.R. Assessing the Impact of Comprehensive Medication Management on Achievement of the Quadruple Aim. *Am. J. Med.* **2021**, *134*, 456–461. [CrossRef]

MDPI
St. Alban-Anlage 66
4052 Basel
Switzerland
Tel. +41 61 683 77 34
Fax +41 61 302 89 18
www.mdpi.com

Pharmaceuticals Editorial Office
E-mail: pharmaceuticals@mdpi.com
www.mdpi.com/journal/pharmaceuticals

www.ingramcontent.com/pod-product-compliance
Lightning Source LLC
LaVergne TN
LVHW070647100526
838202LV00013B/898